NATURAL
DOG CARE

A Complete Guide to
Holistic Health Care for Dogs

CELESTE YARNALL, PH.D.

Foreword by Russell Swift, D.V.M.

JOURNEY EDITIONS
BOSTON · TOKYO

This book is dedicated to my precious granddaughter Gabrielle.

First published in 1998 by Journey Editions,
an imprint of Periplus Editions (HK) Ltd. with editorial offices at
153 Milk Street, Boston, Massachusetts 02109.

Text by John H. Fudens, D.V.M., on pages 169–170 is reproduced by permission.
Special thanks to Nancy Scanlan, D.V.M., for allowing us to use material from her
article entitled "Animal Acupuncture."
Text by Dael on pages 276–281 is from *The Crystal Book* by Dael, © 1983 Dael
Walker, and is reprinted by kind permission of the author.
Illustrations on pages 268 and 281 by Imelda Casper.
Photograph on page 163 by Jeanie Van Loan

Material for this book has come to me over years of study. Every effort has been
made to credit sources, but if any omissions were made, I will be happy to make
the correction once it is made known to me.

Library of Congress Cataloging-in-Publication Data

Yarnall, Celeste
    Natural dog care : a complete guide to holistic health care
for dogs / by Celeste Yarnall : foreword by Russell Swift.
        p. cm.
    Includes bibliographical references and index.
    ISBN 1-885203-47-0
    1. Dogs. 2. Dogs—Health. 3. Dogs—Diseases—Alternative
treatment. 4. Holistic veterinary medicine. I. Title.
SF426.Y37 1998
636.7'089—DC21   98-8453
                                                      CIP

Distributed by

USA   **Japan**   **Southeast Asia**
Charles E. Tuttle Co., Inc. Tuttle Shokai Ltd.   Berkeley Books Pte. Ltd.
RR 1 Box 231-5   1-21-13, Seki   5 Little Road #08-01
North Clarendon, VT 05759   Tama-ku, Kawasaki-shi   Singapore 536983
Tel.: (802) 773-8930   Kanagawa-ken 214, Japan   Tel.: (65) 280-3320
Fax.: (802) 773-6993   Tel.: (044) 833-0225   Fax.: (65) 280-6290
                             Fax.: (044) 822-0413

First edition
06 05 04 03 02 01 00 99 98   10 9 8 7 6 5 4 3 2 1

Printed in the United States of America

Contents

A Message from
Christina Chambreau, D.V.M.

THE DEMAND FOR new approaches to health for our animals is increasing very, very rapidly. At conventional veterinary conferences in 1995 and 1996, I would have more than 5 percent of the veterinarians attend my lectures on homeopathy for animals. The main reason they were there was that their clients had been asking about homeopathy, and some of them wanted some different approaches to difficult problems they were unsuccessful in treating. Your demand for healthier animals is being heard around the world.

Celeste Yarnall has written a wonderful book to help you have healthy, happy, long-lived dogs. As you read it, you will learn what true health is and how to attain it for your dogs—and yourself, too. Since you have picked up *Natural Dog Care,* you already want to learn more about a different approach. As with every great book, each time you read this book, you will learn something new. By sharing it with your friends and your veterinarian, you can help other people enter the world of full health for their animal companions.

A Message from Christina Chambreau, D.V.M.

When I was a conventional veterinarian, I took care of dogs the way veterinary college had taught me. While many recovered from their problems, some never seemed to be well. I had no idea what to do next to help them. I felt uncomfortable when guardians told me about problems with interacting with their dogs, or just a vague sense of ill health—because I had no way of helping unless there was a concrete problem. I also felt the lack of an underlying philosophy that would help me answer questions about why things were happening to these wonderful animals.

Once I learned the power of homeopathic medicine, a whole new world of health opened up for me. As you learn the power of different holistic approaches, you will find that your dogs can absolutely glow with health. It is good, of course, to start with the holistic approach from early puppyhood, even better yet is treating the parents and grandparents first. Whatever age your dog is, whatever your dog's condition or problem, the holistic approach should be the one to use first. Some may become well merely when their diet is changed to fresh, raw foods. Some may need years of being treated with many of the different modalities so well introduced in *Natural Dog Care*— acupuncture, homeopathy, herbs, nutrition, bodywork, energy work, and more.

You may select a holistic veterinarian to work with you in curing your dog, or start on your own by changing the diet and supplements, adding herbs, or doing energy work. This book contains so many new ideas that you may need to quit work (or sleep) for a few months to absorb even a little of the information!

If you are already feeding your dog a fresh and raw diet, not vaccinating, and using holistic modalities, this is still the book for you. Though I have been in mostly homeopathic practice for ten years, I still refer to *Natural Cat Care* for many details and will be keeping *Natural Dog Care* handy on my shelf as well.

Be sure to read the vaccination section because, in my opinion, this practice is bringing our animals to an intolerable level of ill health. Just being open to questioning current recommendations is very important. What we write today may change some in the ensuing years, but you are learning principles of health that will never change.

Our dogs depend on us to choose the healthiest lifestyles for them. They are here to help us heal the planet, and us. By studying this book and the resources Celeste presents you, you will be moving down the right path. *Natural Dog Care* will help you on the path to developing a cohesive health philosophy. Then you and your dogs can experience vibrant, creative, long-lasting health.

Thank you, Celeste Yarnall, for taking the time to share with dog owners what you have learned throughout the years.

Foreword

SINCE I WROTE the foreword for Celeste Yarnall's first book, *Natural Cat Care,* the demand for holistic alternatives has continued to expand rapidly. I am amazed and delighted with the shift that is taking place. The world (perhaps the whole universe) is changing. People are increasingly aware that we all have a higher purpose. Most of us are still struggling to find it. It is evident that Celeste Yarnall is one of the lucky few who has found it; she has set her sights on improving the quality of life for animal companions on a very large scale. I am excited to see that she is staying on target.

Natural Dog Care is the result of extensive research and study. Ms. Yarnall has managed a difficult feat; she has made easy reading of understanding difficult concepts and healing systems. It is a must-read for dog lovers and those involved in animal care. I am especially impressed by the amount of detail given to the history and development of the various systems. The chapter on vaccinations is articulate and convincing. It is hard to believe that *anyone* with a reasonable level of intelligence could read it and not have second thoughts about this modern medical "miracle." Ms. Yarnall's discussions on homeopathy and acupuncture are clear and concise. Anyone, regardless of his or her level of expertise, will gain from reading *Natural Dog Care.* This book would be an excellent primer for a veterinary college course in alternative medicine. I hope to see the day that such a course is routinely taught.

I am certain that by the time this book is published, holistic medicine will have moved even further into the mainstream (rapidly becoming a trickle). While many conventional practitioners are opening their minds to alternatives, others are becoming more vehemently opposed than ever. The so-called quack blasters are very concerned because they see their cash cow being led to slaughter. In response, they spread odious misinformation about holistic options and practitioners without compunction. Health care consumers are more confused than ever by the mixed messages they are receiving. As "modern" medicine continues to collapse because of ever increasing costs and ever decreasing results, genuine health practitioners look for answers. They will find them in nutrition and energy medicine. Those who are interested in money, status, or holding on to old ideas because they are afraid to change or admit they were wrong will be crushed under the weight of the medical dinosaur as it plummets into extinction. Books like *Natural Dog Care* serve to educate scores of people who will act to bring that day closer.

The next decade promises to be exciting. When medicine understands that physical healing depends upon spiritual growth, degenerative disease will be nothing more than an ancient memory. In writing this book, Celeste has committed a great act of kindness toward companion animals and people. These are acts that elevate our souls and improve the universe for everyone. Celeste Yarnall has the merit of two such books to her credit. I hope she is granted the strength to maintain her convictions and actions in the face of increasing opposition.

—Russell Swift, D.V.M.

Acknowledgments

FOR THEIR INVALUABLE contributions to this project I would like to thank:

My devoted friend Imelda Casper for her assistance in the preparation of this book.

Marina Zacharias—a dear friend who has contributed so much to this work.

Pat McKay, author of *Reigning Cats and Dogs,* for her valuable contribution to animal nutrition.

Barry Sears, Ph.D., author of *Enter the Zone,* who gave me the rules and the tools to feed myself as well as my companion animals.

Christina Chambreau, D.V.M., for giving so much of her time and providing so much valuable information.

Russell Swift, D.V.M, of Pet Friends, for sharing his expertise and many contributions to the field of holistic veterinary medicine.

Charles Loops, D.V.M., for his useful input and guidance.

Richard Pitcairn, D.V.M., Juliet de Bairacli Levy, Wendy Volhard, Kerry Brown, and Diane Stein for laying the foundation for this book with their own excellent ones.

Sis Sewall, *Healthy Pets, Naturally,* and *Natural Pet Magazine* for their continuing contribution to the cause of holistic health care for animals.

The late John Craige, V.M.D., and Joy Birdsall Craige, O.M., for information regarding therapeutic sound and dowsing.

John Fudens, D.V.M., Nancy Scanlan, D.V.M., and Ron Silver, D.V.M., Marc Bittan, D.V.M., Holistic Veterinary Healthcare, and David B. Nielsen, D.V.M., my animal companions' veterinary dentist, for their insights.

Wayne Perry, of Sound Touch Therapy Center, for his contribution through healing with sound.

Gail Daniels and Bill Volbrecht of Best Friends.

Systemic Formulas, Inc.; Lydia Hibby, Animal Communication; and John Lowry, Energy Balancing, for assistance in their areas of expertise.

Yolanda LaCombe for her considerable knowledge of flower essences.

Jim McMullan for giving me the confidence to present this material to the world.

To Siegfried, Roy, and Lynette, who have inspired me to make my dreams a reality.

Isabelle Bleecker and Deane Norton, my editors, for their patience and for always being there to help me.

My mother, Helene Yarnall, for teaching me to shoot for the stars.

My daughter, Camilla Forte, for her endless encouragement throughout this project and, indeed, my life. My son-in-law,

Steve Forte, for his help and guidance. My granddaughter, Gabrielle, the newest addition to our family.

The companion cats of my family, friends, and colleagues—among them my mother's Ariel, Teddy, Tiffany, and Cassie; Cami's Aladdin and Charlie; and Imelda's Clawed Monet and Tiger Lily—for the love and inspiration they offer every day.

My special companion animals—Celina, Romeo, Colette, Jasmine, Jacqueline Rose, Dominique, Dandy, Dewey, Bamboo, Snow, and all the precious kittens and cats I've had the privilege to raise.

And, lastly, my beautiful collie, Connie.

I am eternally grateful for their enormous contribution to this work, and deeply blessed to have shared my life with them.

Introduction

I LOVE ANIMALS and have chosen to dedicate my life to their well-being. As a holistic health care practitioner in southern California I consult with animal guardians and veterinarians on alternative healing therapies. I specialize in feline and canine nutrition, the fresh raw food diet and supplementation, which you will learn all about in this book. I recently completed my Ph.D. in nutrition and serve as an adjunct professor at Pacific Western University.

I have raised many generations of Tonkinese and Oriental shorthair cats on my natural regime as well as my dog, Connie, who oversees my day-to-day activities. After the release of my first book, *Natural Cat Care: A Complete Guide to Holistic Health Care for Cats,* it was made very clear to me by my dog clients that I needed to write *Natural Dog Care.* They insisted that my canine friends deserved equal time and that all the special holistic health care ideas that I reserve only for them belonged in print. People love to think of themselves as either dog people or cat people, but, truthfully, most of my clients love, honor, and cherish them both, just as I do. So, in the interest of fairness, here goes.

I begin this undertaking with my faithful collie, Connie, as my guide, and helping out with their two cents are my Tonkinese and Oriental shorthair cats who share my home and heart. The only thing my dog-loving friends will have to put up with is an occasional cat story to illustrate a point or two. If you've read *Natural Cat Care,* you may recall that as a child I raised parakeets and had pet lizards, a rooster, and a cat named Dusty. However, I can't forget the dog I almost got to keep as a pet, a beautiful sable and white collie who appeared at my backyard gate. I took him in and cared for him. I wanted desperately to keep him. He had run away from a neighbor family, whose children harassed him something terrible, and naturally he had to go home. So I resorted to watching every episode of *Lassie.* Sometimes you just have to grow up to get what you want, and so it was with me.

I adopted my own little sable and white collie puppy from a local breeder. I named her Lonnie, and she became the love of my life. We went to obedience school together, and I read every book I could get my hands on about collies . . . how to feed them, groom them, and train them. She went everywhere with me. She competed in novice obedience trials, where she performed like a bright young star. All she ever wanted was to please me. Back then, we lived with "make-believe" kitties. Every morning I'd ask Lonnie, "Where's the kitty?" She'd patrol the house and come back and tell me we didn't have one! Boy, have things changed!

As a young starlet, I did a feature film with Elvis Presley

entitled *Live a Little, Love a Little.* After Elvis separated from Priscilla (and I had separated from my first husband), Elvis invited me to Las Vegas for a visit. I didn't go, because I didn't want to leave Lonnie! Perhaps you think I'm crazy, but I have always put the needs of my companion animals ahead of my own, and Lonnie would have been miserable in a kennel. Elvis somehow muddled through without me.

One of the most exciting memories I have of Lonnie is her introduction to Lassie (who was actually a male) at the Malibu home of the late Rudd and Betty Weatherwax. They agreed to a breeding, as they thought Lonnie was magnificent. The stud fee would be a puppy back to them if a little male were to be blessed with the famous white blaze that is the trademark of all the Lassie dogs. Lassie courted Lonnie for almost a week. Rudd, Betty, and I watched this tender union, and Lonnie gave birth to two adorable pups two months later (a female named Misty, and a male with a white blaze, whom we named Alphie). The Weatherwaxes were so taken with both of them, they purchased the female from me as well.

It was not long after that Lonnie developed a little lump on the outside of her right knee. I thought it was a bee sting and applied compresses. I kept expecting it to go away, but it didn't. I took her to the veterinarian. The doctor kept her in the examining room for what seemed an eternity. I waited patiently, and my mother and daughter, Cami, waited out in the car. The doctor finally came out with tears in his eyes and told me that Lonnie had terminal bone cancer and had very little time left to live. I was devastated. I don't think I've ever felt so helpless in my life. I wanted to do something—anything—but the doctor said it was too late to even consider amputation because the cancer had metastasized throughout her body. He said all we could do was to love her and help her through to the end, and it was at the end that she was put to sleep. She was barely five years old.

Now I know that the canned and dry-food diet that she subsisted on did nothing more than sustain her life. With all I've learned today, I hope to spare you this kind of grief by sharing with you a better way . . . a return to nature that will do more than just allow your dog(s) to get by, but to truly enjoy abundant, glowing health.

No, I can't bring Lonnie back, or any of the other precious animal friends I've had the pleasure of knowing and loving who have passed on—like Pixie, our little Sheltie, and Bonnie and Laddie, a pair of sable and white collies, all of whom died far too young.

I do not pretend to practice veterinary medicine. I am not a veterinarian, but I can share with you and your veterinarians all the holistic health care tools to help you find your way through the myriad of alternative healing therapies. I would have given anything for this information before, but all I can do is share it with you and use it today.

Connie is doing beautifully on my program. She is not a young dog. However, she looks and acts like one. She has a job to do and feels needed, whereas Lonnie was an inside dog and slept at the foot of my bed. Connie loves the outdoors and guards the property. She loves to come in and visit the cats and kittens, who respect her (they probably think she's a great big cat), but she can't wait to go outside again and patrol the property and play, play, play. She has a very puppylike attitude . . . a kind of canine joie de vivre! I can't imagine my home without her collie smile.

I started Connie on the natural diet when she was seven

years old and have raised six generations of kittens on this program as well. There are many natural-rearing dog breeders on their seventh generation. All you can do is try it and see for yourselves what a difference it makes. I welcome you to the wonderful, healthy world of *Natural Dog Care*.

A Note of Caution

THIS BOOK IS not intended, nor should it be regarded, as veterinary medical advice. Prior to administering any therapeutic course, please consult a doctor of veterinary medicine or a holistic veterinarian. It is their function to diagnose your dog's medical problem and suggest a course of therapy.

Because my approach to dog care is considered to be alternative by definition, many of the ideas expressed herein have not been investigated or approved by any regulatory agency. National, state, and local laws vary regarding the application or use of these therapies. Accordingly, the reader should not substitute them for treatment by a doctor of veterinary medicine, but rather may use them in conjunction with veterinary care. Always discuss alternative approaches with your doctor of veterinary medicine before embarking upon them. An increasing number of veterinarians are utilizing alternative therapies, and you may wish to consult one or more of them regarding the treatments they offer. Ultimately, you must take full responsibility for the health of your canine companion.

The author and the publisher expressly disclaim responsibility for any adverse reactions or effects resulting from the use of information contained in the following pages.

Chapter One

Getting to Know Your Dog

A BRIEF HISTORY OF THE DOG

WHEN INTRODUCING PEOPLE to my health regimen for dogs, I'm often asked, "Aren't our domestic dogs different from their wild ancestors?" So, before covering the various holistic methods of dog care and feeding, let's look at the history of this magnificent animal.

The modern canine descended from a branch of carnivorous mammals that shared the distinction of having four carnassial teeth. Examining fossilized remains reveals how these teeth evolved from being for crushing and chewing to being for cutting through flesh. These meat eaters (prevalent 38–54 million years ago) were called Miacis. As the number of herbivore animals increased, so did the number of carnivores. Many believe that the dog's closest relatives lived in North America and belonged to the now extinct Hesperocyon family (26–38 million years ago). *Cynodictis* followed (19 million years ago). This successful carnivore belonged to the genus *Amphicyon* and developed independently around the world. By the Myocene period (about 12 million years ago),

• 1 •

Tomarctus appeared on the scene with the beginnings of the modern dog's dentition. By this time, approximately forty-two different genera of canines had developed. Two million years ago, the forty-two genera of canines were consolidated into the ten genera we have today. *Canis,* the largest genus, includes wolves, jackals, coyotes, and dogs. The next largest group, *Vulpes,* includes twelve species of fox.[1]

As human beings shifted from being nomads to living in fixed communities, the wolf joined them and, in doing so, changed his ways. Thus, selective breeding was born, and so was the domestic dog.

All canines share many of the same characteristics. They all have a scent-making gland on the dorsal surface of the tail, which allows them to leave a scent whenever or wherever they choose to wag their tails. They also share a body language that enables them to communicate with one another—for example, how the tail is positioned and how its hairs move. They have long skulls that house strong cheek muscles to hold on to prey— ultimately killing and devouring it. They have semirigid hind legs that provide them with excellent endurance. Their front limbs have a "locked" radius, and ulna bones that cannot rotate, providing them with stability when running.

Equipped with large brain capacity, unique teeth, excellent hearing, compact feet, and fur coats, dogs evolved into social hunters. A pack relationship enabled them to bring down much larger animals.

It is commonly accepted that the ancestry of today's domestic dog is the wolf, for surely wherever humans lived, the wolf followed and learned to scavenge our leftovers. The process of taming probably began when humans adopted orphaned wolf cubs.

Throughout the ages dogs have been involved in warfare, sports, hunting, and farming; today we also find them in police work, art, literature, and films. Their role in human society evolves and expands as we do. But most people share their lives with a dog because of his unconditional love, trust, and companionship. Bruce Fogle, D.V.M., refers to them as "furry comforters," a trait of dogs that anthropologists have observed to trigger a desire in humans to feed and comfort them. The old expression "a three dog night" reminds us that the dog has kept many of us warm on cold, cold nights.[2]

The early canines must have been very intelligent opportunists who learned that when prey was scarce, all they had to do was guard campsites and assist in hunting to get a handout. It wasn't difficult for this pack animal to become a willing member of a human pack. However, now we are responsible for providing him with creature comforts!

The needs of the domesticated dog are not that different from those of his wild ancestors. He remains a carnivore with twelve small incisors, four canines, sixteen premolars, and ten molars. He eats raw meat but can also nibble on grass and roots.

THE MODERN DOG . . . THEN AND NOW

IT'S NOT DIFFICULT to imagine that our ancient relatives loved their canine companions much as we do today. We know that dogs were ultimately treasured by their human friends: recently excavated neolithic burial sites show that people laid out their dogs' bones in a neat and orderly fashion.

When our ancestors realized that a tamed dog could be useful for hunting and other tasks, it seems likely that wild puppies were caught and that selection for special traits began. This was accomplished by identifying desired physical and behavioral traits and tendencies, thus making dogs better suited for the tasks at hand. Centuries later, there are approximately 350 man-made breeds, with their distinct characteristics, recognized by the Federation Cynologique Internationale (FCI), whose headquarters is located in Belgium. Today, however, many national kennel clubs are not members of the FCI, and the total number of recognized breeds is closer to 500. Each breed has an official standard, which causes us to reflect on how far they have come from those first wild dogs that our ancestors domesticated.

Parent breed clubs for seven groups of dogs have mapped out standards that cover how the dogs are to be judged in the showring. Judging criteria include general appearance, temperament, conformation (head, body, tail, limbs, coat, coloration, and so on), gait, size, and penalizing faults.

The seven groups are broken down as follows, and I've listed some, but not all, breeds in these categories:

1. Herding group *(collie, Shetland sheepdog, border collie, briard, and Old English sheepdog).* Early human beings captured wild animals, corralled them, and used them for agriculture and livestock farming. They did not wish to have these animals run away and be eaten by predators, so they devised a way to protect them. The early sheepdogs were bred and trained for such a purpose. Human needs were met by having these animals protected in order to use their talents.

2. Working group *(German shepherd, Alaskan malamute, Siberian husky, Saint Bernard, Leonberger, mastiff).* The working dogs have an innate ability to warn people of impending danger (for example, a trespassing enemy). Thus, the guard dog was born. This group includes military (police) dogs, dogs who pull loads (referred to as pack dogs), gentle lifesaving dogs, fighting dogs (once bred to battle other dogs), those beloved companions of the deaf and blind, and sled dogs.

3. Sporting group *(American cocker spaniel, Irish setter, Labrador retriever, weimaraner).* The sporting dogs are known for their incredible sense of smell. They can alert people to the whereabouts of birds that have been shot down. They are also capable of retrieving them. Many can swim and will retrieve from the water.

4. Hound group *(Afghan, borzoi, greyhound, basset, beagle).* Hounds are classified in two groups: sight hounds and scent hounds. The sight hounds are spotters who can see far away and chase their prey until it drops from exhaustion. Scent hounds are used extensively by the police to search for drugs and bombs. Hound dogs can run about thirty-five miles per hour. Racing hounds are an example of this group's speed and agility.

5. Terrier group *(fox terrier; Airedale; Kerry blue, Welsh, and Jack Russell terriers).* The word *terrier* comes from the Latin *terra,* meaning "soil." These dogs can hunt prey that hides in burrows. Large hunting dogs are referred to as hounds and small ones as terriers.

6. Toy group *(Pekinese, Chihuahua, Yorkshire terrier, Maltese, papillon, bichon frise, pug, Pomeranian).* There are some hounds, sporting dogs, and terriers who fall into the toy group because of their small size. People love them as companions, and they are just plain cute. They live nicely in small quarters, such as city apartments.

7. Nonsporting group *(keeshond, dalmatian, chow chow, poodle, shar-pei, Lhasa apso, schnauzer).* This group lumps together dogs suited for specific work but not related to dogs in other groups. They are found in circus acts, as ratters, or as excellent guard dogs.[3]

All dogs have an amazing ability to find their way home with their five senses. They also love to be clean, preferring not to defecate where they sleep or eat. Mom teaches them their good habits young. Soon they learn to play hide-and-seek and fetch.

Dogs' loyalty is generally unchallenged. They bring us unconditional love and teach us responsibility. I adopted Lonnie, my collie puppy, the year before my daughter was born. Caring for her needs and learning to be unselfish helped prepare me for motherhood. When a dog needs to be fed and walked, it's irrelevent whether you are tired or don't feel well. His needs must be taken care of, just like a child's. What could be better than teaching a young child the responsibility of caring for an animal? If more people learned to put the needs of other living things above, or at least equal to, their own needs, this world, this planet that is our home, would be a better place.

The dog, just like the cat, helps us psychologically. We know conclusively that petting and walking one, and having one as a companion, helps speed recovery, comforts the elderly, and helps make amazing breakthroughs with retarded or handicapped individuals. A dog not only is a best pal but improves the quality of our lives. They have my eternal respect and gratitude.

See "Resources" for several excellent books on various breeds.

A HOLISTIC APPROACH TO DOG CARE

WHAT IS HOLISTIC health care and how does it relate to your dog? To me, holistic care means treating the whole person or animal as a unique individual, a perfect living thing. In the course of upsetting the delicate ecological balance of our planet, we humans have upset the ecology of animals, both wild and domestic.

The term *holistic* was coined in the 1960s by H. Ray Evers, a medical doctor concerned about chronic diseases for which there were no cures and about the growing use of drugs to treat various complaints. Dr. Evers felt many of the "wonder drugs" prescribed by *allopathic* (conventional) physicians suppressed symptoms (which he saw as the body's way of expressing itself) that would only resurface later, sometimes in more severe forms. He believed that certain drugs caused side effects that are worse than the original disease. While studying the New Testament, he discovered the Greek word *holos* (whole); both Saint John and Saint Paul mention it in reference to the whole person—body, mind, and spirit.[4]

Evers began working from the belief that there was more to illness than just germs and the endless quest to annihilate them. He felt that imbalances and stresses were the roots of disease. The cure was not in drugs, but in rebalancing patients' bodies and returning them to peace and harmony with their environment. This philosophy could also be used by patients as a powerful tool for self-healing.

It's vital to understand what true health means. Certainly, a healthy dog would have no obvious diseases. Just as important, he'd be free to express himself creatively, to be humorous, playful, angry, sad, happy, exuberant, clever, and agile. In the last few decades we've tolerated many symptoms in our dogs that we believe aren't real problems but that actually reflect ill health. The following are early warnings that your as-yet-undiseased dog should be treated preventatively by a holistic practitioner.

EARLY SIGNS OF DISEASE IN DOGS

CONDITIONS

Doggy smell

Attracting fleas

Dry, oily, or lackluster coat

Excessive shedding

Chronic ear problems (wax)

Eye discharge

Tearing, or matter in the corner of the eyes

BEHAVIOR PROBLEMS

Fear of loud noises, thunder, wind

Excessive barking

A too suspicious or timid nature

Constantly licking self

Fear of people or things

Irritability

Indolence

Eating dog or cat stool (it actually may be normal for dogs to eat horse, cow, and rabbit manure)

Sensitivity to handling

Aggressiveness at play and destructiveness

Digestive upsets such as mucus in stool

Tendency to diarrhea with smallest change in diet

Obesity

Bad breath

Poor appetite

Cravings for weird food

Source: This list was provided by Christina Chambreau, D.V.M., and was compiled by Drs. Richard Pitcairn, Jeffrey Levy, Christina Chambreau, Charles Loops, and Don Hamilton, seminar, October 31, 1995, Orange County, Calif.

Also be alert to a dog who is stiff when he gets up or is sensitive to temperature changes and has low-grade fevers (101.5 degrees is considered to be the normal temperature for both dogs and cats). However, I recommend establishing a baseline norm for your animal when he is healthy. You are then equipped to recognize a significant change that might indicate a need for a veterinary workup.

If any of these symptoms are present—or any others that make you ask yourself whether something is normal—please call a holistic veterinarian immediately rather than waiting for your dog to get so sick that you have no doubts. Early, deep, energetic treatment may extend and enhance the quality of your animal companion's life.

Holistic practitioners offer a myriad of approaches: nutritional therapy, herbs, homeopathy, flower essences, and aromatherapy; chiropractic, acupuncture, and other hands-on modalities; and energy, light, sound, crystal, and magnet therapies, among others. I also include astromedicine, the study of the twelve sun signs as a guide to understanding the needs and behavior of our dogs. I believe that in treating the whole being, we should make use of everything nature has to offer.

Finding the right practitioner is a basic part of providing your dog with the right care. The "Resources" section provides information on finding holistic veterinarians in your area. You can contact the American Holistic Veterinary Medical Association (AHVMA) for referrals and information. The AHVMA will give you a list of member veterinarians in your area but offers no information about their skill or training in a holistic modality, or even their current interests.

You must ask each practitioner about his or her philosophy, watch how he or she is with your dog, and evaluate your dog's response to therapy (see Chapter 5, "Natural Remedies"). Only you can determine the right practitioner for your precious dog. Don't be afraid to interview several or to change practitioners if you're not satisfied. Ask as many questions as necessary to be sure you understand what is involved before you agree to any treatment.

THE DOG AND YOU

IF YOU'RE ABOUT to adopt a dog, I urge you to read this book in its entirety and to ask yourself the questions below. If you answer no to any of them, you could well be in for some sleepless nights and many lessons learned the hard way. If you're already living with a dog, perhaps considering these questions now will help you improve the existing situation. In any case, I hope to spare you and your beloved canine companion the heartache of hazards that could claim his life.

Am I prepared to treat the dog as a member of my family? Nobody really owns *an animal, be it a dog or cat. You become his companion, his friend, or maybe even the alpha wolf. You may dominate or control him, but without love as the dog's reward, the relationship becomes pointless.*

Am I prepared to be responsible by providing the dog with his own yard or run and/or take him for daily walks to provide ample daily exercise?

Am I prepared to civilize my dog and teach him basic obedience, to come when called, and heel on a leash?

Am I prepared to pick up and properly dispose of his stool?

Will I be responsible and have the dog spayed or neutered unless he or she is in a supervised breeding program?

Am I quite certain the animal's health and characteristics necessitate breeding? If so, do I have responsible homes for the puppies prior to mating? Far too many unwanted dogs and puppies have found a cruel and bitter end at animal shelters. As responsible guardians and/or breeders, we walk a fine line when choosing to breed or not. Ask yourself, Am I certain this line should be continued, and will this litter be healthier, happier, and genetically predisposed to enhance the breed?

Am I prepared to feed one to two (or in the case of puppies, several) fresh, raw, natural meals with supplements, or will I use ease and convenience as an excuse to continue the dangerous practice of commercial feeding?

Am I prepared to, at all times, provide fresh, pure water?

Am I prepared to provide veterinary checkups for routine dental care, fecal exams, diagnostic blood work, and so on? These tasks can be costly and time consuming.

Am I prepared to hire a pet-sitter when I go away to continue my natural feeding regimen and exercise?

Can I really make a commitment to holistic health care for the animal's life span?

Am I prepared to be legally responsible if my dog bites someone, even if that person provoked or beat my dog?

Look, I know how adorable a new puppy can be, how they come to you at shelters, pet stores, or kennels. The question is, Will you be good for and to the puppy? We are not talking about a bowl of tap water and a plate of canned or dry food. We are talking about excellence and optimum health here. A stuffed toy requires no care or feeding. A puppy is as close to having a child in responsibility as you can get—without nine months to think about it.

Before examining the various ways to get your dog healthy and keep him healthy, seriously determine whether or not you are up to the task.

Chapter Two

Interacting with Your Dog

NONVERBAL COMMUNICATION

NONVERBAL COMMUNICATION IS a gift that all life-forms share, one you'll need to reawaken to better interact with and care for your animal companion. Most dog lovers already possess a good working knowledge of canine body language. Through nonverbal communication, you can actually begin to see things through your dog's eyes and become his voice. You can learn the basics simply by taking a class (see "Resources").

I studied nonverbal communication with my friend Lydia Hibby, who received her training from Beatrice Lydecker, the author of *Stories the Animals Tell Me.* I highly recommend this book, as well as *Kinship with All Life,* by J. Allen Boone, the grandfather of this communication technique. Boone explains how long before we had language, we were able to communicate among ourselves and with animals.

Those of us fortunate enough to have been raised with animal companions "talked" to them—and they "talked" back—

without words. You've probably chalked up your own memories of such experiences to an overly active imagination. Or perhaps you once played with a set of twins who told you they each knew what the other was thinking, or you heard your mother say she had "woman's intuition" or "just knew something was wrong." Have you ever had an image of a friend come to mind and then received a phone call from that very person saying, "I was just thinking about you and wanted to say hello"? These are all examples of nonverbal communication.

Try it now with your dog. Start by listening to your heart instead of to your mind. Close your eyes. Remember every detail: the feeling of his lovely coat, those deep, trusting eyes staring up at you. Try to visualize him walking toward you. Often, even the first time you try it, the dog will be by your side before you know it, so happy that you've communicated with him in his own way.

Always communicate in positive terms—what you want your dog to do rather than what *not* to do. Dogs live fully in the moment, so don't ask them if they want to go to the groomer. They don't know how they'll feel until they get there.

When you say, "Don't jump on the couch," your dog sees an image in your mind's eye of his jumping on the couch. He'll think it's okay to jump on the couch, but your yelling at him sends a mixed signal. Better to say in a stern tone, "No! Go to your bed!" Even better is actually taking him to his bed, to reinforce the positive behavior.

It's impossible to hide your feelings from dogs. They can even take on your stresses, fears, and frustrations. In *Behaving As If the God in All Life Mattered,* Machaelle Small Wright suggests that you avoid arguing in front of your companion animals.[1] It's too stressful for them. It's not fair to treat them as if they're not in the room when we lose control of our emotions. Their sensibilities must be respected.

So try visualizing positive, loving pictures rather than negative, worrying ones. Do you ever wonder why what you worry about happening often seems to happen? Practice positivity, and you'll find it spilling over into every aspect of your life.

You can practice heart-to-heart communication skills with a brand-new dog at a dog show or shelter. I like to begin by learning the dog's name, if possible. Try saying the name in a sweet, soft, "feminine" (high-pitched) voice. In the animal world the female voice is nonthreatening—the lower sounds conjure up fear. If you're a man, or a woman with a deep voice, raise your pitch and speak gently.

Animal communicator Cindy Wood recommends getting down on the floor, at the animal's eye level.[2] Imagine the dog sitting on the floor of your own home. You may get a picture of what his home looks like from his point of view (perhaps you can distinguish the outlines of a bed or a coffee table from underneath), and what the dog sees from that perspective. Your image may look like a black-and-white negative.

If you don't get a picture, it doesn't mean you're not doing it right. The dog may just be telling you he's not allowed in the bedroom. Continue to listen with your heart. Read the feelings you do get, and go on. He may be trying to tell you something about what he likes or dislikes. Or he may be content exactly where he is right now. Keep going.

What do his floors look and feel like? Do the cold, slippery floors make him nervous as he skids on them? Now visualize the dog's feeding area. Does he eat dry or moist foods? Do you taste or feel any textures in your mouth? What about clean, fresh water? What has he smelled recently? He may change the picture you get to reflect his truth.

Are there other animals where he lives? Send him a picture of one of your animal companions. What does he say to that? What does he like to play with—a ball, a Frisbee? Give him these images and see what you get back. Ask his human companion questions to help you assess your images.

As you read the visual images your animal friend sends, along will come feelings of space and expansion if he has room to play and places to rest in—or feelings of contraction if he's been caged or otherwise too restricted.

Perhaps you may feel he's trying to tell you about an aggressive person. This person may not necessarily be a man; it could be a woman or child with a strong personality—dogs sense human beings as personalities, not as men and women. Ask the dog how he likes this person. He may wish the person would leave him alone, or he may enjoy playing with the person but can't understand why he gets scolded for playing too roughly.

One way to analyze the overall well-being of an animal is through a body scan. Just look at the animal, starting with the head and working down the back to the tip of the tail. How do you feel compared with how you felt before scanning? If you feel anything unusual as you continue your scan, you know you're on to something. Ask the dog, using his name, how he feels as you move along his body with your eyes.

Once when I was at a holistic animal clinic, I met a woman who didn't have any idea what was wrong with her ailing animal companion. While nonverbally communicating with this animal, I felt that his mouth was hurting him, so I told the woman to have the veterinarian check it. Sure enough, he had a severe gum infection.

Lydia Hibby tells a story about consulting with a woman whose snake wasn't eating. Lydia communicated with the snake and asked the woman if there could be any reason to suspect that paint was the problem. In fact, she had recently painted a tiny screw in the snake's habitat. As soon as she removed the screw, the snake began eating again. The paint fumes had made the snake lose its appetite.

As you practice, your skills will improve. When doing a body scan, you may feel discomfort in certain parts of your own body. If so, simply release the feeling and say to yourself, "This animal's feelings are his own. I release them." In your mind's eye, wrap the dog in a healing white light or say a prayer or blessing. Then simply turn off the pain, much as you would the TV when it transmits images that upset you. In any event, don't be the recipient of this pain.

Nonverbal communication seems to come most easily with other people's animals. It's sometimes difficult to practice with our own because we've become so emotionally involved with them, but gradually you'll develop a proficiency. I do my best communicating with my own animal companions through play. I talk to them about their day. Sometimes they compete to communicate with me all at once.

Before I touch someone else's dog, I always ask his guardian if it's okay, and then I ask the animal's permission. Actually, petting the dog's aura is more subtle. Using this indirect way of laying on hands (the space around the body is referred to as the etheric double), you can often feel the animal's energy. This is a valuable avenue of communication and diagnosis, and through it you can offer much healing, especially when you use love as the catalyst.

Nonverbal communication can greatly expand your relationship with animals, but some dogs are reserved, just like certain people are. They simply don't want to converse. Don't be discouraged. And some people never get pictures, only feelings—and that's fine. Trust yourself and proceed with imagination and confidence. You're on your way to being a nonverbal communications expert!

TRAINING AND PLAY

YOU PROBABLY ENJOY some verbal communication with your dog as well, especially if the two of you have attended obedience classes. There you learned how to train and handle your dog. These sessions are fun and create a mature respect and deep bond. An excellent book on dog training is *Mother Knows Best—The Natural Way to Train Your Dog,* by Carol Lea Benjamin. Dr. Benjamin graduated from veterinary school in 1966 but felt ill equipped to adequately answer questions from clients regarding their animals' behavior. Dogs' behavior (such as house guarding, aggression, flea biting) could lead to an early demise as surely as some life-threatening disease or accident. Such behavior is even probably a subtle sign of underlying disease. It also reflects on our domesticated animals' relationships with their own mothers, their siblings, and—just like our companion dogs' wild ancestors—the rest of the pack (your family members, be they animal or human).

Before you graduate from obedience training to play (as a reward or just for fun), your dog needs to understand his place in your "pack." This will not be new to him but is a part of the natural order of things. This understanding bridges nonverbal communication, verbal communication, obedience training (civilization), and, ultimately, play. I call this work *play*, because it should be fun for both you and your dog.

As our canine companions evolved, they created, with our help, a mutually beneficial partnership. We learned together that they had abilities we could benefit from, and we had "stuff" that made their life a little more comfortable. And so human and beast trudged along through the millennia helping each other. He helped out perhaps in the hunt, warned of intruders, and shared meals. Just as those ancient ancestors of ours played games in their caves, so do we in our homes, yards, parks, and beaches.

The dog innately respects the group leader, the alpha wolf, and the alpha wolf's mate, too. Once upon a time, humans' and dogs' needs were not too different. Each wanted to enjoy a hearty meal; a warm, dry place to sleep; a chance to reproduce; and the ability to play outside without getting eaten by predators. They were a family who depended upon each other. Eating, playing, and escaping were full-time jobs.

You may argue that it's not so different today. However, life has clearly become more for us than a hunk of raw meat, a bone to gnaw on, a warm animal skin to cover up our nakedness, and a safe, clean cave to live in. Now we have stress, thank you very much. Life is complex. We have language and means of communication across vast distances of time and space. We don't read our old pals' posturing and moods quite like we used to. So guess what? Man's best friend is stressed, too.

There is a gap between us, something like a generation gap. If we don't bridge this gap, enter the undesirable behaviors—and the dog is all too often disposed of. Let's not let that happen. (See the discussion on flower essences in Chapter 5, "Natural Remedies," if stress is an overwhelming problem.)

Let's turn to mom for a moment. She is where it all starts, unless you took on this job because of the loss of the mother dog. Watching a mother dog raise her puppies is truly something to behold. She trains, praises, corrects, feeds, grooms, and relates—twenty-four hours a day. And it all translates as love to the little ones.

What is amazing about mom, with all her wisdom, is that there is an economy to what she does, and she rarely has to repeat a command or reprimand. She means to enforce her actions. Her patience is overwhelming and reminds us of what a wonderful virtue it is. Good old Job. Mom knows exactly what to ignore and what to correct. She has great timing (and sharp teeth!). Mom, in a few short weeks, accomplishes some miracles that you, as the new mother, shouldn't let puppy forget. So remember to teach and love at the same time, but don't forget your role. Male or female, you are now mom. You must encourage the behavior you want and discourage the behaviors you don't want. You may prefer to use your own methods. A little poetic license here is good. As Dr. Benjamin mentions, you may prefer the taste of vichyssoise to dog fur, so mouth-on corrections may not be for you (she does have a charming and humorous style).

If you listen to the mother dog's verbal sounds, they're not too difficult to understand. There are sounds of love, which are a sort of coo; some that call the pups to come; those warning of danger and the need for protection; others that are angry and sound a little snappy and, if you'll pardon the pun, bitchy.

If you are able to watch mom do her physical thing, you'll

see the nipping and body slamming she does with her tail or front paws, as well as the pups' trying to earn back mom's favor.

The dog's pack instinct survives whether he was bred to point, retrieve, or protect. Puppy nuzzles under mother's chin just as he will do with you. She speaks back with a bite across the muzzle just to remind him who's the boss. Now all this is still deemed play. But mom, God bless her, is still in total control.

No matter what happens, mom will never deny her baby nourishment. If she can help it, her puppies do not go to bed hungry. However, she doesn't do treats beneath the kitchen table or offer dessert! We have eating. We have educating. Mother never uses food as a reward. We can reach some level of dog training by using treats, but it's only mediocre and not nature's way. Mom doesn't do it. She knows that in the presence of rare roast beef or raw filet, pups can't think. Robotlike, they just perform the same task, like Pavlov's dog, to get the desired reward. Your dog performs his obedience lessons for love. This is not true for any other species that I know of.

We want to teach this animal how to concentrate. All the good information contained in Chapter 4, "Nutrition," as well as Chapter 5, "Natural Remedies," on homeopathy, herbs, and flower essences will help him be healthy enough to be able physically to concentrate. When you attend obedience class or practice at home, you'll see the delight your praise, both verbal and physical, brings your dog. The tone of your voice will remind him of his mother. "Good boy. That's a good dog" will make him tingle and wiggle and wag his whole body. Just figure out how much praise is adequate, so he doesn't venture "over the top."

Remember, when mom corrects, it's for a behavior she has observed. Dogs live in the here and now. Think of rewards for good behavior: a "good dog," a pet, loving eye contact, or a smile. "Very good dog" behavior can include play, hugging, "What a gooooood, good dog." You can branch out from there and make up all kinds of fun.

When the puppy is bad, we can say sharply, "no" or "out" ("out" sounds a lot like mom's reprimand) in a low voice. Stop the pup with a tug on his collar and leash. Give a warning look that says, "Don't even think about it!"

We must remember that mother dogs don't hit their pups with rolled-up newspaper. She might grasp the pup by the scruff of the neck and shake him. She might roll him onto his back, growl, and give harsh eye contact. It's respect we are teaching, not brute force. There is a fine line of distinction here.

I have always used a chain collar made of large stainless-steel links and a six-foot leather lead. My early dog training was in the Koeller method, which many deem to be harsh. However, is it harsh to train your dog to "come" when a truck is barreling along toward him? I lovingly put my collies through my own home course of dog obedience . . . a loving, gentle version of the Koeller method. Once, when off leash, Lonnie broke and headed for the street and that truck was a reality—coming straight at her on a collision course from hell. I yelled, "Lonnie come!" as loud and as sharp as I could, and she heard me, stopped on a dime, turned, ran back, and sat in front of me looking for that "good dog" she always heard when I was happy with her behavior. This time I was so emotionally overcome that I slumped to the ground, cried a torrent of tears all over her—so glad I had not succumbed to wishy-washy training methods. I was her mom, her alpha wolf, her whole world. She was thrilled she had pleased me, and I was just grateful she was still alive. I didn't have

Dr. Benjamin's book to guide me, but I did the best I could at the time.

Books can teach the basics of novice obedience in a wonderful way. They are a must—along with proper housebreaking and other good dog manners. Obedience is more than a series of commands; it is also showing your dog that he must do what you tell him, where you tell him, when and for as long as you say he should—so that if that truck ever comes his way, you and he will know what to do.

In essence, each learned action and command forms a chain of learning—and learning, pleasing, and being rewarded are some of the stuff your dog loves best.

After a lesson, games are a great reward. You can play tug-of-war with a store-bought or homemade toy. You can teach your dog to overcome his aversion to look you in the eye (an act of dominance in the wild) by getting down on the floor with him, making a little noise to get his attention, and trying to get him to look at you. Each time you do it, his attention span gets longer. This is a good game after you've played ball or Frisbee, or had a long lesson or run. Dogs love to mimic and copy facial expressions. You can play copycat and mimic his actions, too. You can pant, play bow (like the Japanese do), lie down, roll over, offer him your paw, or sneeze (which dogs do to clean their nose for a new scent or when they're happy). Watch and see if he sneezes back. Above all, stay in tune with eye contact, with words and touch.

You can play "catch me if you can." When you have a collie, this feat is easier said than done. Mine can get me every time. You can play "speak." You can even roughhouse a little. When a puppy gets hurt, he cries. If your little guy goes too far, feign tears, crying, and whimpering sounds or say "out" or "enough" in that "I really mean it" tone. Think active rather than rough.

Above all, remember that you are the guardian, the caregiver, not the owner. We don't really own anything in this life, let alone another living thing. Your dog is his own being, totally unique. He is not your possession or your slave. He is your friend, and you want him with you because he loves you, not because you own him or he has no choice . . . more like mother was.

Finally, always be gentle and include lots of love in your sessions. This is the magical ingredient in all holistic therapies. As children, we loved to play. Who's to tell us we can't still be children with our dogs—they won't tell anyone!

Chapter Three

The Dangers of Conventional Care

VETERINARY VISITS AND LAB TESTS

IF YOUR VETERINARIAN (holistic or allopathic) recommends a thorough physical examination (including a complete blood count, serum chemistry profile, urinalysis, and fecal analysis), the first question that should come to mind is, Why does he or she want to do this? My dog seems healthy. What will this tell us? Veterinarians are taught to recommend these procedures so that normal baselines can be established. For example, most dogs' normal temperature (cats', too) is around 101.5 degrees Fahrenheit. If your dog's temperature goes above 103 degrees, it's reasonable to assume that veterinary care is needed as soon as possible. However, if your dog's normal temperature is 102.5, a half-degree increase is not a cause for alarm. This examination and ultimate laboratory testing may be quite useful (especially when working with a holistic veterinarian) in creating a relationship between you, your veterinarian, and your dog.

Besides taking the dog's temperature, your veterinarian evaluates your dog's general attitude and appearance and checks his eyes, nose, teeth, mouth, skin, and musculoskeletal, respiratory, heart, nervous, digestive, genitourinary, and circulatory systems. A homeopathic veterinarian asks you to fill out or discuss a detailed list of mental or physical "guide symptoms"; goes over the dog's current diet; makes recommendations for converting to a fresh food diet and natural supplementation; and discusses which vaccinations the dog has been given and what reactions were noticed, no matter how subtle. He may want to run a CBC test, which is a complete blood count, a routine profile to analyze the quantity and quality of the cells in the blood.

If your veterinarian is not holistically inclined, you may elect to have copies of all diagnostic tests sent to your holistic veterinarian. Since many consult long-distance via phone or fax, I recommend keeping copies in your own files as well. After all, you are paying this professional, and these tests belong to you. (My holistic veterinarian, Dr. Charles Loops, is in Pittboro, North Carolina, and I am in Los Angeles. We work together to support allopathic treatments when necessary.)

If a chem screen or chem s screen (serum chemistry profile) is ordered, you get an extensive database to evaluate your dog's current condition that can serve as a normal baseline or help diagnose a (potential) problem. Usually a dog must fast for twelve hours prior to the test.

A urinalysis examines your dog's urine to reveal the health of the genitourinary system and to reflect the state of a variety of diverse processes involving other organs.

A fecal examination, a test of a stool sample, reveals the presence or absence of parasites. It can also show undigested food particles, which indicate whether your dog is able to break down and digest his food properly.

It is important to tell your veterinarian that you want the same lab used unless a second lab test elsewhere is required. Each laboratory establishes its own norms, and sometimes human labs are used because they are less expensive. But they can also be inaccurate because their instruments are not calibrated for animal blood. Also keep in mind that blood values change day by day. A high value one day may be normal again for months afterward. Some animals appear fine for years with high blood values.

Feel free to ask questions. Your veterinarian works for you. You are hiring him or her to spearhead this diagnosis. Be an active partner in your dog's health.

I recommend Wendy Volhard and Dr. Kerry Brown's *The Holistic Guide for a Healthy Dog* for a complete discussion and explanation of these diagnostic tests (see "Resources"). I refer to it often if my dog needs blood work, so I am able to at least follow the very complicated language of the CBC test. The book also includes a valuable glossary of terms and a discussion on the merits of testing for heartworm before having a worming medication prescribed for your dog.

Be sure to ask your veterinarian whether the results of your dog's blood chemistries are normal for your particular breed of dog. Also note that simply changing your dog's diet to the fresh raw method should produce a pronounced change for the better after at least a thirty-day period. This one simple change often puts a dog who seems to have health problems back into balance and ensures that whatever treatment is selected will work optimally.

Most of all, don't react in haste to whatever the lab tests reveal. Many times—more often than you can imagine—false positives and negatives occur. Many tests on young puppies are inconclusive. Always seek a second, and possibly a third, opinion, as I know of many animals who were put to sleep on account of a laboratory error or veterinarians who simply did not take the time to explain alternative therapies. Animals, like people, have a tremendous desire to live and be with their human companions. Give them a chance to prove this. Spontaneous remission occurs in animals just as it does in people. In Deepak Chopra's 1991 book *Perfect Health,* he explains that "Nature is like a radio band with infinite stations. The reality you are now experiencing is only one station on the band, completely convincing as long as you stay tuned to it, but masking the other choices that lie on the other side."[1]

Dr. Christina Chambreau suggests, "Before using the conventional veterinary cadre of 'anti' drugs (antibiotics, antihistamines, anti-inflammatories, etc.), try several holistic modalities first. Use conventional treatments if you feel completely 'stuck' or the dog becomes more ill."[2]

Before you allow anyone to vaccinate your dog, your cat, your children, or even you, be aware of the potential consequences and then make an informed decision. Believe me, there is nothing routine about vaccination. This simple act, which we have been brainwashed to believe protects us, is not necessarily safe. There are risks that must be evaluated *prior to* vaccinating, not after.

The only way laws (such as mandatory vaccination) can ever be changed for the good of all living things is by our rising up and protesting through legislative action. In order to accomplish this task, we need to be informed. Those who profit by this procedure would rather we weren't informed and just proceeded on blind faith and custom. Great scientific breakthroughs have historically occured when custom is challenged, not simply accepted. The next section on vaccination suggests that now is the time for "customary procedure" to be more closely evaluated and rethought.

VACCINATION

THOUGH VACCINATION HAS become a highly controversial subject, those who challenge the concept are still treated as if they are against apple pie and motherhood. I consider conventional vaccines to be extremely dangerous. Many veterinarians agree that vaccination is one of the most harmful things we do to our animals because of the severity of potential allergic reactions (both short and long term)—many of which are fatal.

Why do we vaccinate? We're afraid our animals will get certain diseases. If we were offered a single vaccine to protect our dogs against any possible ailment, we would welcome it without question. Christina Chambreau, D.V.M., questions the practice of vaccination: "What are we doing to the whole animal, the whole immune system of our animals? Why are dogs and cats becoming more unhealthy, living shorter life spans, and having smaller litters? New diseases have appeared even since we started vaccinating so heavily."

We need to examine three aspects of vaccination: (1) Are vaccines safe, or do they cause harm? (2) Are they necessary and effective? (3) What are the alternatives to vaccinating against specific diseases?

Most veterinarians recommend that dogs be vaccinated for canine distemper, hepatitis, adenovirus cough, parainfluenza, parvovirus, and leptospirosis. Many also encourage injections for Lyme disease, corona virus, and Bordetella. Local law requires rabies vaccinations. These combinations of shots are repeated every year until the dog dies. "Where in the natural order of this world do we get more than one infection at a time?" asks John Fudens, D.V.M.[3]

W. Jean Dodds, D.V.M., well known for her research at Cornell University College of Veterinary Medicine, states, "Recently, polyvalent [containing different viruses] vaccines have been shown to induce suppression of absolute lymphocyte responsiveness. Previous studies have shown a reduction in platelet count. Can antigenic overload from single or combination vaccines overwhelm the host's immune system? If so, can immunosuppression result?"[4] Dr. Dodds raises the possibility that inoculating our dogs with all these different viruses at one time may weaken their overall health.

Vaccinated dogs also "shed" after being inoculated with modified live vaccines. Dogs (and cats) actually shed the viruses through their skin and feces for ten to twenty-one days. If one of your other dogs has an autoimmune disease, exposure to this shedding can be extremely dangerous.

Richard Pitcairn, D.V.M., received a Ph.D. in immunology and has done extensive research with tissue samples. He reports that when overpopulation has occurred in the wild, there have been rabies epidemics or distemper epidemics, but never both at once. Few people get both diphtheria and measles at the same time, yet we vaccinate for both simultaneously. How would you feel if your internist recommended that you be vaccinated for all the childhood diseases as well as influenza and hepatitis every year for the rest of your life?

Do vaccines cause harm? Dr. Pitcairn states that the majority of problems facing veterinarians today stem from vaccines. (The

term used in homeopathy for this condition is *vaccinosis*.) He
cites case histories of seriously ill animals that improved when
given a homeopathic remedy known to treat vaccinosis. In fact,
says Pitcairn, the animals did not respond to other remedies until
given the one that counteracted the damage done by vaccines:
"The effect of vaccination, besides the physical effects of stimulating an antibody response, is to establish a chronic disease . . .
resulting in mental, emotional, and physical changes that can, in
some cases, be a permanent condition."[5]

Dr. Pitcairn has also shown that in each animal, vaccination
causes a chronic condition with different multiple symptoms.
When faced with these symptoms, we often think our dogs have
contracted a disease or developed a problem, rather than identifying the ailment as vaccinosis. Pitcairn says that such symptoms
include laziness or inaction; finicky or ravenous appetite; poor
grooming; vomiting or cough; cystitis; nephritis; inflammatory
bowel disease; chronic upper respiratory infections; increased
sexual desire; aggression; destructiveness; excessive licking; and
seizures. He warns, "If I may venture to make a prediction, it is
that fifty to one hundred years from now, people will look back
at the practice of introducing disease into people and animals for
the purpose of preventing these same diseases as foolishness . . . a
foolishness similar to that of the practice of bloodletting and the
use of toxic doses of mercury in the treatment of disease."[6]

If you knew, asks Dr. Pitcairn, that by giving a vaccination,
you might save an animal from an acute disease but would also
be sentencing him to a lifetime of chronic disease, would you
still vaccinate? C. Edgar Sheaffer, D.V.M., has said that "vaccinosis
in animals is a true disease state."[7] My own research leads me to
believe that some vaccines prevent acute disease by presenting a

chronic disease in its place and that the disease will come back in a form that modern veterinary medicine is incapable of curing.

Drs. Pitcairn and Chambreau, as well as many other veterinarians, feel that poor nutrition and vaccinations are the primary causes of all chronic and most acute health problems our animal companions experience today. They also believe that with optimal nutrition, the number of animals succumbing to infectious disease would decrease dramatically in three to four generations. This would virtually eliminate the pressure to develop and rush vaccines to market.

According to Volhard and Brown, "Immunologists are finding a direct correlation between the increase in autoimmune and chronic disease states and the overuse of vaccines. Breeders have had entire litters wiped out after using parvo vaccines. Some breeds (notably rottweilers) who were subjected to weekly doses of parvo vaccine in the late 1980s were riddled with bone cancer and died around the age of four years. The Lyme disease vaccine is thought to have been responsible for the collapse of some dogs' immune systems, and a recent study at Cornell University suggests that treating the disease is less risky than getting the vaccine. Some European veterinarians now believe that the benefits of many vaccines are outweighed by the risks, and that the dog is better either not being vaccinated or being vaccinated only for distemper and parvo."[8]

Why do our doctors recommend vaccinations so vehemently? Why must we be forced to settle for chronic conditions in place of optimum health? Western medical and veterinary schools indoctrinate their students in a single belief system, that of allopathic medicine. Graduates of these institutions truly believe vaccines help keep disease under control. In addition, the very schools that teach drug and vaccine therapies are funded by the petrochemical and pharmaceutical industries, which manipulate the human and animal population in order to maximize profits.

Indeed, many veterinarians no longer believe in the practice of vaccination but are afraid to buck the system. A few brave souls have condemned the practice in print, but the public is still largely unaware of the dangers associated with vaccines.

As a direct result of vaccination, humans have had to deal with cancer, leukemia, multiple sclerosis, autism, lupus, mental retardation, blindness, asthma, epilepsy, cerebral palsy, encephalitis, paralysis, tuberculosis, sudden infant death syndrome (SIDS), arthritis, meningitis, allergies, hyperactivity, mild to severe chronic ear infections, learning disabilities, and damage to the liver, kidneys, and pancreas. Our dogs are affected by many of these same things, as well as by parvovirus, renal disease, hyperthyroidism, and innumerable other syndromes. No two dogs are alike; what may be tolerable to one may be toxic to another.

Are vaccines effective? Let's look at some frightening facts regarding vaccination of human beings. A study published in the *American Journal of Public Health* "demonstrates that there is a 7.3-fold increase in cases of sudden infant death syndrome in the interval between zero to three days after immunization with the DPT vaccine."[9]

What about the smallpox vaccine? Smallpox (along with other infectious diseases, including diphtheria and scarlet fever) declined with sanitation reforms instituted in the latter half of the nineteenth century. Government health records from all over the world show that during the most intensive periods of vaccination, the incidence and death rate attributed to smallpox increased, though the disease was actually on the decline when vaccination began.[10]

Before 1903 smallpox was almost unheard of in the Philippines (less than 3 percent of the population was affected, and then only with a mild form). Then the United States military went in and began vaccinating, and by 1905 the Philippines had its first major epidemic. The mortality rate became the highest in cities where vaccination was most intensive. Japan adopted compulsory smallpox vaccinations at a time when the Japanese people had experienced only a few cases. By 1982 they had the largest smallpox epidemic in their history: 165,774 cases and 29,979 deaths. Australia banned the smallpox vaccine after two children died as a result of inoculation, and in the following fifteen years only three cases were reported. The smallpox vaccine was discontinued in the United States after Dr. Henry Kempe reported to Congress in 1966 that fewer people were dying from the disease than from the vaccination.

In 1987 a front-page article in the London *Times* headlined SMALLPOX VACCINE TRIGGERED AIDS VIRUS reported the spread of AIDS through intensive vaccination promoted by the World Health Organization (WHO) in Africa and Brazil. Though this story reached the Associated Press, United Press International, and Reuters news services in the United States, it was never reported to the American public.[11] In 1978 the hepatitis B vaccine was given to thousands of homosexual men in major cities throughout the United States. According to Dr. William Campbell Douglas, the hepatitis B vaccine "exhibits the exact same epidemiology as AIDS," and "homosexual males between twenty [and] forty years of age who were not monogamous were targeted for vaccinations."[12] (For an excellent understanding of the AIDS crisis, read *Inventing the AIDS Virus,* by Peter H. Duesberg. See "Resources.") And what about polio? Here is a sampling of evidence from 1958 and 1959:

Tennessee	119 cases of polio before compulsory shots
	386 cases of polio after compulsory shots
Ohio	17 cases of polio before compulsory shots
	123 cases of polio after compulsory shots
North Carolina	78 cases of polio before compulsory shots
	190 cases of polio after compulsory shots [13]

By the time the Salk vaccine was replaced by the Sabin oral vaccine, the epidemic had been on a downswing for many years, even in areas where no vaccination centers had been set up. In June 1985 the *Los Angeles Times* reported that the only cases of polio occurring in the United States were being caused by the Sabin vaccine.[14]

Both the Salk and the Sabin vaccines were "cultured" in monkeys, and macerated monkey kidneys constituted an ingredient of the vaccine. Consequently, cancerous brain tumors containing genetic material from the SV-40 monkey virus have been discovered in people who were vaccinated and in children born to mothers who received the polio vaccine during pregnancy.[15]

Viera Scheibner, Ph.D., a retired principal research scientist with a doctorate in natural sciences and author of *Vaccination: A Medical Assault on the Immune System,* has summarized the results of orthodox medical research on vaccines and their long- and short-term side effects, including brain damage and death. The research proves the ineffectiveness of vaccines in preventing infectious diseases, as shown by epidemics in fully vaccinated populations and the causal link between DPT and polio vaccines and crib death.

Dr. Scheibner developed, along with electronics engineer Leif Karlsson, a breathing monitor for babies thought to be at risk for "cot death" (crib death, or SIDS) called cot watch. They noticed that the alarm sounded when babies suffered various stresses; vaccination was found to be the most prominent stressful event. The link between vaccine injections and cot death became painfully obvious. Her book is dedicated to the babies and their parents who suffered from vaccination.

Dr. Scheibner studied some thirty thousand pages of medical papers dealing with vaccination and found no evidence of the effectiveness and safety of vaccines. Vaccines are highly noxious. Neither the sum nor any of their parts should ever be injected into human beings (let alone our cats and dogs, who are considerably smaller than we are). They erode the immune system and alter the immunological response to diseases. The appearance of many new autoimmune diseases, such as asthma, childhood leukemia, cancer, the upsurge in the incidence of cerebral palsy, infantile convulsions seen in children of vaccination age and not before, should all be taken as serious warnings that medicine should focus on treating the infectious diseases of childhood (and puppyhood) rather than attempting to eradicate them.

Infectious diseases of childhood are beneficial when contracted at the right age and allowed to run their natural course. These diseases serve to prime the immune systems of animals and children.[16] When people contract the measles, their overall immune system is strengthened in response to the mild challenge of this simple disease (death as a consequence of measles is generally seen only in undernourished populations). When doctors started routinely vaccinating children against the measles, we started to see babies contracting the disease at a dangerously early age because vaccinated mothers were not able to pass on an immunity. And what was the medical community's solution to this dilemma? Vaccinate infants for measles even earlier!

Might the whole business of vaccinations be a scare tactic perpetrated on the world's people? According to a report presented by the British Association for the Advancement of Sciences in 1971, deaths from diphtheria, whooping cough (pertussis), scarlet fever, and measles had declined by 90 percent from their peak in 1860 by the time DPT shots were in common use around 1940. After French children had been inoculated in 1941, diphtheria rates rose dramatically to 13,795 cases by the end of the year. By 1943 the number of cases had increased to 46,750.[17] The power of medical science has been based on instilling fear of contagious diseases. Without this atmosphere of fear, they'd be out of jobs. Besides, the big bucks are in discovering new microbes, new vaccines, and new test kits!

But what about vaccination in animals? After all, that's what this book is about! Whereas humans are vaccinated only a few times in their lives, animals are so treated once or twice a year for life. Pamphlet #3 of the Florida League for Humane Progress in Saint Petersburg, Florida, quotes the Delson Chemical Company as stating that compulsory inoculation of your dog is unconstitutional, not to mention unnecessarily troublesome and expensive. The League has concluded that inoculations for canine diseases can be extremely dangerous and are at best unreliable. Vaccinated dogs frequently develop paralysis, blindness, and convulsions; some even die.[18]

And J. E. R. McDonough, F.C.R.S., has written: "Immunization with an attenuated virus [modified live vaccine] cannot prevent distemper. The author has treated many dogs which have developed distemper despite two to three injections of the preventative agent. He is of the opinion that fits, chorea hysteria, etc., in dogs have become more frequent since the use of distemper vaccine. Successful prevention will never by achieved by inoculation."[19]

The English homeopath C. E. I. Day, M.A., Veterinary M.B., M.R.C.V.S., tells us that "there is an awakening recognition among veterinarians of the connection between immunization and various illnesses" and conditions, including bloat, stained teeth, ulcers, chronic gastroenteritis, and seizures. After conducting controlled studies of the effects of both vaccinations and homeopathic immunizations for kennel cough in dogs, Day has concluded that its vaccine is not an advantage but a health risk.[20]

Many other articles have been written over the years about the relationship between vaccinations and immune system diseases. (See "Resources," particularly articles by Day, Dodds, Rude, Oehen, Tizard, Wilford, McDonald, Phillips, Bastide, and Frick.)

Most people with chronically ill animal companions believe the animals were always sick, but often the problems can be traced to the time of vaccination (or to their parents' having been vaccinated). Vaccinosis does not afflict all vaccinated animals; some are lucky enough to have very strong immune systems. But you take a risk every time you allow your animals, your children, or yourself to be vaccinated. Remember, it's your decision, unless the laws in your state complicate your freedom of choice.

Ron D. Schultz, D.V.M., Ph.D., of the University of Wisconsin School of Veterinary Medicine (professor and chair of the Department of Pathobiological Services), is recognized as a pioneer in clinical immunology and vaccinology. Dr. Schultz feels there has been a tremendous overuse of vaccination and antibiotics.

In both human and veterinary medicine, often no immunity develops, or so-called vaccine breaks occur, whereby the stimulation of antibodies isn't sufficient to protect against the natural disease. Conventional medicine blames the body. Dr. John Fudens states, "It is the fault of the vaccines, as conventional vaccination treats all humans and animals the same."[21] All dogs, for example, get the same number of virus particles in the vaccines, regardless of the animal's weight or age. They (and we) all get inoculated with the same combinations of viruses, on the same schedule, and then get the same boosters whether they need them or not.

Even when injectable vaccines do create antibodies, the body still pays a high price. Tissue damage may be caused by massive amounts of *adjuvant* (the substance used to stabilize the vaccine) and *antigen* (the actual virus particles, which allopathic practitioners believe stimulate immunity) overloading the system. When large quantities of antigen combined with particles of the carrying agent (usually aluminum hydroxide) enter the body, cysts and tumors often form at the vaccine site and become cancerous.[22] This has become a very serious condition in cats.

Holistic veterinarians and others have raised many additional questions: How can you declare a vaccine safe with a test group of only fifteen animals? Are booster vaccinations needed annually? Is it safe to vaccinate geriatric animals? Drs. Ron Schultz and Tom R. Phillips, writing in *Kirk's Current Veterinary Therapy* (a book even your conventional veterinarian will have on his shelf), say:

A practice that was started many years ago and that lacks scientific validity or verification is annual revaccinations. Almost without exception there is no immunologic requirement for annual revaccination. Immunity to viruses persists for years or for the life of the animal. Successful vaccination to most bacterial pathogens produces an immunologic memory that remains for years allowing an animal to develop a protective anamnestic (secondary) response when exposed to virulent organisms. Only the immune response to toxins requires boosters (e.g., tetanus toxin booster, in humans, is recommended once every seven to ten years), and no toxin vaccines are currently used for dogs or cats. Furthermore, revaccination with most viral vaccines fails to stimulate an anamnestic (secondary) response as a result of interference by existing antibody (similar to maternal antibody interference). The practice of annual vaccination in our opinion should be considered of questionable efficacy unless it is used as a mechanism to provide an annual physical examination or is required by law.[23]

(For instance, certain states require annual revaccination for rabies.)

Dr. Schultz vaccinates his puppies for distemper and parvo, then tests their titers (a quantitative measure of the concentration of an antibody or antigen in the bloodstream) annually; he has found that the dogs still have titers in their old age. He does not revaccinate his dogs, except for rabies. Even the rabies vaccine, though legally required every three years (or annually, in some states), is probably good for a longer period—laboratories have not challenged animals with the rabies virus over a long period of time to see if the vaccine would be good for as long as ten or even twenty years. Because these tests haven't been conducted, veterinarians continue to vaccinate every one to three years for the life of the animal. It is my opinion that we are playing Russian roulette every time an animal is either vaccinated or given a booster shot. Remember, for dogs, the rabies vaccine is the only one required by law.

If you have a dog that has had a bad reaction to the rabies (or other) vaccine, or you know your breed of dog is susceptible to vaccinosis, get a veterinary certification. Most states honor it, at least for a few months. If your veterinarian gives you a hard time about not vaccinating for distemper, for example, suggest testing titers as Dr. Schultz does to see whether your dog has retained protection against distemper or other diseases. A blood sample is sent to a lab, which measures the amount of antibodies present against a disease. These antibodies may have been formed either as a result of vaccination or owing to healthy, natural exposure. Many people report that their animals have maintained titers against distemper for as many years as they've been tested.

Dr. Schultz reminds us that we don't know what level of antibodies (what titer) is needed for an individual's protection. Some need just a few antibodies; some need many more. Says Dr. Chambreau, "The best thing to do is to boost your pet's overall health by feeding fresh raw food and supplements as described in this book and not to worry."[24] Unfortunately, we have a system that pressures us, legally, to give our dogs chronic disease via injectable vaccinations.

Most holistic veterinarians recommend alternatives to conventional vaccination, such as monitoring serum antibody titers. (It is very important to ask for vaccine-related immunity and to start at low dilutions when ordering the tests—otherwise, the lab will test for the active virus, and the results will be distorted.)

Avoid the common practice of multiple, simultaneous vaccination. Research indicates that this practice is not only minimally efficacious but produces unacceptable side effects. If you choose to vaccinate, avoid vaccination thirty days prior to estrus onset (heat cycle in females), during estrus, pregnancy, or lactation. Vaccination should also be avoided entirely in geriatric animals, sick or debilitated patients, and immunocompromised animals.

The following are a few examples of vaccinosis related to me by Dr. Chambreau. She tells of a golden retriever who developed severe ear problems that lasted longer and longer after every annual set of immunizations. When he was six, she started treating him homeopathically. The ear responded very slowly, and two years later had been clear for thirteen months. Then he received his mandatory rabies vaccine, and the ear relapsed, taking another six months to be healed again.

Many dogs develop problems within a few weeks or months of vaccination that respond to homeopathic medicines known to counteract the negative effects of vaccines. Dr. Chambreau told me about a poodle who would go in for vaccines and develop an infection somewhere in the body two weeks later—ears one year, vagina another year, between the toe pads another year. After antibiotic treatment, the infection would be gone, but the dog would become lethargic, irritable, have a dull, dry coat, shed a lot, not let her nails be trimmed, and want to eat dog feces. This would last six months and then she would be fine (though less healthy year after year) for a month or two, until her next vaccination. Homeopathic treatment and ceasing vaccination cured this dog.

Dr. Chambreau recalls that a collie kennel that stopped vaccinating discovered that its collies would successfully have puppies for four years longer than before.

Allopathic veterinarians claim that vaccine reactions are rare, but I'm hopeful that eventually they'll recognize, just as holistic veterinarians have, that the possible long-term effects (such as chronic disease) are just as dangerous as the diseases the vaccines are meant to prevent.

To understand the concept of vaccination, imagine my handing you a glass of bovine urine to drink and telling you that it would keep you from getting sick. This is, in effect, what we're doing by subjecting our animal companions to these suspicious substances. The vaccines we so readily inject into our animals' bodies (and our own) may contain any of the following noxious ingredients: decayed animal or animal embryo proteins, pus, blood, diseased mucus, urine, feces, formaldehyde, acetone, mercury derivatives, aluminum, carbolic acid, glycerine, and even antibiotics (to protect the virus particles from bacterial contamination). And to think this is what we've been convinced produces protection against disease!

The bottom line is that "unhealthy animals should not be vaccinated, and healthy ones don't need to be because they can probably resist infection, or may be successfully treated holistically even if they do get infected. This is not, of course, a 100 percent guarantee. But vaccines don't provide 100 percent guarantees or protection, and with them, as you've seen, come long-term consequences to overall health."[25]

When we build a state-of-the-art office building, we install elaborate warning and safety systems. We test them periodically to be sure they work. The same is true with inflammatory responses that test our immune systems. The common cold virus in people, dogs, and cats is a perfect example of testing the immune system to see if and how it functions. Orthodox medicine advocates vaccination—a futile attempt to prevent the immune system from functioning by not allowing our children and animals to contract childhood diseases. We have an irrational fear of illness. The truth is, childhood illnesses create immunities to many diseases we could contract as adults. Many individuals who have developed cancer and degenerative diseases report that they had few infectious diseases as children.

Do you actually know what vaccines you, your children, or your animals have been injected with? When shopping for a car or a computer, we investigate the manufacturers, their integrity, their warranties, their maintenance and service policies, what it costs to insure the car, and what it takes to keep it running. But when it comes to our own bodies and those of our precious animals, do we ask for the credentials of the pharmaceutical company? What's in a medication? What are its side effects? How was it tested? How long has it been in use? What are the alternatives? What are the chances that our animals will get these diseases if we don't vaccinate?

Isn't it time to take responsibility not only for our own health but for that of our companion animals? Every medical system since prehistory has acknowledged the power of a higher being, of spirit, and of the life force. But have the American Medical Association, the Veterinary Medical Association, the American Dental Association, the National Institutes of Health, the Centers for Disease Control, the World Health Organization, the pharmaceutical companies, and the Food and Drug Administration become our new gods? Perhaps all living things were put on this earth with everything they need for survival. Where did we get the idea that we know better and can tamper with something as precious and complex as the immune system? After all, we can't get drugs and vaccines out of our blood once they're there. Only through deep homeopathic treatment or other holistic modalities can we ameliorate the effects of drugs and vaccination gone wrong.

Perhaps we can have healthy animals simply by making lifestyle changes (fresh raw foods, purified water, natural supplements, fresh air, regular exercise, proper hygiene, reduced exposure to stress and pollutants). With such a regimen, who'd need vaccines? We'd actually have immune systems operating at their peak!

I hope by now you're at least willing to question the practice of vaccination, especially the whole idea of massive, repeated (booster) vaccinations. I encourage you to find out as much as you can, not only for your own sake but for the sake of our animals, our children, and future generations. If we just continue to accept the practice of vaccination and do not speak out when we see the effects of vaccinosis, a new and safer system (such as the use of immune boosters rather than immune suppressors) will never be developed. I feel we're on the right track when we work holistically to keep both ourselves and our animals healthy in the first place. What a concept—a healthy immune system simply supported to do the job for which nature designed it, to keep us well naturally!

There are still many questions to be answered: Would my veterinarian continue to examine and treat my animals? Could they be boarded or groomed? Should I isolate them at home? How do I help my already vaccinated animals? How could I protect them with homeopathic vaccination or *nosodes* (homeopathic substitutes for conventional vaccines)? If a rabies vaccine must be administered by law, is there any help I can give my animals?

Guidelines for Vaccination

FIRST, AS ALWAYS, I recommend that you become the client of a holistic veterinarian. Interview several to find out their philosophy regarding treatment and vaccinations. Let them know you want to do the absolute best for your animal and ask what they recommend. After this process, if you still wish to vaccinate, please make sure the animal is as healthy as possible at the time and that he does not receive any other treatment, such as surgery, a bath, or even teeth cleaning, during the same visit. If your dog is taking antibiotics or steroids, these drugs suppress the immune system, so do *not* vaccinate then.

If you choose to vaccinate, I recommend only the vaccines required by law. Discuss using killed-virus vaccines rather than modified live ones, and don't use combination vaccines. Use homeopathic remedies for any side effects that may occur, and keep in mind that a vaccine is supposed to provide lifetime protection. Further boosters, as previously mentioned, are of little or no benefit and may undo whatever antibody protection you've created. I've found most veterinary clinics automatically want to update vaccinations when animals are brought in for their annual visits, so you must tell your veterinarian why you wish to stop this practice. Make sure he or she puts a note to this effect in your animal's records. Remember, you are the caretaker of this animal . . . not them.

If you must bring a sick animal to a new veterinarian who wants to vaccinate, I urge you to refuse, reminding him or her of the manufacturer's instructions accompanying the product that it is to be administered to healthy animals only.

Do not vaccinate animals during any time of stress on the immune system, such as when you have to board your animal at a kennel. Even the simple act of bathing lowers the body temperature and thus creates stress.

To me, there is no safe time. How do we know whether our animals are incubating a disease or are immunosuppressed? I can only suggest that you consult with a practitioner well versed in veterinary homeopathy and other alternative healing therapies and then weigh the risks. I hope this information helps you make your own decision, rather than having one forced upon you—out of fear, habit, or ignorance—by your breeder or veterinarian.

If you do vaccinate for rabies, use only a killed-virus vaccine. Drs. Chambreau and Pitcairn highly recommend giving the homeopathic nosode Lyssin 30C two hours after the rabies vaccine has been administered, but only if the animal isn't under deep homeopathic treatment. Again, be sure the animal is as healthy as possible at the time of vaccination.

What about animals that have already been vaccinated? Some may not have been negatively affected at all. Most show subtle signs of energy imbalance. And many are obviously ill with any of several ailments. It's best to contact a holistic practitioner as soon as you see a problem.

And even if you become certain that vaccination made your animal ill, don't feel guilty. Remember that you did your best, based on the advice of experts, the veterinarians to whom you entrusted the care of your animal, and that they, too, were only doing what they were taught was appropriate.

NOSODES

IF YOU FEEL your dog needs immunization but are now fearful of conventional vaccines, consider *nosodes,* homeopathic remedies made from diseased tissues or discharges from an infected but unvaccinated and untreated animal. Many people think of nosodes simply as homeopathic vaccines (see Chapter 5, "Natural Remedies"), but this is not their only function. Nosodes can be administered either *therapeutically* (in order to treat a disease) or *prophylactically* (in order to prevent a disease).

Though nosodes do contain a causative organism, their efficacy doesn't depend on the presence of the organism itself. It is the substances formed by the animal's immune system in response to invasion by bacteria or viruses that make nosodes effective. In homeopathic terms, the substance in the nosode was taken from an animal suffering from a disease that manifested itself in a certain symptomatic picture, so the nosode is administered to an animal whose condition resembles that picture. For instance, the nosode distemperinum may be used to treat distemper.

Many nosodes have been proved and have an established drug picture, but most veterinary nosodes have only recently been developed, and there have been no *provings*.[26] These nosodes are used solely for the prevention of a given disease or in its treatment. In some cases, the use of nosodes has brought out symptoms of a latent disease, but I don't know of their ever having produced the disease itself.

As with conventional vaccines, nosodes should be administered only to healthy animals when used preventatively. When they are given to sick animals (even those with only subtle symptoms such as thirst, a red line on the gums, or a dry coat), *some may actually exhibit deeper signs of existing illness.*

Currently nosodes are controversial for several reasons: Should nosodes be used at all? Should they be administered in combination, or one at a time with a break in between? Should they be used routinely for prevention, only after exposure to a particular disease, or as a remedy when the animal has actually contracted the disease? For how long do they protect the animal? Much more work needs to be done to evaluate and standardize the use of nosodes.[27]

You may want to consult via telephone with a holistic veterinarian (see "Resources"). Some practitioners advise that you boost immunity with nutrition and supplements only. Others prefer homeopathic treatment. And some promote the use of nosodes not only as being perfectly safe but as being the best alternative to conventional vaccination. Of course, nosodes are not always effective—but neither are conventional vaccines.

The homeopath C. E. I. Day has shown that homeopathic vaccines may protect against kennel cough.[28] An outbreak of kennel cough among forty dogs showed the use of conventional vaccination to be ineffective. Eighteen of the forty dogs had been previously vaccinated with P13 and Bordetella before the outbreak. Every one of the vaccinated dogs became ill with a cough (100 percent), but only nineteen of the remaining twenty-two unvaccinated dogs developed symptoms (86 percent). The symptoms were severe, and the owners decided to try the kennel cough nosode. Over the next several months, a total of 214 dogs were treated with the nosode and observed. The incidence of kennel cough decreased in the previously unvaccinated dogs.

Historically, nosodes and homeopathic remedies have been most successful in the midst of human epidemics, which is probably when to best use these remedies in animals as well. Dr. Chambreau suggests the following scenario:

You've put your new dog on a fresh food diet consisting of raw meat, raw vegetables, cooked grains [see Chapter 4, "Nutrition"], and supplements. Your holistic practitioner has treated the animal with homeopathy or other holistic therapies in order to eliminate any of the subtle signs of underlying energy imbalance. You have not undermined the system by immunizing them. Then you go to a dog show or bring home a stray you've rescued and soon after you hear of an outbreak of distemper at the show or in the neighborhood. You give one 200C dose of the nosode for distemper as well as herbal or dietary supplements to stimulate the immune system, and wait to see if any symptoms develop. If they do, you treat them homeopathically with the help of your holistic veterinarian. Unfortunately, the notion of using nosodes on an ongoing basis is slipping into our modern rationale of "protecting the body because it can't be healthy enough to protect itself." But far better than using vaccines or even nosodes—supposedly to prevent or control disease—is to have your dog be so healthy that you don't feel the need to protect against any specific disease.[29]

Indeed, there's a trend among many holistic veterinarians to use nosodes in place of vaccines. I feel they're far less risky than conventional vaccines as a preventative protocol. Most often given orally, they may be injected as well; however, I'm opposed to the all-too-common practice of injecting things into the body. If you decide to use nosodes prophylactically, contact your homeopathic veterinarian for recommendations as to how and when to administer them.

Even though Dr. Pitcairn seems to have had no problems with using nosodes in combination, he admits that single nosodes are probably a better bet.[30] Drs. Loops, Hamilton, Chambreau, and others recommend that ascending potencies (30C, 200C, and 1M in puppies) of individual nosodes be given

at eight weeks of age or older, according to the following protocol (one dose is three granules given orally):

- One dose of 30C twice in one day.
- One week later, one dose of 30C.
- One week later, one dose of 200C.
- One month later, one dose of 200C.
- One month later, one dose of 1M.
- Six months later, one dose of 1M. [31]

Another alternative is to use only the 30C potency on the
same timetable. Yet another protocol Dr. Loops is pioneering is
to work only with LM (50 millesimal) potencies on a more frequent basis for the first five to six months of the dog's life, but
these potencies should only be prescribed by very experienced
homeopathic veterinarians.

This schedule may be "boostered up" every six months if
your homeopathic veterinarian feels it's necessary or used only
after potential exposure. Your veterinarian will advise you about
what the best regimen is for your particular case and which
nosodes to use.

I advise against combination nosodes. Start with distemper
and wait until step 3 before adding any other nosode.

Warning: I've heard that some holistic veterinarians have recommended oral administration of nosodes, with follow-up doses
put in the water bowl. This can be a very dangerous practice.
Nosodes are not food supplements but extremely energetic
remedies. They should be used, if at all, only under the strictest
guidelines, so seek a second opinion if this manner of administration is suggested to you. When used haphazardly or on a long-
term basis, nosodes may cause an *aggravation* (symptoms that
actually mimic the remedy, that is, look like the disease you're

trying to prevent), as can any homeopathic remedy. Dr. Loops says this would be unlikely to occur when using LM potencies.

Keep reading the holistic animal care magazines (such as *Wolf Clan, Natural Pet,* Marina Zacharias's *Natural Rearing Newsletter,* Sis Sewell's *Healthy Pets, Naturally*) to get updates on nosodes. I've found that all the practitioners in the holistic community care deeply about the welfare of companion animals. Feel free to share information with them and to network actively. If you experience a problem with nosodes, report it to Drs. Pitcairn, Chambreau, Loops, or Hamilton, or to the American Holistic Veterinary Medical Association (AHVMA) (all telephone numbers and addresses are listed in "Resources").

Remember, the jury is still out on nosodes. Opinion is deeply divided right now. To repeat my feeling about using any substance, conventional or not: A healthful lifestyle, with plenty of fresh food and proper hygiene, is what keeps our immune systems at their peak. Let's encourage research dollars to be spent on natural ways to build up the immunity of both ourselves and our companion animals so that we can, at long last, prove the efficacy of holistic health care!

A BLOOD BANK FOR ANIMALS

A LIFESAVING TREATMENT worth discussing here is transfusion medicine. This practice has undergone a tremendous growth in the last five years. Until now, animal blood components have not been readily available. Consequently, many vets may not be familiar with their use. Transfusions can be helpful in some instances.

Marina Zacharias provides us with the following information:

Dr. Jean Dodds has set up a lab service called "Hemopet" (see "Resources" section). Its purpose is twofold. First, it is a rescue service for racing greyhounds. Secondly, those dogs that pass rigorous blood screening tests are kept for a short time as "blood donors." During their stay they are, of course, kept in the most gracious of conditions with an enriched environment, exercise, and personal attention. They are then adopted out to good homes. Screening for blood-borne diseases is crucial, and all are tested for brucellosis, Lyme disease, heartworm, Valley fever, and many others. Hemopet provides a variety of blood donor products, including canine whole blood and canine fresh frozen plasma, available to any veterinarian across the country. Currently, many vets do not perform transfusions due to the high costs of individual collection and screening. Where community donors are available, most are screened only once a year, leaving the safety of the blood in question. Most owners are less concerned with costs when compared to the safety and efficacy of the transfusion. Many hospital stays can be shortened when receiving a blood component, so the actual overall cost can also be justified. Fresh frozen plasma is one of the most important products Hemopet produces, and it has a variety of applications. It can be used to control serious bleeding diseases, such as hemophilia and Von Willebrands disease. It is generally indicated for the replacement of albumin, globulins, electrolytes, and other nutrients of plasma. It has been essential for helping orphaned puppies or kittens and for those neonates who received only a minimal amount of colostrum. Given within the first forty-eight hours, it provides the neonate with the necessary immunity it needs to survive. The plasma is then repeated at about ten days and again at three to four weeks of age (transfusions would be given more often for sick neonates). One of the most important uses of fresh frozen plasma is in the exposure to acute viral diseases such as parvovirus. Dr. Dodds reported at the AHVMA conference that a drastic reduction in death from parvo is seen when the plasma is used. A clinic in Winnipeg has reported 100 percent recoveries and shorter hospital stays on all parvo cases while using the plasma. Transfusions of fresh frozen plasma also happens to be helpful in cases of acute pancreatitis and in burn patients, according to Dr. Dodds.[32]

TOXINS IN YOUR HOME AND GARDEN

THERE ARE MANY reasons to create a nontoxic environment in your home—obviously, health of self, family, and companion animals being at the top of the list. Over time, exposure to toxic chemicals can contribute to cancer, birth defects, genetic changes, allergies, and other disorders and illnesses, to say nothing of a generally weakened immune system.[33]

Another reason to detoxify your home is expense. The use of toxic chemicals in the home indirectly costs billions per year—about $1 billion in medical bills and $5 billion in lost work time. Furthermore, many household items on the market lack adequate warnings.

Owing to their size and physiology, children and animal companions are the most vulnerable to toxicity. They inhale more air per their body weight than do adults because their respiratory rate is 10 percent higher. Many pollutants are heavier than air and are therefore found in greater concentration lower to the ground, so children and animals receive much higher exposure. Finally, their bodies are not as well equipped as adults' to process toxic chemicals.

Cleaning products are among the most hazardous materials found in the home. The following is a list of potentially toxic substances. Check your local health-food store for safe products.

Partial List of Potentially Toxic Substances
Air freshener (especially those in aerosol dispensers)
Ammonia

Antifreeze
Chlorinated water
Dangerous plants
Dishwasher detergent
Disinfectant
Dog treats, like hooves and ears, that are heavily preserved
Fabric softeners
Flea and tick medications
Fluoride
Formaldehyde (new carpets produce formaldehyde fumes)
Furniture polish
Garden chemical sprays
Glass cleaner
Insecticides
Lawn chemicals
Lead paint
Liquid dish detergent
Pesticides
Rawhide chew toys that contain propylene glycol
Scouring powder
All heavy-duty chemicals

Pottery and brightly colored dog dishes can contain heavy metals in the bright paints used to decorate them. Pottery not fired at a high enough temperature or for the right amount of time can leak lead. Use stainless steel; it's safer. Other sources of lead include batteries, linoleum, putty, tar paper, golf balls, fishing sinkers, drapery weights, shotgun pellets, and water from lead pipes in old houses or buildings with brass faucets. Eating lead-based paints creates toxic symptoms. Pressure-treated lumber contains arsenic and can be deadly if your dog chews it. Any unusual symptom that your dog shows should prompt you to do a complete survey of your animal's environment.[34]

Please note that many companion animals' levels of toxic metals have reached dangerous proportions. If you wish to have a heavy metal or mineral analysis (by atomic absorption rather than by flame photometry, which is not as exacting) done on a sample of your companion animal's fur, contact Analytical Research Labs (see "Resources").

Warning: Be sure to read labels on everything that goes into your companion animal's mouth. For instance, the preservative sodium benzoate, which is added to such products as Stat and Nutrical as well as many brands of aloe vera juice, can be toxic to pets. Look for brands free of this dangerous preservative.

I also highly recommend the use of an air purification system to minimize airborne contaminates.

In her book, *Natural Healing for Dogs and Cats,* Diane Stein provides this list of common plants that are poisonous to pets as well as humans (so be certain to keep them out of reach of children too!): bittersweet (bark, leaves, and seeds), dumb cane (including berries), poison hemlock, ivy (English and Baltic), jimson weed, thorn apple, marigold, marsh marigold, hemp, mistletoe, oleander (all parts), philodendron, poinsettia, poison ivy, potato (unripe tubers and sprouts from tubers), and rhubarb (leaf blades). Poisoning symptoms include vomiting, diarrhea, convulsions, coma, dizziness, loss of muscular control and coordination, disordered vision, intense thirst, rapid pulse, swollen mouth and throat, and itching, redness, and blistering of skin.

Here's a summary of basic steps for getting started on your holistic regimen.

1. Make contact with a holistic veterinarian, either a telephone consultant or someone who practices near you, or both. Dr. Chambreau suggests that "If you choose a telephone consultant, find a sympathetic local veterinarian. Take him or her to lunch (get away from the office environment) and see if he or she can work with you on your holistic terms. If not, move on to the next vet on your list and take him or her to lunch!"

2. Start feeding your dog the fresh food diet (see Chapter 4, "Nutrition") as soon as possible.

3. Use stainless-steel bowls.

4. Research the vaccination issue thoroughly before inoculating your animal. Remember, you can't undo a vaccination.

5. Instead of annual vaccinations (unless required by law), visit your veterinarian for a checkup. Think prevention. You can do blood workups, including titers and fecal exams.

6. Use baby soap (like Ivory Snow) to wash pet bedding if your dog has skin allergies or problems, and don't use fabric softeners, as they can cause damage to the central nervous system.

7. Use gentle shampoos and conditioners from herbal sources (fleas drown in soapy water) to bathe your dog.

8. Don't use flea collars unless they are 100 percent herbal. If you have a flea or parasite problem, it's the animal's immune system that's to blame. Feed your animal the fresh food diet and you'll see an amazing difference. If you see fleas, treat the environment with natural flea products.

9. Eliminate household cleaners and kennel disinfectants and use chlorine bleach (1/4 cup per gallon of water) or 3 percent hydrogen peroxide (H_2O_2) and disinfect often. Lysol and Pinesol are typical household cleaners that are toxic to animals. Before disinfecting, remove the animals, and rinse the area thoroughly after disinfecting.

10. Check your or your gardener's sprays and fertilizers. Could they cause harm to your dog? Don't use snail pellets.

11. New carpet, carpet cleaners, reupholstery, construction work, glues, dust, and pollens can all be toxic. Consider the

Second Wind air purifier and Rainbow vacuum system.

12. Think about the consequences to your animal with anything new introduced into your environment, including microwaving. Use bottled water and think natural!

WHAT ARE WE FEEDING OUR COMPANION ANIMALS?

DIANE STEIN RECOUNTS her some six years of testing pet food, bottled water, and some human foods routinely fed to animals both at home and in veterinary clinics.

Her work began when her own cat became ill. She sent a sample of fur to Analytical Research Labs. The deranged mineral levels that were detected prompted a heavy-metal screening test. The lab found heavy levels of lead and mercury and also extremely high levels of aluminum (.45 ppm [parts per million]; .05 ppm is the allowable level in humans). It was amazing that the animal was still alive under such conditions.

The cat's food and water were then tested. It turned out that the popular prepared food Stein had been feeding, which was highly touted as being both complete and natural, contained several thousand times more aluminum than was allowable for humans! She treated her cat with homeopathically prepared substances and started making her own food, and the cat recovered.

To be sure, aluminum is a very serious cause of chronic degenerative diseases; for example, it has been found in the brains of victims of Alzheimer's disease. Stein found high levels of aluminum in Gerber's[35] baby food (veal, chicken, and beef varieties), Starkist tuna, and every dog and cat food marketed during 1985. The dry food contained the highest levels (even higher than food canned in aluminum) because of the way it's processed.

Stein's study concluded that twenty-eight of the sick dogs and cats she tested had toxic levels of aluminum. She reported finding central nervous system symptoms such as chewing wall boards and doorknobs, trying to catch imaginary objects in the air, and aggressive, violent behavior; a suppressed immune system; chronic dermatitis; coryza; nasal discharge; and endocrine dysfunctions such as hypothyroidism, hyperactivity of the parathyroid due to lowered calcium levels, and adrenal hyperfunction as continued chemical stress influenced the medulla of the adrenals.

She also found that hypothyroidism, diabetes, a lack of pancreatic digestive enzymes, and lowered hydrochloric acid in the stomach (needed for protein digestion) resulted in signs of poor nutrition such as dry, lusterless hair and coat; dry, flaky skin; increased intestinal fermentation; constipation; dehydration; low-grade fever; and liver, kidney, and heart pathologies. Blood tests showed increased BUN (blood urea nitrogen) and creatinine levels (indicating kidney damage), decreased platelets (needed for blood clotting) in the circulating blood, and elevated cholesterol levels (indicating liver and pancreas damage).[36]

Following her strict detoxification program supported by homeopathic treatment, Stein was able to restore balance and health to the tested animals. For four years she tried to share her findings with the Food and Drug Administration (FDA), but to no avail.

Commercial Pet Food

ONCE YOU BEGIN challenging what's in commercial pet food, you'll be amazed at what you'll find. One of the things that convinced me to begin preparing the fresh food diet (see

Chapter 4, "Nutrition") for my animals was the video *Holistic Pet Care,* in which Joanne Stefanatos, D.V.M., tells of a visit to a meat-packing plant, where she saw tumors being cut out of animal carcasses, then placed along with the diseased organs and anything else not salable for human consumption (so-called meat by-products) into a separate container. When she asked what that was all about, plant personnel told her not to worry because this material was only going to be sold to pet-food manufacturers![37]

We have all heard the horror stories of pet food containing contaminated ingredients. There is a darn good reason why your dog may not like his kibble! Ann Martin, author of "Does Your Dog Food Bark? A Study of the Pet Food Fallacy," has stated that she was able to document through government investigators the trek of euthanized dogs and cats in her hometown of London, Ontario, Canada. These animals were sent from veterinary clinics to rendering plants in Quebec and sold as meat meal and digests for livestock and pet food. I think we all find abominable the use of companion animals in pet food, but don't forget the pathogens, pesticides, heavy metals, and drugs that withstand the rendering process. The sodium pentobarbital used to euthanize companion animals withstands the rendering process without undergoing degradation. Ann Martin has devoted the past five years to investigating the pet-food industry in Canada and the United States, the industry's use of a disgusting array of ingredients, and the lack of regulations governing it.

She describes the vegetable proteins contained in dry food— yellow corn, wheat shorts and middlings, soybean meal, rice hulls, and peanut meal—as nothing more than the sweepings and offal from milling-room floors. The removal of the oil, germ, bran, starch, and gluten from these grains eliminates the essential fatty acids and many fat-soluble vitamins and antioxidants. The animal proteins (besides the euthanized companion animals) come from diseased meat, roadkill, contaminated matter from slaughterhouses, and fecal matter. Dead-stock-removal operations provide the "4-D" animals (dead, diseased, dying, or disabled). Most died from unknown causes and had been treated with a wide array of drugs or had been given a lethal injection. These animals then make their way to a receiving plant, where the hide is sold to a tannery; after being completely covered (blackened) by charcoal, the skin, fat, and meat are removed to be used by the pet-food industry. Of course, by then it is unfit for human consumption. If the animal arrived at the receiving plant in a state of decomposition, it is then transported to a rendering plant along with such appetizing foodstuffs as roadkill too large to be buried by the side of the road. Now animals that die on the way to slaughter, along with diseased animals or animal parts, diseased blood, extraneous matter such as hair, feet, heads, mammary glands, carpal and tarsal joints, or any part of the animal condemned for human consumption, can be rendered for pet food.

The slaughterhouse "denatures" these animal parts (thank the Lord), which means that they are doused with chemicals to prevent them from getting back into the human food chain. Ms. Martin states that in Canada the chemical used is Birkolene b. According to the Department of Agriculture, Animal, and Plant Health Inspection Services, the composition of this chemical cannot be disclosed. In the United States a number of agents can be used, including carbolic acid, fuel oil, kerosene, and citronella. For me, the most gruesome statement she makes is that the dogs and cats euthanized at clinics, pounds, and shelters are sold to rendering plants, rendered with other materials, and sold to the pet-food industry. A small rendering plant in Quebec was rendering ten *tonnes* (eleven tons) of dogs and cats per week. You'll hear the pet-food industry vehemently deny these facts. However, the Ministry of Agriculture in Quebec, where a number of these plants are located, advised Ms. Martin that the fur is not removed from dogs and cats and that dead animals are cooked together with viscera, bones, and fat at 115 degree Celsius (236 degrees Fahrenheit) for twenty minutes.[38]

If you don't think your favorite brand of pet food is part of this problem, consider this (and again I quote Ms. Martin): "One large pet food company in the U.S. with extensive research facilities used rendered dogs and cats in their food for years, and when the information came to light claimed no knowledge of it."[39] The Food and Drug Administration's Center for Veterinary Medicine (CVM) in the United States is aware of the use of rendered companion animals in pet food and has stated, "CVM has not acted to specifically prohibit the rendering of pets. However, that is not to say that the practice of using this material in pet food is condoned by CVM."[40] The Association of American Feed Control Officials (AAFCO) guidelines state that there are no restrictions on the type of animal that can be used in meat meal, tankage, digest, and so on. The AAFCO further allows sprays of dried blood, hydrolyzed hair, dehydrated garbage, calf carcasses, dried poultry litter (animal waste products composed of a processed combination of feces from commercial poultry and litter that was present in the floor production of poultry), dried ruminant waste, dried swine waste, and undried processed animal waste products (animal waste products composed of excreta, with or without litter from poultry, ruminants, or any other animal except humans). These guidelines and definitions apply to both livestock feed and pet food.

Now, after all this, what do you think of the veterinarian who tells you "no table scraps"? Ms. Martin worked on this project for more than seven years. Would you eat pet food if your life depended on it? So why would you want to feed it to your animals? Their lives do depend on it!

The *Los Angeles Times,* in an article entitled "Elephant Deaths Draw Spotlights' Glare" reported that two of Circus Vargas's elephants died of tuberculosis.[41] The necropsy showed that one of the elephants' lungs was infected with either cancer or tuberculosis. Her body was then taken to a rendering plant to be processed into animal food. Have you ever seen elephant meat listed on a can or bag of pet food?

Moldy grains and other rancid foods, such as spoiled processed meats, are also used. At one time a particular pet-food company used as a source of fiber peanut shells contaminated with fungus that produced a lethal toxin. In 1983 researchers at the University of California, Davis, alerted veterinarians to be on the lookout for a potentially serious skin disease traced to consumption of several generic dry dog foods in supermarket chains.

A ground-up array of disease-ridden tissue containing high levels of hormones and pesticides (which may have contributed to the animal's death) wind up in a concoction called meat meal. P. F. McGargle, D.V.M., a veterinarian and federal meat inspector, observes that feeding such waste products to animal companions increases their chances of getting degenerative diseases and cancer.[42]

Many people use the term *starvation diet* to describe this

nutritional nightmare. How can anyone consider this to be a healthy diet for our animals? It doesn't remotely resemble the food they'd eat in the wild!

Why, then, have we been feeding our domestic animals such an inferior diet? For years pet-food manufacturers have worked to convince us that only they possess the proper formulas to give our companion animals a balanced diet. That's like telling you that you're not qualified to prepare a nutritious meal for your own child (which is exactly what the baby-food companies try to do!). The pet-food industry turns a profit of some $9 billion a year[43] (although I have heard it was up to $11 billion in 1996), and we Americans have been spending twice as much on pet food as we do on cereals and grains for ourselves, and four times as much on pet food as on baby food[44] (you can make your own baby food, too, by pureeing organic fruits and vegetables in the blender).

Today you need to be a chemist just to identify half the ingredients in a can or bag of pet food. Since I'm not, I'd rather prepare food for my animals from scratch. At least I know what's in it! At first this seemed like a lot of work. Now I enjoy it and feel a tremendous sense of satisfaction in knowing that my animals are eating quality natural food.

Raw Food Versus Cooked Food

PET-FOOD MANUFACTURERS cook their meat to sterilize it and supposedly to prevent disease (they also add chemicals to sterilize and preserve the meat), but this is necessary only because they're using inferior and spoiled animal remains. However, when animal fat is cooked, it becomes grease—which isn't any better for your animal's arteries than it is for your own!

Furthermore, restaurant grease has become a major component of feed-grade animal fat over the past fifteen years. This grease is often held in fifty-gallon drums for weeks and months on end, in extreme temperatures, and kept outside with no regard for its safety or future use. Dogs and cats need the essential fatty acids found in raw meat and cold-pressed oils. Cooking also destroys many of the valuable enzymes found in raw meat and vegetables.

Enzymes break down foods and also play a specific role in the process of absorption of substances. Several enzymes are essential transporters of nutrient substances. Most commercial dog and cat foods are essentially "dead" and rely totally on the animal's own digestive enzymes for nutrition. When the digestive enzymes are overworked, the body identifies the incompletely digested food molecules as foreign *antigens* ("bad guys"). Metabolic enzymes are then called upon to mobilize macrophage *leukocytes* ("good guys" that come in to clean up the garbage) to digest the food. The problem is that these guys are taken from their immune system duties, and as a result the immune system is weakened.

As Douglas Kappstatter, D.V.M., states, "The value of a raw food diet lies in its content of enzymes undamaged by the heat of cooking. Enzymes are responsible for every metabolic reaction that takes place in your body, whether it be the blinking of your eye or the functioning of your liver. Thus, when you're out of enzymes, you're out of vitality . . . in fact, you're out of life."[45] Dr. Kappstatter further explains, "We're all born with a checking account filled with enzymes. A judicious person would contemplate every check written very carefully. When you eat an apple turnover at McDonald's, you're virtually writing a very big check. When you eat an apple, you're writing a much smaller check."[46]

Scientific research justifies the time needed to prepare a fresh food diet. In 1932 Francis M. Pottenger, Jr., M.D., began a ten-year experiment in which he fed a diet of two thirds raw meat, one third raw milk and cod liver oil to a group of cats. (Dog people need to hear about this study, as it is just as important to canine health as it is to feline health.) The study showed that generation after generation of cats on this raw meat diet maintained regular broad faces with prominent malar and orbital arches, adequate nasal cavities, broad dental arches, and regular dentition; inflammation of the gums was seldom seen. The male skull remained differently formed than the female's; in fact, throughout their bodies, each sex maintained its distinct anatomical features. The animals' tissue tone was excellent, and their fur of good quality, with very little shedding. The calcium and phosphorus content of their femurs was consistent, and all internal organs were fully developed and functioned normally.

Over their life span, the cats were resistant to infections, fleas, and various other parasites; they showed no signs of allergies. They were gregarious, friendly, and predictable in behavior. They produced healthy litter after litter, with few miscarriages, and the mothers nursed their young without difficulty.

Dr. Pottenger fed another group of cats a diet of two thirds cooked meat, one third raw milk and cod liver oil. Those cats produced offspring in which each kitten in the litter had a different size skeleton. There were almost as many variations in the faces and dental structures of the second and third generations as there were animals—the effects of a deficient diet were literally written all over these kittens' faces. In addition, their long bones tended to increase in length and decrease in diameter, with the hind legs longer than the front ones. The internal structure of their bones became coarser, and they showed evidence of calcium loss.

By the third generation, their bones had become as soft as rubber, and bone infections were common, as were heart problems; near- and farsightedness; marked irritability; parasites, skin lesions, and allergies; underactive or inflamed thyroids; infections in the respiratory system, kidneys, liver, genital organs, and bladder; arthritis and inflammation of the joints; inflammation of the nervous system; paralysis; and meningitis. By this time the cats were so physiologically bankrupt that none survived beyond their sixth month, thereby terminating the strain.

Some of the cooked-meat-eating females were dangerous to handle, including a trio nicknamed Tiger, Cobra, and Rattlesnake, with their proclivity to bite and scratch. The males, on the other hand, became more docile, often to the point of being unaggressive, and their sex drive was "slack or perverted." This diet seemed to have caused a role reversal, with the females becoming the aggressors and the males becoming passive; there was also evidence of "increasingly abnormal activities between the sexes." Such sexual deviations were never observed among the raw-meat-eating cats.

The average weight of kittens born to cooked-meat-eating mothers was 19 grams less than the raw-meat-nurtured kittens. Diarrhea and pneumonia took a heavy toll on the cooked-meat group of kittens, who developed all kinds of allergies. They sneezed, wheezed, scratched, and were irritable. Autopsies revealed that the intestinal tract of cooked-meat-eating cats measured 72–80 inches long (six feet or longer), whereas the normal length for an average cat's intestines is 48–49 inches (approximately four feet).

Dr. Pottenger concluded that the elements in raw food, which activate and support growth and development in the young, appear easily altered and destroyed by heat processing and oxidation. Just one year on a diet considered adequate for human consumption could so reduce the vitality of cats that it could take them as long as three years to recover, if ever. It took three or four generations on the raw meat diet to reverse these problems genetically.[47] (It is true that if that study were repeated today, all kinds of vitamin and mineral supplements would be added to the cooked diet to make up for some of its difficiencies. And, yes, there are now antibiotics today that might have saved or prolonged those nutritionally deprived cats' lives by suppressing the symptoms of disease.)

So we can't blame genetic deficiencies and chronic diseases simply on luck. We have a responsibility to provide each new generation with what it needs to be better than the last, or we won't have our animal companions around much longer.

At the time of Pottenger's research, the nature and composition of the vital elements in raw food was not then known, but it was understood that ordinary cooking denatures proteins, making them less digestible to carnivores. The modern pet-food industry would argue that all the essential amino acids destroyed by cooking are added back in the form of supplements. However, the supplements used are the cheap, synthetic type (see the section on vitamins and minerals in Chapter 4, "Nutrition").

Necessary Nutrients

YOU CAN'T IGNORE that carnivores benefit from raw meat in ways they can't from cooked, bagged, or canned foods. For even if a cooked food diet could provide essential nutrients, it doesn't necessarily follow that those nutrients can be absorbed by the body. They may have been rendered unabsorbable by excessive heat in the presence of sugar and fat, protein may have been exposed to strong alkaline solutions or oxidized when stored with polyunsaturated fat—means by which the pet-food industry routinely processes ingredients.[48] It's a tricky business trying to replicate the structure of a living thing, and living things (raw whole food) is what carnivores were designed to hunt and eat. When a can of cat food boasts 78 percent moisture and 10 percent crude protein, we know cats will be malnourished eating it.

How can we trust the feeding of our beloved companions to an industry driven by profit? Robert Pett of Pett Foodco says one of the reasons commercial and veterinary pet foods are nutritionally bankrupt is economic competition. Keeping the price competitive dictates cheap ingredients, whose appeal is enhanced by chemicals (artificial colors and flavors). You save money in the short run, but ultimately the veterinary bills are enormous.[49]

My research has shown that the majority of commercial pet-food companies label their products misleadingly, referring to corn husks and peanut shells as "vegetable fiber," and hydrolyzed chicken feathers as "poultry protein products," the sweepings off the milling-room floor as "rice [or wheat] middlings." The percentage of protein, fat, and carbohydrates listed on the labels provides no useful information on biological values (the actual utilization quality of ingredients). Alfred Plechner, D.V.M., author of *Pet Allergies: Remedies for an Epidemic,* makes this challenge: "Can our animals really use this so-called food? Can they even digest it and process it into the necessities of life?"[50]

If our pets keeled over and died after they ate a single can of commercial food, there would be no doubt about its danger. But since it takes years to develop cancer and other degenerative diseases, most allopathic veterinarians just blame these occurrences on fate. They'd certainly never blame their own, expensive veterinary brands. These foods may sustain life, but they don't promote wellness, let alone optimum health.

How quickly pet-food manufacturers and veterinarians have forgotten about a taurine deficiency causing eye problems (lesions and central retinal degeneration) as well as reduced reproduction in breeding female cats, reduced growth of kittens, and dilated cardiomyopathy in cats all over the country.[51] More cats suffer from this disease than dogs do because of their bodies' higher demand for this amino acid. However, it does occur occasionally in dogs fed commercial pet-food diets.

There are ten essential amino acids that dogs require in their daily diet: arginine, histidine, isoleucine, leucine, lysine, methionine, phenylalanine, threonine, tryptophan, and valine. There are also sixteen nonessential amino acids: alanine, asparagine, aspartic acid, carnitine, citrulline, cysteine, GABA, glutamic acid, glutamine, glycine, hydroxyproline, ornithine, proline, serine, taurine, and tyrosine. L-carnitine and taurine supplements, for example, have been helpful to dogs suffering from cardiomyopathy. These twenty-six amino acids are not listed on pet-food labels. They are all obtained primarily from animal proteins and some plant proteins. Taurine, however, is found only in animal protein.[52]

All amino acids, both essential and nonessential, are heat sensitive. So why cook in the first place? We must stop imposing our dietary restrictions on carnivores. They were designed to eat their meat raw, even though pet-food companies would like to convince you that your dog is a kind of "wimpy" creature that can't survive without their processed products.

These companies can use ingredients not fit for human consumption and still claim that their food is nutritionally complete because a governmental body called the National Research Council (NRC), which defines nutrient levels in pet food, says so. These levels are established on the basis of studies using isolated nutrients. Differing diets are fed to animals; the results are observed and recorded. If a particular diet seems to prevent disease from nutritional deficiencies, it's used to establish minimum levels of nutrients that must be present for a food to be considered complete.[53] Another group, the American Association of Feed Control Officials (AAFCO), performs a feeding trial in which a so-called complete diet is fed to animals for a few weeks in order to determine if it prevents obvious diseases or malnutrition.

State and national regulatory bodies permit foods that have passed these two tests to be advertised as nutritionally complete. Another test determines the digestibility of a pet food by measuring the nutrients ingested and then eliminated in the stool. By this means companies try to prove that their food contains nutrients that are digested and absorbed into the body to a degree believed to be adequate.

Many feeding trials are performed by the manufacturers themselves, so we see only the studies they want us to. Besides, the duration of their tests is insufficient to prove anything. Just because an animal doesn't get sick or die during a few weeks' time doesn't mean the diet is good for the animal. It's the subtle deficiencies that occur over the long term that concern me. And how about the excretion test? Is nutrition now a lesson in subtraction—the difference between what is eaten and what is excreted? Many substances, including outright toxins, may be absorbed by the body. Simple digestibility is not an adequate test for nutritional value.

The NRC levels seem ridiculous to me because more than forty nutrients are known to be essential, and another fifty are under investigation. How then can commercial pet food be truly complete? Minimum levels represent the bottom of an average. Would you be satisfied eating no fresh food, but only a processed ration that met NRC levels?

So, once again, we're expected to turn over responsibility for the well-being of our companion animals to someone else, just as we've done with our own medical care and nutritional needs. R. L. Wysong, D.V.M. (a well-respected pet-food manufacturer), calls us the "turn-it-over society," because our habits make promoters of fast food for both humans and animals rich. When huge financial concerns are at stake, we can't trust that our individual best interests are being served.

Dr. Wysong's company has had the courage to admit that its pet food, and every other manufacturer's, is incomplete without the addition of fresh raw meat and vegetables, grains, and supplements. The Wysong Institute has put out a pet health alert to the human companions of dogs and cats, warning that veterinary research has shown that thousands of animals have become ill and suffered needlessly from improper nutrition. In the booklet *Fresh and Raw* (see "Resources"), Dr. Wysong tells us there's no such thing as a complete and balanced commercial pet food, whether bagged or canned, and that supplementation to such food is an absolute necessity.

The Wysong Company recommends, of course, that you buy

its brand of food and supplements. Dr. Wysong admits that cooking destroys, alters, or depletes many vital nutrients and that heat can initiate chemical reactions that turn food into toxins and carcinogens. He states that the ideal protein source in the wild is "prey" animals, and that for domesticated animals, muscle and organ meats are the best substitutes. [54]

Pet-Food Additives

HERE IS A partial list of the most common pet-food additives, provided by the Animal Protection Institute of America's investigative report. Although some ingredients on this list may sound harmless, in combination with others they may form toxic compounds. They may also cause allergies in some animals.[55]

Antioxidant Preservatives
- Ethoxyquin
- Butylated hydroxyanisole
- Tertiary butylhydroquinone
- Propyl gallate
- Rosemaric acid/rosmarequinone

Antimicrobial Preservatives
- Citric acid
- Hydrochloric acid
- Phosphoric acid
- Sorbic acid
- Fumaric acid
- Pryoligneous acid
- Propionic acid
- Sodium propionate
- Calcium propionate
- Potassium sorbate
- Sodium nitrite

Humectants
- Sorbito

- Corn syrups
- Sucrose/dextrose
- Cane molasses

Coloring Agents/Preservatives
- Artificial colors
- Azo dyes (tartrazine [FD&C yellow No. 5], sunset yellow [FD&C yellow No. 6], alura red [FD&C red No. 40])
- Nonazo dyes (brilliant blue (FD&C blue No. 1), indigotine [FD&C blue No. 2])
- Caramel color
- Sodium nitrite
- Sodium eythrobate
- Titanium dioxide
- Iron oxide
- Sodium meabisulfate

Flavors/Flavor Enhancers
- Digests
- Artificial flavors
- Monosodium glutamate
- Natural smoke flavor

Palatability Enhancers
- t-Lysine
- Onion powder/oil
- Garlic, garlic powder/oil
- Phosphoric acid
- Hydrochloric acid
- Sucrose, dextrose, cane molasses
- Acidified yeast

Emulsifying Agents, Stabilizers, and Thickeners
- Glyceryl monostearate
- Monoglycerides (of edible fats and oils)
- Diglycerides (of edible fats and oils)
- Glycerin
- Modified starch
- Gums (hyrocolloids)
  - Exudate gums (gum arabic)

- Seed gums (guar gum)
- Microbial gums (xanthan gum)
- Chemically modified plant materials (sodium carboxymethyl cellulose)

Miscellaneous Additives
- Mineral oil (reduce dust)
- Charcoal
- Polyphosphates
- Sodium tripolyphosphate
- Disodium phosphate
- Tetrasodium pyrophosphate

If you really want to see your companion animal's health improve, get him off this "nightmare" in bags and cans and feed him fresh food! I personally could never return to feeding any commercially prepared food after learning what's in it. The results I have seen over the past years from feeding fresh, raw food are nothing short of spectacular!

Never Microwave Anything!

STATISTICS NOW INDICATE that something very serious happens to food heated in microwave ovens, an appliance many people use every day to warm their animals' meals. A recent study indicates that human consumption of microwaved milk and vegetables is associated with a rise in cholesterol and a decline in hemoglobin levels, and low levels of hemoglobin are associated with anemia (which may result in rheumatism, fever, and thyroid insufficiency).[56] The study also concludes that eating microwaved vegetables is associated with a major drop in *lymphocyte* (a type of white blood cell) counts, showing that the subjects tested responded to the food as if it were an infectious agent.[57] The subjects' radiation levels of light–emitting bacteria were higher as well, which indicates that microwave energy is transmitted from food to person. Stanford University Medical Center no longer uses microwaves to warm breast milk, and Minneapolis Hospital tells new mothers not to microwave their babies' milk, as it has been found that microwaved breast milk loses 98 percent of its immunoglobulin A antibodies.[58]

Clearly, a pathological change occurs in human blood when microwaved food is consumed—to say nothing of the nutritional damage done to food when it is vibrated 2.5 million times per second. In September 1993 a rumor circulated at the AHVMA conference about a study done on microwaved food with cats as subjects. All the cats in this supposed study were said to have died after a short period of eating only microwaved foods. The experiment was allegedly funded by a microwave manufacturer, which, when the results proved disastrous, shut down the study and buried the data.[59]

Fact or fiction—who knows? But what is clear is that the powers that be in the food industry want to turn us all into fast-food junkies. Millions of dollars are spent convincing us we can't live without this or that modern convenience, without regard for the consequences to our health. The microwave is high on the list of these lethal "conveniences."

Chapter Four

Nutrition

NUTRITION AS PREVENTATIVE MEDICINE

HOLISTIC MEDICINE FIRST departed from allopathic medicine in the area of nutrition, which became the foundation of all alternative healing therapies. Twenty-five hundred years ago Hippocrates said, "Thy food shall be thy remedy." In 1965 Henry G. Bieler, M.D., echoed this principle in his landmark book *Food Is Your Best Medicine.*

Barry Sears, Ph.D., author of *Enter the Zone, A Dietary Roadmap,* tells us that "Food . . . is a potent drug that you'll take at least three times a day for the rest of your life."[1] "Zone" principles also apply to feeding our companion animals.[2] We Americans have been incorrectly guided in our eating habits and consequently have grown fatter and fatter, and so have our dogs and cats; consequently, their health has declined, along with our own.

Food is broken down into basic groups, (glucose, amino acids, and fatty acids), which are then sent into the bloodstream.[3] The food we feed our companion animals has a more powerful impact on their bodies and health than any drug our veterinarian can prescribe. Our dogs' food needs to be administered appropriately in the proper ratios (protein, carbohydrates, and fats) at the proper time (for growing puppies, several times per day; for adult dogs, one or two times per day).

Food, like drugs, has a therapeutic zone. Too much or too little in the bloodstream at any one time can bring about toxic reactions. Every meal and every snack you feed your dog needs to be a proper balance of macronutrients (proteins, carbohydrates, and fats). These proper combinations produce favorable hormone responses in terms of glucagon, insulin, and eicosanoids. The term *eicosanoid* (pronounced "eye-kah-sah-noid") may be new to you, even if you have a medical background. Eicosanoids are powerful hormones that number in the hundreds.[4] Dr. Sears states that they are among the most powerful substances in the body and act as "master switches" controlling virtually all body functions including the cardiovascular system, the immune system, and the system that controls how much fat we store. They are the molecular glue that holds the body together. Restoring and maintaining a proper balance of eicosanoids through nutrition might just become a primary treatment for disease as well as its prevention.

Through balanced nutrition, we can achieve not just wellness but optimum health for both ourselves and our companion animals. But how do we do this? First of all, we need to discard many of our preconceptions about food, including pet food. For many years nutrition experts have repeated what we all instinctively know, that "we are what we eat." We humans know it's good for us to order a salad (raw vegetables) with our dinner.

Even if we don't do so, we know we should; and none of us has to eat exclusively out of cans or bags all our lives. So why should it be different for our dogs?

Dogs are carnivores, and supermarket dog food and expensive veterinary brands are not what nature intended them to eat (see "What Are We Feeding Our Companion Animals?" in Chapter 3, "The Dangers of Conventional Care"). Canines in the wild eat rabbits, birds, reptiles, insects, mice, fruits, and vegetables. They don't carry around little Bunsen burners to cook their meals. They don't nibble all day on bits of kibble. They nibble on grass, bark, and berries.

As the caretakers of our animal companions, we can ensure their long life, optimum health, and resistance to disease. I'm not suggesting that we provide them with rabbits and birds, but rather that as closely as possible we duplicate in our kitchens the dog's natural diet. Basically, we must try to re-create a rabbit! Wolves that hunt in the wild eat the whole animal, bones and all, and get a ration of predigested vegetable matter from the innards of their prey.

This is Nature's plan, and a whole cadre of holistic veterinarians agree. Dr. Christina Chambreau says, "A natural diet consisting of raw meat and vegetables, cooked grains, natural supplements, and pure water is so necessary for overall health that it's difficult to cure an animal if a raw diet is not being fed."[5] This combination is the foundation of what I refer to throughout this book as "the fresh food diet."

There are very few physiological differences between our domesticated dogs and their wild relatives. A diet of raw food makes sense for all dogs because they have sharp tearing teeth, short small intestines, and highly acidic systems to protect them from most of the parasites and bacteria in raw meat. Meat eating is deeply ingrained in the canine nature, causing the bodies and emotions of all dogs to be the way they are today, even among domesticated breeds. Deprive your animals of their birthright, and you'll have ill-tempered, sickly companions.

Everyone knows that food is made up of proteins, carbohydrates, and fats—the macronutrients. But did you know that they generate complex hormonal responses every time we eat them or feed them to our dogs (or cats)?[6]

Caloric Composition of a Zone-Favorable Diet for People and Dogs by Dr. Barry Sears.

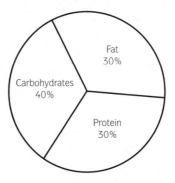

From Figure 7-3 of *The Zone,* p. 71

The diet depicted in the chart may, at first glance, look like a high-fat diet. However, the protein sources are raw, lean meats and poultry, and the fat recommendation is only 2 tablespoons of a light olive oil mixture per each pound of meat in our diet. Fat calories are two and a quarter times greater in density than protein calories. There are 9 calories per each gram of fat and 4 calories per each gram of protein. Remember, to fatten cattle, you feed them plenty of low-fat grains. The absolute value of fat in this diet is not a lot. It just looks higher because the carbohydrate calories have been reduced to a moderate level.

Let's examine carbohydrates. Sugar, starch, vegetables, and fruits are carbohydrates. They are all forms of simple sugars linked together in polymers. Dr. Barry Sears refers to them as something like edible plastic.

The body needs a continual intake of carbohydrates to feed the brain, which uses glucose (a form of sugar) as its main energy source. However, any carbohydrate not immediately used by the body will be stored in the form of glycogen (a long string of glucose molecules linked together). The body stores glycogen in the liver and muscles. The glycogen stored in the muscles is accessible to the brain, and the glycogen stored in the liver can be broken down and sent back to the bloodstream to maintain adequate blood-sugar levels. We eat and feed our dogs carbohydrates so that the liver's glycogen reserve can be maintained.

The question is what amount of carbohydrates to feed a carnivore. Feed it too much (once the glycogen levels are filled in both the liver and the muscles) and these excess carbohydrates get converted into, you guessed it, fat! Fat is then stored in the adipose tissue (fatty tissue), and we have fat dogs (fat cats, people, and kids, too).

The type of carbohydrates we feed our animal companions is also critically important. Our own genes and those of the modern carnivores haven't changed in 100,000 years. Eight thousand years ago grains were not farmed; there was no bread, or pasta—the foods we commonly eat and feed our animals today. The evolution of our digestive system, as well as theirs, was based on a diet of low-fat protein and low-density carbohydrates (that is, fruits and fiber-rich vegetables). We need to go back to eating like cave dwellers, and our dogs and cats need to eat like wolves and tigers! Genetically, none of us has evolved to a stage that allows us to consume excessive amounts of grain products without adverse biochemical consequences.

Any meal that is high in carbohydrates generates a rapid rise in blood glucose. To adjust to this rapid rise, the pancreas secretes the hormone insulin into the bloodstream, and the insulin then lowers the levels of blood glucose. Insulin is essentially a storage hormone that evolved to put aside excess carbohydrate calories in the form of fat in case of future famine.[7] The problem is that these increased levels of insulin tell the body to store carbohydrates as fat and not to release any of it. See why dogs, cats, and humans are getting fat on high-carbohydrate foods and commercial pet foods? By taking in too many carbohydrates, the body releases too much insulin. Too much insulin takes you and your dog out of what Dr. Sears calls "The Zone"—optimum health and a state of well-being.

Don't get me wrong. We all need carbohydrates. The solution often lies in the glycemic index. The glycemic index is the entry rate of a carbohydrate into the bloodstream. The lower the glycemic index, the slower the rate of absorption.[8] You may not want to hear this, but refined table sugar has a lower glycemic index than the typical breakfast cereal, not to mention the low-quality grain used in commercial pet food. To make it easy, virtually all fruits (except bananas and dried fruits) and fiber-rich vegetables (except carrots and corn) are low-glycemic carbohydrates. All grains, starches, and pastas are high-glycemic carbohydrates.

"Complex" carbohydrates still need to be broken down into simple sugars for absorption. Glucose is the most common of these sugars, followed by fructose and galactose. Glucose is found in grains and starchy vegetables, fructose in fruit, and galactose in dairy products. Because they are so high in glucose, grain products virtually gallop back to the liver. Fructose has a much slower re-entry rate compared with galactose-containing carbohydrates.

What about fiber? Fiber is a nondigestible carbohydrate and is not absorbed. Therefore, it doesn't affect insulin levels. It acts more like a set of brakes on the absorption rate of other carbohydrates into the bloodstream. High fiber equals slower entry. Remove the fiber (as pet-food companies do), and the rate accelerates.

It's interesting to note that humankind has shrunk in height. Neopaleolithic men were about five feet ten inches and females were about five feet six inches. After the introduction of grain, the average height of both shrank about six inches. It's taken ten thousand years to get those six inches back, and we just recently made up for it in the twentieth century.[9] This is because food in general, and protein specifically, has become more abundant. But with our fast-food mentality—process it, preserve it, denature it, and bag it—we widen out and get fatter and fatter, and sicker and sicker, as do our animal companions.

The significant difference between humans' and dogs' need for carbohydrates lies in dogs' difficulty in digesting carbohydrates. Just look at their jaws and mouths. All forty-two of those teeth were designed to tear flesh from bones. Dogs also eat as fast as they can, swallowing food nearly whole. No digestion takes place prior to their food hitting their stomachs. Human digestion begins in the mouth; we grind our food between our thirty-two teeth and our saliva has enzymes that help us break down food.

When carbohydrates form a large part of your dog's diet, he performs more poorly because of the greater time and energy spent digesting his food. He also produces large amounts of stool from eating a high-carb diet. Many dogs are so protein deprived that they become sick as a result. Dogs do much better on diets containing more protein from animals than grain. Think back on the wolf's diet once again—a whole animal carcass containing everything needed to survive, including predigested vegetable matter in the intestinal tract of the prey.[10]

John Briscoe, a senior animal keeper at the Los Angeles Zoo, says that they feed their carnivores raw meat and bones every day, supplied in five-pound feeding tubes supplemented with vitamins and minerals.

The dog needs to eat raw meat just like the cat, the snake, and the birds of prey. Why? Because they're wolves underneath it all. And, no, they aren't different physiologically just because they come when you call them and sleep at the foot of your bed. Your dog requires raw meat protein.

Another danger stemming from the use of grain in pet foods is mycotoxicosis—the toxic effects of fungal growth in grains and foodstuffs that have been exposed to moisture and heat. These toxins can be deadly to your dog, according to Wendy Volhard and Dr. Kerry Brown, and are detectable only by laboratory analysis. They are not killed by heat. Cancer, mutations, and suppressed immune function are but a few of the dangers caused by feeding dogs food composed primarily of grains.[11]

Even if the finest ingredients money could buy were used, grains are an incomplete source of protein, lack various vitamins and minerals, and contain fat. Cooked proteins are not what carnivores were designed to eat.[12] The grains I include in my dog's diet are barley and oatmeal (slow-cooked for at least thirty minutes). The grain portion of the fresh food diet has become a controversial subject. I have not experienced problems with my animals on grains, but again, I use small amounts of oats and barley flakes. The carbohydrates I recommend are fruits and vegetables with a low glycemic index mixed in with sweet potatoes or yams.

Now, let's take a close look at protein. Proteins are the basis of all life. Protein is more plentiful in the body of mammals than is water. Muscle, skin, hair, eyes, and nails are all made up of protein. Protein is the main structural ingredient of our cells and the enzymes that keep them running.[13] The immune system is essentially composed of protein. Amino acids, the building blocks of protein, are the foundation of life, and we in the holistic health care field, along with numerous animal nutritionists and veterinarians, feel that carnivores need to eat their protein raw. Carnivores are not like us. If you have doubts, just look at their teeth! The following chart lists essential amino acids and the food sources. [14]

Essential Amino Acids in Dogs	Food Sources
Arginine	*Animal protein, peanuts*
Histidine	*Animal and plant proteins*

Isoleucine	Animal protein, soy, beans, legumes
Leucine	Animal protein, soy
Lycine	Animal protein, garbanzo beans, comfrey
Methionine	Egg yolks, some animal protein, grains
Phenylolinine	Milk, grains, liver, fish
Threonine	Some animal proteins, grains
Tryptophan	Fish, chicken, eggs, beef milk, soybeans, corn
Valine	Parts of liver, chicken, some fish, parsley, milk, wheat, yeast
Non-Essential Amino Acids	**Food Sources**
Alanine	Avocado, beef, pork, turkey, cheese, wheat germ, oats, yogurt
Aspargine	Most protein sources, asparagus
Aspartic acid	Most protein sources
Carnitine	Animal protein sources only
Citroline	Protein sources
Cysteine	Animal protein, wheat gluten, egg yolks
Gaba	Animal and vegetable protein
Glutamic acid	Animal and vegetable protein
Glutamine	Animal and vegetable protein, beet juice
Glycine	Protein sources
Hydroxyproline	Gelatin made from animal bones
Ornithine	Animal protein
Proline	Eggs, milk protein (casein), blackstrap molasses, glucose, meat, wheatgerm
Serine	Animal protein, wheat gluten, peanuts, soy
Taurine	Animal protein sources only

Protein is composed of amino acids. Of the twenty-five known amino acids, ten or eleven are essential and cannot be produced by the dog's body. They must be included in the dog's diet. Amino acids are altered by heat, cooking, and canning. Extruding (the process used to make dry pet food) denatures the protein, causing the finished product to be deficient in amino acids. So please feed your animal companion raw meat and poultry graded for human consumption. You may use the sterilization method offered on page 118.

Besides protein and carbohydrates, you and your dog need fat! Everyone seems to be "fatphobic" these days. Virtually every shelf in the supermarket is loaded with fat-free everything. The truth is fat is necessary to provide energy as well as supple skin and good hair coat.[15] Fat is needed to transport fat-soluble vitamins such as A, D, E, and K through the body. It is essential in the digestion of vitamin D, which is needed for the use of calcium in the body. Fats keep cells strong to protect them from invasion from microorganisms and damage by chemicals. They are needed in the manufacturing of steroids and sex hormones. They play an important part in the function of the nervous system. Fat protects the vital organs from trauma and temperature change by providing padding and insulation. It also helps regulate body temperature.

Dietary fat does not make us fat unless it contributes too many calories, so it is important to learn the proper ratio of fats and the differences in fats. There are two kinds of fat: animal fat (saturated fat) and fats derived from plants (polyunsaturated fats).

We need to provide our dogs with enough fat for energy and performance, but a high-fat diet will cause the animal to eat less, consequently depriving him of other essential nutrients. A neat fact about fat, according to Dr. Sears, is that fat in a meal causes the release of a hormone called cholecystokinin (CCK) from the stomach. This hormone tells the brain you are satisfied and to stop eating. It is always wise with dogs to practice portion control. They should not overfill their stomachs.[16] Again, balance is the key. Remember, once fat is cooked, it turns to grease. The fat content in raw meat and poultry should be kept to a minimum.

Everyone who has been introduced to the fresh food diet initially protests: "But my dog has been eating this inferior commercial diet all his life. What can I expect if I start feeding him raw meat? What about the effects of microbes such as salmonella on my animal, who hasn't had the opportunity to develop the 'right stuff' in his digestive tract?"

John Briscoe wasn't at all concerned about any danger from raw meat, and Rich Freitag of Spectrum Foods (suppliers of raw feline and canine food to the majority of American zoos) says that the only animals he would worry about are those who have been fed sterile diets or animals with highly compromised immune systems. Dr. Christina Chambreau even finds that feeding raw meat to very sick animals who are also under holistic treatment helps them recover much faster. She says it's safer to use naturally raised meat because the animals from which it came were not filled with steroids or forced to live and breed in deplorable conditions, and therefore they were more resistant to parasites. You may ensure the safety of the fresh food diet by taking the necessary precautions to guarantee freshness. Make sure you know about the techniques of proper refrigeration and kitchen hygiene, and use the meat-sterilization technique detailed in "How to Prevent Contamination and Spoilage," on page 118 for perhaps the first year your dog is on this diet (though you may continue to sterilize indefinitely if you wish).

Russell Swift, D.V.M., told me that even though commercial processing with heat destroys many harmful parasites and bacteria in pet food, a healthy dog's digestive system possesses a strong, naturally occurring defense mechanism capable of destroying these organisms on its own. Feeding dogs cooked meat products weakens this system, making the animal more susceptible to parasites and infections from such sources as tapeworms (transmitted by fleas)—those who fear what's in raw meat should be more concerned about what's in those cans and bags! Remember, your veterinarian may not have this information. He or she has been taught that good health is dependent on declaring war on viruses and bacteria. Only healthy immune systems can do that job, and the only way to have a healthy immune system is to build it up with fresh, raw food.

When we feed a dog fresh food, his intestinal tract remains clean and strong. The digestive secretions are potent, and the environment within the bowel is inhospitable to worms, salmonella, and other parasites and diseases. In fact, the entire body is healthier as a result of improved nutrition and is thus more resistant to all disease.

Raw meat, Dr. Swift says, contains enzymes that help dogs digest it.[17] Cooking destroys these vital compounds, so the animal's pancreas must secrete more of its own enzymes to compensate. Such artificially created stress is a precursor to a great number of chronic and acute health problems. Cooking also reduces the water content and alters the protein structure of meat, making it more difficult to digest, further damaging the animal's health and vitality. Dr. Sears says that cooking meat degrades arachadonic acid. Arachadonic acid is vital to our animals' health and well-being.[18] I hope by now you can see that proper nutrition through fresh, raw food is the best preventative medicine—the key to your dog's good health!

THE FRESH FOOD DIET

Before You Begin

AT THIS POINT you may be considering the idea of adding fresh foods to your dog's commercial diet, thinking it might help at least a little. If you wish to add fresh foods to commercial ones, says Dr. Nancy Scanlan, it's vital to prepare the complete diet (meat, vegetables, grains, and supplements in the proportions shown in the chart on pages 96–97).[19] Note that dry dog food stays in the stomach fifteen to sixteen hours before all of it passes into the small intestine. Canned or semimoist food stays in the stomach eight to nine hours. Raw food stays in the stomach four to five hours; it breaks down the quickest and can be detected in the small intestine within thirty minutes.[20]

Many people start by mixing their current commercial food fifty-fifty with the fresh food diet and then wean their dogs to all fresh food. See the section on bribe foods (page 104) for more about helping your dog make the transition. This is a short-term solution, however. For the best results, feed your dog 100 percent fresh food. You will not truly reap the rewards of this diet until the animal has been detoxed and converted to 100 percent fresh food. For me, it has been well worth the effort. When you see the results in your companion animals, it is to be hoped you'll make "Zone-favorable" choices in your own diet so you can be around to enjoy your animal's good health and long life.

There are hundreds of books promoting a variety of nutritional approaches and claiming theirs to be best. You know that you stay healthy by eating a variety of fresh foods and no doubt have learned what is best for you as an individual. Dr. Chambreau reminds people that they need to find what works best for each of their dogs. Some may need a bit more meat, more grain, no grain—or even to avoid certain foods until they are cured.[21] You will find the combination that works best within the guidelines. Please feel free to let me know your discoveries on this path to optimum health or ask questions about getting started. My phone number is listed in "Resources."

Nutritional Checklist

I HAVE PUT together a checklist to help you keep track of the components that are so important to your dog's health—proteins, vegetables, and grains/potatoes (for more detailed information on each of these items, see the sample weekly meal plan and shopping list that begins on page 101). Let's review the macronutrients. Remember, each dog is an individual and may require slight variations. Therefore, you may need more or less of the following ingredients:

Protein: Raw meat should be the cornerstone of your dog's diet. But too much of a good thing—that is, a meat-only diet—overworks the kidneys and liver and might push your dog into ketosis (an abnormal increase of ketone bodies in the body). Ketosis occurs when we have insufficient carbohydrate stores in the liver to meet the requirements of the body and brain. Ketone bodies are abnormal biochemicals that accumulate from an extremely high-protein/low-carbohydrate diet. Excess thirst and increased urination are symptoms, as well as weight loss. Follow the proportions given on pages 96–97. For dogs older than five months of age, milk products should be given in moderation, if at all. See below for information about other protein sources.

Carbohydrates: Whole grains are an important part of the diet and a good source of energy. Refined sugar, corn syrup, malt, white flour, or other refined grain products, all of which are found abundantly in commercial pet foods, are not. I use a lot of raw vegetables and some fruit. I use barley and oatmeal (slow-cooked for thirty minutes).

Fats: Cooked fat clogs arteries. But the fat in raw meat and in cold-pressed oils supplies highly beneficial essential fatty acids. Dr. Sears recommends an EFA (essential fatty acid) oil mixture consisting of light olive oil, salmon or cod liver oil, borage oil, and vitamin E oil.[22] (See "The Basic Homemade Fresh Food Recipe" for instructions on mixing, page 95.)

Fiber: In the wild, dogs get fiber from plants, feathers, hair, beaks, and so on. Their stool thus has ample volume, preventing them from developing anal gland problems, as the gland is squeezed every time they have a bowel movement. Fiber supplements such as bran are okay to use occasionally as a colon cleanse. However, routinely including in the diet food-processed raw vegetables, fruits, and grains is preferable. Most pet-food companies use cheap and indigestible sources of fiber such as cellulose (wood pulp, beet pulp, or peanut hulls) and even feathers and beaks. Yes, it's true that these may be a part of the wolf's nat-ural diet, but who wants to find it disguised as meat protein?

Vitamins: Most vitamins are destroyed in cooking, so pet-food manufacturers add back synthetic substitutes (see "Vitamins and Minerals: A Guide to Nutritional Supplements," page 124). Chemical farming has robbed our soil of more than seventy trace minerals, so most vegetables and fruits are picked before they're ripe and often reach our markets overripe or rotten—not to mention the dose of carbon monoxide they get while being transported by truck. Therefore, we must supplement our own and our animal companions' food because it simply doesn't con-tain all the necessary micronutrients. The pet-food industry can't afford to use quality supplements.

Minerals: Minerals act as coenzymes; without them, vitamins don't work. Chelated plant minerals and colloidal minerals are the most useful. There are some seventy-odd essential trace min-erals of major importance. You won't find many of them in canned or bagged pet food.

Enzymes: We know that enzymes are not a part of the bagged or canned fare, because heat and processing inactivate them. Dogs manufacture enzymes naturally from the basic raw materials in the fresh food diet, and the simple addition of enzymes to sick or geriatric animals' food often leads to signifi-cant improvement. I recommend Dr. Swift's Florazyme food enzymes when I suspect digestion or assimilation problems.

Air: Air, of course, is an essential nutrient because without oxygen, we cannot survive. Yet, in major cities, owing to pollu-tion, we have 40 percent less oxygen to breathe than our grandparents had. Molds, dust, pollens, ammonia, and chemicals contaminate our air. Air filters, such as the Second Wind purifier, can help provide a steady flow of clean, contaminant-free air in our houses and businesses. I have installed this system in my home, and reportedly it attacks and destroys 93.7 percent of airborne contaminants and pet odors. It's unfortunate that many of us must confine our animals indoors for their safety. However, your dog must have fresh air and exercise every day. So get outside and take that walk. It's good for you, too. Try to aim for forty-five minutes to one hour daily.

Electromagnetism: A nutrient is defined, in part, as any substantial particle, and electromagnetic currents are considered particles by modern physics. The earth has a natural resonance we're deprived of when we spend our time indoors with microwave ovens and television radiation, which dose us with harmful human-induced electromagnetic particles. When we touch the earth barefoot or in leather-soled shoes and take our dogs out on a leash, we get the benefit of the earth's natural resonance.

Light: The need for full-spectrum light for health and reproduction was documented by John Ott, of Walt Disney stop-motion photography fame. Scientists tell us that the pineal gland needs a minimum of fifteen minutes of sunlight daily. Most hardware stores carry full-spectrum lightbulbs, which I place strategically in my house for an extra boost. Once you try them, you'll feel their benefit. I make certain my stud males and kittens get ample amounts of full-spectrum light every day. Many natural-rearing dog breeders recommend doing this as well.

Water: Distilled, purified spring water or Willard water (catalyst-altered water) is the only way to go in a world where our water has become so chemically polluted.

Love: Without love, babies and animals die, so prepare the fresh food diet with love. Your dog might be finicky at first, but wait and see what happens when he finally digs in! With a little extra time spent on your dog's behalf and lots of love and patience, you can provide him with the best. He deserves it, doesn't he? Make today your day to begin anew!

The Basic Homemade Fresh Food Recipe

IF YOU'RE LIKE me, not prepared to provide your dogs with fresh prey, the fresh food diet comes as close as possible to what they would catch themselves in the wild. What's more, it's fun once you get the hang of it, and you'll be delighted with the results!

Let's look at the basic components of the fresh food diet: fresh, lean raw meat or poultry, naturally raised whenever possible; organically grown, food-processed fresh vegetables (if you can't get naturally raised or organic components, supermarket foods are still much better than what's in commercial pet food); cooked organic oatmeal or barley; and natural supplements. The ratio of raw meat to carbohydrates is extremely important.

The following is the basic diet. All the meats I use and recommend pass inspection for human consumption. I prepare the very same vegetables and grains for myself, my dog, and my cats. The supplements I give them, albeit in different proportions, are of a quality fit for humans. And I use only purified or distilled water, with Willard water for mixing the ingredients together (see "Pure Water and Catalyst-Altered Water," page 120). Why feed your dog something you wouldn't eat yourself? Please try to obtain organic ingredients, especially if your animal is ill. I know this isn't always easy, but do the best you can. Consult with your holistic practitioner, animal nutritionist, or holistic veterinarian before changing your animal companion's diet.

Please note: Whenever you prepare and serve fresh food, make sure to follow all storage and hygiene precautions outlined in "How to Prevent Contamination and Spoilage," pages 118–120. No matter how good your raw ingredients are, if you don't handle them properly, you can make your dogs ill!

Feed your dog this food once or twice daily. Your dog will soon tell you, as he adjusts to his new diet, how much food he requires. Please don't overfeed him at any one meal. Calorie control is always important. Overeating makes us all fat!

The recipe is for normal adult dogs.[23] You may need to adjust the proportions for puppies and pregnant or nursing mothers. The ratio of protein, carbohydrate, and fat is that recommended by Dr. Sears. Supplementation to this recipe is also based on adult needs (see "More About Supplements—Some Good, Some Bad" on page 138 and "Resources" for further information on the vitamins, minerals, and enzymes included; see "Pure Water and Catalyst-Altered Water," page 120, for the types of water that are safe to use).

(These amounts apply to fifteen- to thirty-pound dogs. Increase or decrease amounts to accommodate larger or smaller dogs' appetites.)

½ lb.	Raw meat (beef, chicken, turkey, or lamb and organ meat [organ meats at a ratio of two parts organ to four parts muscle])
⅔ cup	Slow-cooked oatmeal or barley (optional—if dog is allergic to grain)

1 tablespoon	Essential fatty acid (EFA)* oil mixture (combine 4 ounces of light olive oil, one 1-gram capsule of borage oil [containing 240 mg of GLA], 2 teaspoons [10 ml] salmon or cod liver oil [containing 1 gram of EPA (eicosapentaenoic acid)], and 1,000 IU of vitamin E oil). Refrigerate all oils after opening.
1/2 tablespoon	Bonemeal or vitamin and mineral supplement (containing bonemeal, kelp, dandelion, trace minerals, garlic, vitamin C, and so forth)
2/3 cup	Food-processed raw vegetables (sprouts, dandelion greens, broccoli, cauliflower, zucchini, cabbage, parsley, squash—double the amount if grain is omitted and add food-processed raw or cooked sweet potatoes/yams). If you can't add a medley of vegetables or grains, try 1/2 tablespoon of spirulina, barley grass juice, or other green powder and include minced alfalfa sprouts.
1/2 teaspoon	Superfood supplement, if not included in basic supplement (that is, sea vegetables, bee pollen, chlorella, barley or wheat grass, spirulina, rose hips, Super Blue-Green Algae)

Sterlize the meat or poultry in 1 cup of distilled water to which four drops of standardized extract of grapefruit seed has been added. Mix the solution thoroughly into the meat (use just

*If you prefer to use only cold-pressed (expeller-pressed) oils, substitute 1/2 tablespoon of cold-pressed sunflower oil.

enough to saturate the meat, but don't turn it into soup—you want the consistency of thick chili). Add the food-processed vegetables and cooked grains. Serve or freeze in serving-size containers. I don't like to freeze my supplements in the meals; I always add them at feeding time. Some dogs may also require Dr. Swift's food enzymes—Florazyme EFA or LP. Slowly introduce new food into your dog's diet in small increments to allow him to get used to the change in diet (one quarter new food to three quarters old food for the first week and increase by one-quarter increments each week thereafter).

You may make up large quantities and freeze serving portions. I use a measuring cup for the vegetables and grains. You can make up much larger batches, of course. Thaw frozen meals overnight in the refrigerator before using them.

There are several different variations to the fresh food feeding plan. Each of us needs to find what works for our individual lifestyle. The *Natural Rearing Breeders Directory* contains listings of a wealth of folks who are happy to help with specific breed issues. I also highly recommend the *Natural Rearing Newsletter* as well. (See "Resources" for information.)

The Grain Controversy

A CONTROVERSY OVER grains was brought to my attention by Dr. Russell Swift. While attending the 1996 AHVMA conference, he found that he was not alone in questioning whether grains belong in carnivores' diet. As Dr. Sears has pointed out, carnivores and human beings preexisted grain farming.[24] In the true natural setting, grains hardly exist in carnivores' diet today. Therefore, the argument that wild cats and dogs eat prey animals that have grain matter in their digestive tracts doesn't hold up to scrutiny. Animals living near farms or other civilized areas are likely to have access to grains, but this is not the true wild diet.

The beneficial nutrients of grains can be found in other foods; B vitamins are found in organ meat, and trace minerals come from bones and vegetables. (Modern agriculture has stripped the soil of its trace minerals, so we must supplement a dog's diet to be sure we are not causing deficiencies inadvertently.)

Dr. Swift feels that carnivores cannot maintain long-term production of the quantity of the amylase enzyme necessary to properly digest and utilize carbohydrates. The proteins in grains are less digestible than are animal proteins. As a result, the immune system becomes irritated and weakened by the invasion of foreign, non-nutritive protein and carbohydrate particles. The animal's system does its best to keep up with the demand for amylase, but over a lifetime, this type of pancreatic stress may lead to problems. Consequently, grains are optional in a carnivore's diet. If you choose not to use grains, double the vegetable ratio and include some starchy food, like yams. I have taken a middle ground and include only barley and oatmeal in my animals' diet because they are wonderful sources of GLA and soluble fiber. You will find that holistic practitioners have slight differences of opinion. Experts have for many years advocated whole grains in the carnivore diet, in particular Juliette de Bairacli Levy and her Natural Rearing devotees who have for decades gotten excellent results (I recommend her book, *The Complete Herbal Handbook for the Dog and Cat*). You can find what works best for your dog with a little feeding trial of your own.

Liver Shake

HERE IS A special recipe for a cleansing replacement meal that many nutritionists recommend, in at least some form, be used once or twice a month, or as needed. You'll need a blender and juicer because everything needs to be fresh so that your dog can get the maximum benefit.

8 ounces	raw, naturally raised beef, lamb, chicken, or turkey liver (if you cannot get naturally raised liver, you may substitute heart meat)
4 ounces	distilled water and 4 drops standardized extract of grapefruit
8 ounces	freshly made organic carrot juice with a heaping tablespoon or two of fresh parsley added to it
2 teaspoons	aloe vera juice
2 teaspoons	kelp, Super Blue-Green Algae, spirulina or barley grass powder
1 tablespoon	super B-complex liquid syrup
2 teaspoons	apple cider vinegar
1 teaspoon	freshly minced rosemary
1 tablespoon	EFA oil mixture (Combine 4 ounces light olive oil, one 1-gram capsule of borage oil [containing 240 mg of GLA], 2 teaspoons [10 ml] salmon or cod liver oil [containing 1 gram of EPA], and 1,000 IU of vitamin E oil. Shake well and refrigerate after opening.)

Blend ingredients on a slow speed and serve one cup immediately. Freeze the rest for another serving. You may syringe-feed sick animals this broth, but do not cook or microwave it—serve it at room temperature. Don't overfeed when force-feeding; the animal may throw up. Disinfect the blender after use.

My Sample Weekly Meal Plan

THE FOLLOWING PLAN is meant only as a suggestion and to give you an idea of what you can do with the fresh food diet. Rotate foods often within each food group (see "Suggested Shopping List" on page 103 for suggested variations). Don't forget: variety is the spice of life! Be sure to add the appropriate supplements in the proper proportions.

You may feed the same combinations of carbohydrates several days in a row as long as you have included a wide variety. To begin with, feed only one protein source at a time, to determine whether your animal companion has any particular food allergies. (Allergies are often confused with deficiencies. The inferior ingredients in commercial pet food have caused many veterinarians to think that an animal is suffering from allergies, when it's really toxic reactions and deficiencies in the animal's diet.) If not, you may experiment with combining meats, poultry, cheese, eggs, and dairy products.

WEEKLY MENU

Day	Raw Protein	Raw Vegetables*	Grains/Potatoes
Monday	ground chuck (beef), beef kidney chunks	dandelion greens, celery, parsely	oatmeal
Tuesday	ground chicken backs, necks (pulverized)	zucchini, apples, yellow squash	sweet potatoes
Wednesday	ground chicken, chicken liver chunks	broccoli, cauliflower	barley flakes or millet
Thursday	cottage cheese or coddled eggs, with or without meat	carrots, zucchini, yellow squash	amaranth or barley flakes
Friday	ground lamb, lamb heart, lamb kidney	brussel sprouts	leftover mashed potatoes w/butter or baked potatoes
Saturday	ground beef, beef heart chunks	green beans, alfalfa sprouts, cauliflower	couscous
Sunday**	ground turkey, turkey gizzard/ heart chunks	bok choy or Chinese cabbage	kasha or teff

*Or make a medley of vegetables with barley or oatmeal. If your practitioner wants you to avoid grain, double the vegetable portion and include sweet potatoes or yams (raw or cooked).
**Sunday can also be a "no-meat" day or a "fast-on-broth" day.

Suggested Shopping List

Organic Raw Meats and Other Organic Proteins: Ground chuck (you can grind meat yourself with the meat grinder attachment of your food processor), lamb (ground), chicken (ground and in chunks), turkey (ground and in chunks). Whole or sliced organ meats, such as cubed beef hearts, kidneys, and livers; lamb kidneys; chicken livers; turkey gizzards, livers, and hearts. Ground chicken backs and necks or whole chicken and turkey backs, necks, or wings—dogs need to gnaw! Fertile eggs, raw milk cottage cheese, plain yogurt (from cow's or goat's milk—yogurt helps prevent gas and flatulence).

If you do not have access to naturally raised meat, it is okay to use grocery store meats and poultry, which are far superior to anything found in the cans or bags of pet food, including the so-called health-food brands of pet food. Remember, dogs are scavengers that bury their meat and bones and dig them up weeks later and do just fine. So do not get stressed out if they sometimes eat something less than perfect. Also remember that your supermarket sells its "bad" meat (meat not sold by a certain date) to the pet-food industry, where it gets ground up into the various pet-food "meals." The homemade food you prepare yourself according to this simple recipe, organic or not, is far superior to any pet food you can buy.

Please don't feed your dog pork (even though some breeders advocate its use for a shiny coat). It is high in indigestible fat and will clog his liver and skin. Pork products like bacon and sausage contain cancer-causing nitrates, and Dr. Nancy Scanlan warns that ham can be poisonous to dogs.[25]

Consider ostrich, venison, or buffalo and limit the use of liver to once a week if it is not naturally raised (otherwise, a small portion daily is fine). Raw bones are important for healthy teeth. Allow access to a bone (I like to use turkey necks) for ten to fifteen minutes a day every few days. As your dog adjusts to chewing on bones, you may increase the length of time and frequency of access.

Organic Raw Vegetables: Carrots, pumpkin, zucchini, yellow squash, broccoli, green beans, celery, brussels sprouts, peas, sprouts, sweet potatoes, dandelion greens, and wheatgrass. Frozen vegetables (preferably organic) may be substituted if fresh ones are not available. Carrots are the most palatable vegetables to many animals, but they are high on the glycemic index. You may omit the grains if you are sure your dog has grain allergies, but then double the vegetable ratio. For a fast-food version (if you don't have a food processor), you may even substitute ½ tablespoon of spirulina, alfalfa, or other green juice powder. Follow the directions on the container or simply mince alfalfa sprouts.

Organic Grains: Small amounts of slow-cooked oatmeal (thirty minutes) or barley.

Other Organic Foods: Sunflower seeds, almonds ground in a food processor, or almond or peanut butter (raw and organic, of course). Many dogs enjoy avocados as well. Some dogs like fruit, especially apples, melons, grapes, or raisins. Don't forget to have a fresh bottle of light olive oil on hand.

Bribe Foods: Baby food (lamb, beef, or chicken); water-packed canned chicken, salmon, or mackerel; canned sardines in tomato sauce (they love them!); vegetable, chicken, or beef broth; raw milk butter, raw milk cream, unpasteurized honey. Ripe avocados mixed with low-fat yogurt are a great bribe food and promote a beautiful coat, as do cold-pressed or expeller-pressed oils.

Water and Supplements: Distilled water, purified spring water, or Willard water; bonemeal; vitamin and mineral supplements; expeller-pressed oils and food enzymes (see "Resources" for information on where and how to order).

Raw Meat Treatments: Nutribiotics or Imhotep brand of standardized extract of grapefruit (available at health-food stores or through distributors), or 3 percent food-grade hydrogen peroxide (always dilute 4 drops grapefruit seed extract or 1 tablespoon of 3 percent food-grade hydrogen peroxide in 1 cup of water).

Keep on hand organic honey and apple cider vinegar (1 teaspoon in purified water also helps itchy skin). Lecithin (one capsule in food twice daily) breaks down fats and helps the body to eliminate them. If lecithin is not included in your dog's daily multivitamin-mineral mix, please add it to your program.

Equipment: Food processor or blender (meat grinder is optional).

Shopping will become easier because you won't need to walk down the pet-food aisle (except to buy toys).

SOME GUIDELINES FOR SERVING FRESH FOODS

SOME NUTRITIONISTS RECOMMEND only one protein food per meal. After all, the carnivore in the wild, if lucky, makes one kill a day. You may mix muscle and organ meats, but mix beef with beef organ meats, turkey with turkey organ meats, and so on. You may alternate beef, lamb, chicken, and turkey. I recommend not mixing meat until you are certain the dog doesn't suffer from a sensitivity to a particular one. Avoid veal and never use pork. The fat globules in pork are so large, they can clog your dog's blood vessels. I buy lean cuts of meat or poultry and add essential fatty acids necessary for dogs. However, if your budget is limited, reduce the essential fatty acids but try not to exceed 22 percent fat. Small amounts of organ meats, including kidney, liver, and heart, may be fed daily. Because the liver is the body's "detox central," Dr. Chambreau cautions against feeding your dog liver more than once a week unless it's organic.[26] She and I both feel that heart meat is one of the best protein foods, and I include it in every meal. My animals love a little organ meat in their food. Don't forget, each prey animal comes equipped with glands and organs!

I recommend feeding one to two parts organ meat to four to five parts muscle meat (ground or chunks). A combination of ground meat and chunks mixes well with the vegetable and grain portions of the recipe. If you use only chunks, some dogs eat the meat and leave the rest. Serve chunks on a regular basis to help clean your dog's teeth and keep them free of tartar buildup. All meats must always include bonemeal (1 tablespoon per pound of meat), and don't forget those turkey necks and wings. Dogs love them!

You may use fresh fish. However, a safe source is difficult to obtain. I have used raw or lightly seared organic tilapia, mixed with the usual proportions of carbohydrates and supplements. I call it pet sashimi! Canned mackerel, salmon, and sardines are fine, too, and I include them often, substituting them for part of the meat ration or using them just for flavor for finicky eaters. Reduce the essential fatty acid mixture when including fish.

You may use raw milk cottage cheese from time to time as an alternative source of protein or as a bribe food. Organic plain yogurt (from cow's, sheep's, or goat's milk) is also excellent. If you need another good bribe food, try raw milk butter or raw nut butters. Dr. Chambreau recommends raw milk dairy foods if your dog can tolerate them.[27] I have found many adult dogs that tend to be sensitive to lactose. However, some puppies do great on raw goat's milk.

You may also feed your dog a raw fertile or organic egg yolk, or a whole coddled or soft-boiled two-minute egg. Be careful with raw egg white. Many practitioners recommend that you cook the white; others feel there is no problem serving it raw. I'd prefer that you make an egg white omelette for yourself, and serve only the raw yolks. Use them as a puppy's first food at weaning time, mixed with brown rice baby cereal or oatmeal, minced alfalfa sprouts, and a little raw goat's milk or yogurt. Five weeks old is a good time to then add raw meat.

Dogs require meat or poultry at least five or six days per week. So don't feed dairy products and eggs exclusively to normal adult dogs without the meat ration. Fasting one day a week allows the carnivore's kidneys, as well as other digestive organs, an opportunity to rest and cleanse.

Vegetables may be used in any combination (try using color as a guide, as you would for yourself). Nightshade vegetables (white potatoes, tomatoes, peppers, and eggplant) can be included occasionally and need to be cooked (sweet potatoes and tomatoes are okay raw). Some nutritionists feel that you shouldn't feed nightshades to animals with symptoms of arthritis, inflammation, parasites, respiratory problems, or other conditions marked by symptoms such as swelling or mucus.

You may substitute frozen (preferably organic) vegetables if you can't get fresh ones, but never use canned vegetables—they are very high in salt and/or sugar and have lost their nutritional value through overcooking.

Nuts are a nice addition—grated or finely diced. (Almonds are my favorite. However, my animals do love peanut butter.) Nuts should be fresh, raw, and unsalted. Try grinding them in a coffee grinder. Grasses are also recommended for aiding digestion and cleansing the system. I grow pots of wheatgrass and keep them available at all times for my cats and dogs to nibble on.

I use grain in my animals' diet. I recommend sticking with barley and oats because other grains are difficult for carnivores to digest, and they may promote allergies and digestive upsets. You may omit them and double the vegetable ratio if you suspect allergies, substituting food-processed sweet potatoes or yams for a while.

Your dog really shouldn't have problems with food allergies on the fresh food diet. But if you're dealing with allergies, choose foods you think your dog can tolerate, in combinations of one from each food group at a time. Try starting with ground lamb, sprouts, zucchini, and barley and proceed cautiously from there. I find that food allergies just seem to disappear on this diet. I feel that most animals' allergic reactions have been because of the poor quality of the ingredients used in commercial pet food. As breeders become enlightened about the benefits of the fresh food diet served in rotation, fewer and fewer allergies will be experienced. Work with your holistic veterinarian or animal nutritionist.

Vegetable, beef, or chicken broth is wonderful for binding together the ingredients of the fresh food diet. It's also a good bribe food for the unconverted, and is great for fasting days (see

"Fasting—Voluntary and Involuntary—and More Tips to Get Dogs to Eat Fresh Food," page 115).

Once in a while it's okay to feed your dog table scraps, such as roast chicken and rare beef and lamb. But forget about chocolate, which contains theobromine, a known poison to both cats and dogs. They can become addicted to chocolate, so if you've been feeding it regularly, they may actually suffer withdrawal symptoms. Never leave open boxes of chocolate around your house because your dog or cat could actually die from eating large amounts. Junk foods (especially deep-fried) are taboo. Your dog may beg for a potato chip, but please don't give in.

PLANNING AND PREPARATION TIPS— KEEPING THINGS SIMPLE

I RECOMMEND PREPARING a large quantity of the fresh food recipe ahead of time and freezing it. You may actually save money this way, especially if you can find a wholesale supplier of naturally raised meats and poultry. (If you can't find a reliable local source, check "Resources" for mail-order ideas.) My supplier, Harmony Farms, packs coarsely ground muscle meats and cubed organ meats for me. I stock up with as many one-pound packages as my freezer will hold. If I run out of meat from my supplier, I go to a local health-food store that carries naturally raised meats. I ask the butcher to grind beef or beef heart and to wrap my order in one-pound packages; I do the same with chicken, turkey, and lamb.

I try to buy eggs laid by free-range hens that haven't been given steroids. Don't keep eggs for longer than two weeks, and keep them covered in their original package in the fridge. You can test eggs for freshness by submerging a raw egg in its shell in a bowl of water. If the egg sinks to the bottom, it's fresh; if it floats, throw it away!

At the health-food market, I buy a medley of raw vegetables. We all know organic vegetables are best, but if you can't get them, you may soak nonorganic ones for fifteen minutes in a gallon of purified water with a few drops of standardized extract of grapefruit, or in a gallon of water with 2 tablespoons of apple cider vinegar. Doing so helps remove residue from pesticides and chemical fertilizers. Frozen organic vegetables, which your health-food store may carry, are another alternative if raw ones can't be found; they are okay even though most are blanched prior to freezing. Run them through the food processor partially defrosted just as you would with raw vegetables.

I puree my vegetables as finely as I can, since whole vegetables pass through undigested. I place the pureed vegetables in plastic bags or containers, and freeze or refrigerate them. You may also freeze cooked grains or mix together the vegetables and grains and freeze them. Just be sure to label packages with their contents and weight in ounces so you can mix the fresh food diet in accurate proportions later on.

I also prepare and freeze homemade chicken broth. For convenience, I keep my shelves stocked with beef, vegetable, and chicken broth in lead-free cans, which many health-food stores carry. One tablespoon of raw ground beef and 3–4 ounces of pure water pureed in a blender (you may also make raw chicken broth with 1 tablespoon of ground chicken, 6 ounces of water, and 4 drops of standardized extract of grapefruit) is a great energizing source. Administered with a feeding syringe, this broth is ideal for a sick animal, but you'll need to strain it through a sieve to avoid clogging the syringe.

You can take the chill off fresh food by placing it in a container in a pan of hot water, or warm the food by adding a little heated purified water, weakly brewed herbal tea (such as slippery elm, raspberry, or fenugreek) for flavor or for medicinal use, or chicken broth. Don't cook the food, just make it tepid to the touch. And never use the microwave, as it not only destroys nutrients but may cause other problems as well (see "Never Microwave Anything!" in Chapter 3 "The Dangers of Conventional Care"). I serve my animals their fresh food straight from the refrigerator. If it's too cold, they'll wait a little while before diving in!

I cook my oatmeal or barley in purified water on the stovetop for thirty minutes You should cool grains before adding them to food. You may also substitute chicken or vegetable broth for the water.

Putting a bay leaf in your uncooked grains can keep insects from hatching (but bay leaves are toxic to dogs, so don't let your animals eat them). Store uncooked grains in the refrigerator and cook them within three months if you have problems with little bugs in your cereal.

If your animal nutritionist or holistic veterinarian suggests additional fiber in your dog's diet, try 1 tablespoon of Miller's Unprocessed Bran per each pound of meat. Sometimes a little bran helps pregnant dams, but you'll find that the fresh food recipe produces a more compact stool, with less odor, than does commercial food. Just be sure to add enough water or broth to make the food the right consistency for your animal companion. The rule of thumb is 6–8 ounces of liquid for every pound of meat.

I never use onions, because they are too difficult for animals to digest, but I do include Kyolic aged garlic (see "Resources").

It smells wonderful, as does a pinch of fresh parsley. Remember, this recipe is not complete without bonemeal, a vitamin and mineral supplement, because in the wild, fresh raw bones from prey animals supply canines with calcium and phosphorous in just the right proportions. You must also include vitamin and mineral supplements to offset any nutrients that are depleted through freezing or growing and harvesting practices. Supplementation makes the fresh food diet complete and provides the immune system with an extra boost of antioxidants. This diet is actually better than what animals could forage for themselves in the wild. For further information on other items to add, see "More About Supplements—Some Good, Some Bad" on page 138.

FEEDING SCHEDULES AND QUANTITIES

FOR YEARS VETERINARIANS have been telling us to stick with one food, to open a can morning and night, and to leave the dry food out for our animals to nibble on all day (rather like raising a child on Spam and Cocoa Puffs!). And how would you feel about eating this boring diet left out all day to spoil? Would you ever dream of even tasting it? Of course not. It's not fit for human consumption. With food left out all day to go rancid, some dogs may never show interest in their regular meals. Remember, carnivores are not grazing animals. They need time between meals to fast.

Many adult dogs may be cut back to one meal a day. However, two meals a day is also fine if your dog insists. Fasting is also important (see "Fasting—Voluntary and Involuntary—and More Tips to Get Dogs to Eat Fresh Food," page 115). Dogs that are ill or very old may not fare well with changes in their meal schedule, so consult an animal nutritionist or holistic veterinary practitioner for special problems.

Puppies usually start to eat fresh food containing meat protein at five weeks of age. Once weaned, they need to eat six to eight times daily until they are between eight and twelve weeks old, when they may be cut back to four meals a day. From twenty-four weeks to one year, feed them twice daily; after one year, feed them once or twice daily, depending on health, breed, and so on. Let their appetite and constitution be your guide. I feed my dog once a day, but Dr. Nancy Scanlan, D.V.M., feeds her dog twice daily because it provides a means of loving interaction between them.[28] Pregnant and lactating animals eat more frequently, usually three to four times a day. Check with your puppy's breeder for his meal schedules.

Start by mixing small portions of fresh food into your current dog food. You can begin with as little as one quarter fresh food to three quarters of the old diet and work up from there. Most dogs love it and dive in; others are addicted to their fast-food diets and take longer to convert. Be creative with bribe foods. The slow conversion saves digestive upsets.

How much should you feed your dog at each meal? It's simple: if any food is left in the dish, he's probably had enough. If the dish is licked clean, give him a little more. Appetite may vary slightly from time to time, but his refusing to eat could be a sign of illness. He may need a day to fast and heal, but check with your holistic practitioner first. If your dog has lost his natural "stop" instinct for eating and begs for more, increase play and exercise time—not food.

Leave food down no longer than forty-five minutes per meal. This is a good rule on two counts: you'll guard against spoilage, and you'll get your dog used to being fed at specific times rather than free-feeding on kibble all day long.

GETTING STARTED—SOME HINTS TO HELP YOU MAKE THE TRANSITION

SO, NOW YOU'RE a believer, but you're not rushing out to the health-food store or calling me for supplements. Why not? Perhaps you'd like to improve your dog's diet but are feeling a little overwhelmed.

Okay, let's compromise a little and ease into the fresh food diet. Know that you won't see substantial improvement in your dog's health until you make the switch completely. But you can start right now to improve his diet, the goal being to get to fifty-fifty for starters and increase the proportion of fresh food from there. If you can get that far, the rest will be easy. Holistic veterinarians and nutrition experts offer the following advice to get you started.

Begin the transition to a natural diet by adding the fresh food ingredients to a high-quality canned food. Gradually decrease the canned food. Please do not use dry food. If you insist on using it up, then at least moisten it with purified water or broth. Many dogs are so addicted to their dry food that weaning them may be your toughest job. But as your dog's guardian, you must be compassionately determined. He'll soon learn you mean business. Try adding fresh, raw food to the dry food first, crushing the dry food and sprinkling it on top, or mixing in kibble so it looks like little raisins in an oatmeal cookie.

Switch everybody in your household, including yourself, to purified water. You'll love the taste of spring water or filtered water from which harmful chemicals and heavy metals have been removed. Distilled water may be supplemented with Ani-Minerals.

Use high-quality supplements, starting with small amounts. Add food enzymes to the current commercial food you feed your dog because it is virtually devoid of enzymes. Phase out the canned or dry food as soon as possible. (Once you've read the Animal Protection Institute of America's investigative report, you'll be ill every time you open a bag or can of it!)

Make loving and playing a daily routine, just as with the fresh food diet. Most of all, don't obsess. No one is perfect. Everyone I know occasionally slips up. If your recipe isn't exactly right, you'll make up for it at the next meal. Dogs pick up on our negative attitudes, so program yourself for success with this new regimen. You can do it! Your dogs will love you even more for providing them with the foods nature intended them to eat.

FASTING—VOLUNTARY AND INVOLUNTARY—AND MORE TIPS TO GET DOGS TO EAT FRESH FOOD

AN AGE-OLD practice, fasting is one of the most overlooked yet valuable ways to heal. It relieves the body of the task of digesting foods and allows the system to rid itself of wastes and toxins while encouraging gentle healing. Many holistic practitioners encourage *therapeutic fasting* the first day or two of an illness, especially if there is a fever (or, I would add, diarrhea). This is a type of *involuntary fasting*. Animals in the wild fast when they're ill, instinctively allowing their bodies to cleanse and detoxify.

Many experts recommend routine involuntary fasting once a week. Fasting from breakfast to breakfast can help animals convert to one meal per day and control their weight. I fast my animal companions only when I have time to give them special care—extra love and lots of broth and water. If you choose to have your dog fast, the fasting day is a wonderful time for grooming and playing. Do not have your dog fast when you are not home. He needs the extra attention when deprived of his food!

Healthy wild animals gorge on their fresh prey, then sleep. They may not catch another meal for a day or two. As you switch your dog over to the fresh food diet, you'll probably observe his *voluntary fasting*. You'll put down the food and he'll just sniff it. You can add a bribe food or two until he gets used to the smell of this new food, and smell is what attracts dogs to their food. He'll get the hang of it. It took me two weeks to convert my dog. I just kept decreasing her dry and canned food until she was gobbling up 100 percent raw.

Most animals beg for food and treats because what they really want is love and attention. Holistic physician and author Deepak Chopra, M.D., cites a study done with two groups of laboratory animals. One group was provided daily with an optimum diet by a technician who merely put the food down but never touched the animals. The other group was fed the equivalent of a fast-food diet, but was loved and stroked at feeding time. The animals that got the good food but no love died, and those that got the bad food and the cuddles lived.

Accept a *voluntary* fast for up to four meals (forty-eight hours) unless your dog has a medical condition that warrants special care. At each scheduled mealtime, put down the dish (including bribe foods if you feel you need to) and pick it up and clean the area forty-five minutes later, whether your dog has eaten or not. Show him that you love him but that you also mean business. If he doesn't eat, let him fast. No more junk food! Provide greens and chicken broth for him to cleanse his system. Keep a bowl of fresh purified water down at all times during fasting. Broth is wonderful during fasts. Serve it three to five times a day, but leave it down for only forty-five minutes. You can include a pinch of vitamin C with bioflavonoid complex and food enzymes and a dash of AniMinerals.

Since dry-food eaters are used to nibbling, at first they may not think you mean business when you remove the dish. They think that if they sit by the cupboard where you keep the old bag of kibble (they know you kept it), maybe you'll break down. If you make it through four meals of this siege, you deserve a pat on the back. Most dogs will dive into their fresh food by the fourth meal. You can help by popping a raw "meatball" into their mouths so they get the taste of it. If repeated tries at the new diet fail, Dr. Chambreau thinks that your dog may have an underlying energy imbalance and may be in need of some holistic treatment (such as acupuncture or homeopathy) to develop a good appetite.[29]

If your dog is over seven years old, pregnant, nursing, or seriously ill, most holistic veterinarians recommend that you not allow an extended fast. Get your dog eating as best you can. He will need extra bribes and TLC. If your dog normally gobbles up his fresh food diet and suddenly refuses to eat or shows any other unusual symptoms, suspect an involuntary fast. Consult your holistic veterinarian as soon as possible.

Your holistic veterinarian may want you to force-feed a dog that refuses to eat. Check with your practitioner for guidelines on what to force-feed your dog. I use pureed raw beef liver with bonemeal. You'll need a feeding syringe. I feed this broth every six hours or, again, follow the advice of your holistic practitioner. A raw meat broth is extremely useful for short-term force-feeding: simply puree ground beef and water, strain, and feed by syringe.

HOW TO PREVENT CONTAMINATION AND SPOILAGE

TO ENSURE YOU'RE giving your dogs only the freshest food, you need to follow some basic rules of storage and hygiene. Keep your fresh food mixture no more than three days in the refrigerator, or freeze portions and thaw them in the refrigerator the night before serving. Date the frozen packages and never use them more than six months later. Keep meat out of the refrigerator just long enough to prepare it. Finally, always smell the meat before you feed it to your dog; when in doubt, throw it out! Raw food should be left out no longer than one hour.

Ninety percent of spoiled meat problems happen right in our own kitchens. Besides improper storage, spoilage may occur when cutting boards and other preparation surfaces aren't cleaned properly. Clean areas where your animals eat with a diluted bleach mixture, then rinse thoroughly with hot water.

Standardized extract of grapefruit controls bacteria and acts as a natural preservative. I recommend treating raw meat (both muscle and organ meat) as follows:[30]

6–8 ounces purified water
4 drops standardized extract of grapefruit (liquid concentrate)[31]
1 pound meat or poultry

Dissolve the standardized extract of grapefruit in the water and mix thoroughly into the meat. The antibacterial action on ground meat is immediate; when treating chunks or whole pieces of poultry, marinate them in the solution for an hour in a covered glass bowl in the refrigerator. You may also treat raw egg yolk in this manner, especially if you're worried about your dog's immune system. This method is also safe to use on eggs, meat, and poultry you cook for yourself.

Caution: Keep standardized extract of grapefruit away from eyes and sensitive areas. If accidental contact occurs, flush with water for ten minutes. Irritation is usually temporary but may last up to forty-eight hours.

Dr. Swift recommends as an alternative to standardized extract of grapefruit food-grade hydrogen peroxide. (I have used 3 percent food-grade hydrogen peroxide at a ratio of 1 tablespoon per cup of water.) Pour the solution onto raw ground meat and mix thoroughly. If using chunks of meat or pieces of poultry, marinate them in the solution for one hour in the refrigerator.

Caution: Use only 3 percent food-grade hydrogen peroxide. It also comes in 35 percent, which causes nausea and burning if you use it full strength. You may dilute 35 percent to 3 percent, according to Pat McKay,[32] by adding 12 ounces of purified water to 1 ounce of 35 percent food-grade hydrogen peroxide. I never use more than 4 drops of standardized extract of grapefruit dissolved in 6–8 ounces of purified water or 1 tablespoon of 3 percent food-grade hydrogen peroxide to a cup of purified water—more is not better.

Refrigerate all oils immediately after opening, as oxidation begins upon contact with air.

If you include some canned food in the fresh food recipe, never store the food in the can in the refrigerator, as contamination with lead can be severe. Canned pet food contains as much as 0.9–7.0 parts per million (ppm) of lead, a daily intake that's considered potentially toxic for children. So store canned food in glass containers.

PURE WATER AND CATALYST-ALTERED WATER

KEEP A BOWL of fresh distilled, spring, or purified water available for your animal at all times. I have always used distilled or purified water for both myself and my animal companions. Dr. Henry G. Bieler, author of *Food Is Your Best Medicine,* says that just as you'd never put tap or mineral water in a steam iron, your kidneys appreciate the same courtesy. I personally use distilled water. When mixing distilled water with my animals' food, I add the supplement AniMinerals. There is another school of thought that suggests that distilled water actually leaches out minerals from our system. Follow your holistic practitioner's advice.

Marina Zacharias's article "Chlorinated Water—More Bad News" reports that "animal studies conducted by the Environmental Protection Agency have shown that drinking chlorinated water caused blood cholesterol to switch from high-density lipoproteins (the good guys) to low-density lipoproteins (the bad guys)." She adds that "when water is treated with chlorine, the compound 'hypochlorite' is created. This compound creates free radicals which oxidize essential fatty acids and causes them to turn rancid."[33]

Free radicals being created by chlorinated water decrease the body's ability to get essential fatty acids from food. They also create dangerous toxins that have been directly linked to liver malfunction, weakened immune systems, changes in the arteries, and alterations of cellular DNA. So please give your animal companion fresh, pure water.

One day at my local pharmacy, I happened upon a product called Willard water (catalyst-altered water, or CAW, developed by the late Dr. John Willard, a professor of chemistry). I bought a 4-ounce bottle and a small pamphlet about it.[34] I was told by the pharmacy staff that this water cleanses the intestinal tract and is perfectly safe to drink, bathe in, and mix with food for children, adults, plants, and animals.

Willard water is described in the literature as "wetter," more reactive, and more efficient. After my first sip, the notion of the water being wetter seemed a great description. It really quenched my thirst. I liked the taste, and it gave me a feeling of being centered, as opposed to stressful or sleepy.

Catalyst-altered water has been altered by a silicone colloidal particle called the *micelle,* one of the most powerful reducing agents (antioxidants) for organic substances. Like the living cell, the micelle, under the proper stimuli, will reverse its polarity and act as an oxidizing agent. The CAW micelle has a negative charge on the surface, which helps remove most of the toxins, harmful bacteria, pollutants, and carcinogens from air, water, and foods, which have a positive charge. The micelle takes electrons from the water and atmosphere and therefore has an infinite source of electrons to replenish those lost through its action as a reducing agent. The micelle can speed up a chemical reaction without changing the natural result, a phenomenon that allows plants to grow faster and wounds to heal more rapidly. The micelle acts like a catalyst, which is why Dr. Willard named this substance catalyst-altered water.

Dr. Willard believed there to be two causes of illness, both concerned with water, air, and food: either the body needs something that is not there, or something that is not needed by the body is there. In both instances, the use of CAW has an effect. Rather than a nutrient, CAW (like all water) is the vehicle by which nutrients are carried to the cells and by which waste is carried away. Because it is a more biologically active form of water, CAW does a better job of transportation.

Willard water is available in two forms, the clear CAW and the dark CAWXXX. Reputable labs have tested both kinds of Willard water and have classified them as nontoxic, noncorrosive, noncarcinogenic, and incapable of causing harmful side effects. You can safely drink CAWXXX and use it the same way as clear CAW—just remember to follow the package directions (they differ for each kind).

The clear form contains a larger percentage of the catalyst and so is more reactive. The dark CAWXXX contains not only the catalyst but also lignite organics. *Lignite* is the fossilized remains of plants, trees, and microorganisms that lived long before humans made their debut on the earth. The internal chemistry of these plants enabled them to survive under hostile conditions. Lignite is 60–65 percent carbon and contains hydrogen, nitrogen, and oxygen as well as trace minerals—all invaluable for life processes. There is also evidence of antibacterial, antifungal, and antiviral agents in addition to unidentified growth stimulants for plants and animals. When lignite is treated with Willard water, the valuable nutrients are made available as conditioners and normalizers, and all undesirable components are eliminated.

You can mix diluted CAWXXX with your animal's food in place of normal purified water. It helps quiet nervous and excitable animals, so I even use it to shampoo my animals, adding one part shampoo to nine parts CAW. A rinse with CAW helps reduce itching, and I've also used it to bathe stuffy noses or irritated eyes and wounds (both punctures and abrasions) along with the appropriate homeopathic remedies.

Wendy Volhard and Dr. Kerry Brown suggest keeping some CAW in a spray bottle to treat "hot spot"(itchy spots on your dog or cat).[35] Simply part the dog's hair and spray. They have found that when you catch the spot and spray it before it becomes too hot, there is no need to resort to shaving the dog. You can add a few drops of apple cider vinegar to help further reduce itching.

You can spray Willard water on your dog's paw pad to help heal cuts. It actually helps stop bleeding and relieves pain. It is also used, again, according to Volhard and Brown, for insect stings. You can clean surgical sites and watch CAW promote healing even when the sutures are still in. Once you experience the benefits, Willard water will soon become a part of your daily routine.

VITAMINS AND MINERALS: A GUIDE TO NUTRITIONAL SUPPLEMENTS

BASIC SUPPLEMENTS ARE definitely needed when you feed your dog the fresh food diet (see "The Basic Homemade Fresh Food Recipe," page 95), but do not attempt other than basic supplementation without first consulting with a qualified animal nutritionist or a holistic veterinarian who is well versed in nutrition. From time to time your practitioner may choose to augment your dog's diet with additional supplementation. Find a reliable source for your supplements—you must be able to count on the integrity of the manufacturers. I have created a multivitamin and mineral supplement (see Celeste Yarnall in "Resources") that includes bonemeal, vitamin C, bioflavonoids, dandelion, trace mineral powder with kelp and alfalfa, barley grass juice, and garlic. These supplements are extremely important to ensure that all the necessary micronutrients are present in the fresh food recipe. Modern farming and the stress of our dogs' lifestyles make supplementation imperative.

The key thing to remember when administering supplements is that you're trying to achieve balance in your dog's nutrition. Minerals and vitamins work hand in hand, and both are necessary to maintain a healthy body. Our animals' bodies know best what vitamins and minerals are needed at any given time. All we can do as their guardians is try to make sure all the bases are covered. What the body doesn't need at the moment will be stored or eliminated, depending on the type of supplement.

The safest way to provide minerals is through whole food supplements and other natural substances such as bonemeal, herbs, antioxidants, and trace minerals. Soluble minerals act as

- ionized conductors of the electrical current necessary for all bodily functions;
- catalysts and activators of other nutrients;
- building blocks of enzymes, hormones, and other natural chemicals used by the body to perform specific functions;
- equalizers and balancers of body fluids, fluid pressures, and pH (in the absence of certain trace minerals, certain heavy minerals, such as lead, are more likely to accumulate and cause poisoning); and
- aids to digestion and assimilation.

No single supplement is a cure-all. Don't administer isolated vitamins or minerals on an ongoing basis. Just because a friend tells you to try a particular vitamin for a dog that scratches himself, it doesn't mean you want to give it every day for the rest of your dog's life. The animal may not have a vitamin deficiency. So please don't give megadoses of one vitamin or mineral (unless your holistic veterinarian tells you to) just because it seems to benefit a particular condition. Megadoses of antioxidants, for example, may inhibit good eicosanoids. Your holistic veterinarian is aware of interactions and will advise you as to the correct doses and combinations.

Always use vitamins and minerals from organic and natural sources.

The following chart includes vitamins and minerals that research has found to be necessary. Exact requirements of supplements vary, so using the nutrients in live foods and whole food supplements is a more beneficial option. This list is for informational purposes only. Check with a holistic veterinarian or animal nutritionist prior to supplementing your animal's diet. Basic supplements are included in the fresh food diet recipe, and most are available by mail order (see Celeste Yarnall in "Resources").

VITAMIN AND MINERAL GUIDE CHART

SUPPLEMENT	RECOMMENDED AMOUNTS	HEALTH BENEFITS
Vitamin A	10,000 IU weekly	Prevents cataracts, weakness in hind legs; aids tissue development; promotes healthy skin and fur; gives mucous membranes structural integrity; builds resistance to respiratory disease
Biotin	Exact amount required not known	Promotes thyroid and adrenal health and hair growth, cures feces-eating problem; vital for food metabolism. Early sign of deficiency is scaly dermatitis.
Vitamin C	250–3,000 mg daily (or to bowel tolerance) cut back if stool loosens Ester C, or sodium ascorbate, is less irritating to the gastrointestinal tract and is recommended when using more than 3 grams daily	Promotes healing of wounds; used to treat arthritis, and chronic/degenerative diseases from stress due to high fever, cigarette smoke, pollution; prevents kidney stones

INTERACTIONS	BEST FOOD SOURCE
Caution: Excess is as harmful as deficiency; confirm exact dosage with holistic practitioner before using. Absorption blocked by use of mineral oil, sugar, or cortisone, or through liver disorders	Eggs, cod liver oil, raw butter, yogurt, raw meat. Dogs can convert beta-carotene to vitamin A, and many veterinarians, reports Dr. Nancy Scanlan, prefer beta carotene instead of vitamin A.* Dr. Scanlan advises that it should be used with caution.
Antibiotics decrease production.	Lentils and legumes
Depleted by cigarette smoke, baking soda, high fever	Leafy vegetables, cruciferous vegetables (such as broccoli), lentils, sprouts, most fruits

SUPPLEMENT	RECOMMENDED AMOUNTS	HEALTH BENEFITS
Bioflavonoid	500 mg for each 1,000 mg vitamin C	Supports vitamin C and is essential to its absorption
Vitamin B complex (includes B_1 thiamine, B_2 riboflavin, B_3 niacin, B_5 pantothenic acid, B_6 pyridoxine, B_9 folic acid, B_{12} cyanocobalamin, B_{13} orotic acid, B_{15} pangamic acid, B_{17} laetrile, biotin, choline, inositol, and para-aminobenzoic acid [PABA])	Water soluble and sheds easily, so must be continually replenished Exact amount required not known	Helps hyperactivity; improves appetite; used as flea repellent; helps nervous animals; essential for mental and emotional health; helps prevent heart problems; essential for skin and coat conditions; essential to thyroid and adrenals; aids in flea problems and dermatitis
Vitamin D	Exact amount required not known[†] Daily sunlight; needs to be taken with vitamin A	Prevents rickets and hypocalcemia; essential for normal growth of bones and teeth; helps behavioral problems and endocrine imbalances
Vitamin E	100–400 IU once daily—mixed tocopherol	Maintains balance between oils/fats and amino acids; great antioxidant; slows aging; improves skin, muscles, and nerves; important for healing, especially burns

INTERACTIONS	BEST FOOD SOURCE
	Grapes, raisins, rose hips, white inner skin of citrus fruits
Depleted by cold weather, stress, antibiotics; megadoses of vitamin C and folic acid decrease B_{12} levels and destroy many B complex vitamins; absorption blocked by cooking of fats and oils	Raw liver, organ meats, cottage cheese, sardines I supplement with B complex in its entirety unless my holistic veterinarian prescribes individual B vitamins.
Depleted by excessive or insufficient calcium and phosphorus; deficiency caused by insufficient sunlight	Cod liver oil, raw butter, cheese, eggs, organ meats
Absorption hindered by mineral oil, chlorine, iron, synthetic hormones—check with holistic veterinarian prior to administering, as certain conditions and medications require caution.	Wheat germ oil, leafy greens and other raw vegetables, seeds, whole grains, raw meat

SUPPLEMENT	RECOMMENDED AMOUNTS	HEALTH BENEFITS
Vitamin F	Exact amount required not known	Helps prevent heart problems; essential for skin and coat conditions; essential to thyroid and adrenals; aids in flea problems and dermatitis
Folic Acid—Vitamin B_9	Exact amount required not known	Prevents birth defects, weight loss, anemia, eye discharge. Signs of deficiency are anemia and leukopenia.
Pyridoxine—Vitamin B_6		Essential for metabolism of protein, healthy nervous system, red-blood-cell production, strong immune system
Vitamin K	Supplementation needed rarely	Regulates formation of several factors involved in blood clotting; prevents hemorrhaging; large intake produces hemolytic anemia and therefore can be toxic. Diarrhea and colitis may be symptomatic.
Calcium and Phosphorus[††]	Optimum ratio between 1.2 & 1.4:1 500mg per 100g of meat	Deficiencies lead to nervousness, lameness, muscle spasms, heart palpitations, seizures, bone fractures

INTERACTIONS	BEST FOOD SOURCE
Absorption blocked by cooking of fats and oils	Cold-pressed vegetable and fish oils (cod liver oil); linolenic and arachidonic acids; raw meats and vegetables
Depleted by cortisone, cigarette smoke, antibiotics	Cod liver oil, tofu, wheat germ, sprouts, fruit
Depleted by pesticides, sugar, laxatives, synthetic hormones	Herbs, raw liver and other organ meats, whole grain cereals
Depleted by drug treatment, especially anticoagulants	Obtained through bacterial synthesis in intestine and is usually given as a supplement only in the case of certain types of poisoning
Vitamin D required to activate calcium Vitamin C needed to prevent kidney stones and assure iron absorbtion.	Bonemeal is the most natural source of calcium and phosphorous; mix with raw meat to avoid deficiency. (see "The Basic Homemade Fresh Food Recipe" page 95)

SUPPLEMENT	RECOMMENDED AMOUNTS	HEALTH BENEFITS
Magnesium	Normally obtained in diet—deficiency unlikely	Important for nervous system and enzyme function. Signs of deficiency are heart arrhythmia & depression.
Zinc	With normal dietary intake of iron and copper, concentrations of up to eight times minimum requirement will not produce adverse effects. Minimum requirement for dogs unknown	Enhances skin and coat condition. Signs of deficiency include poor growth, emaciation, testicular atrophy, and dandruff.
Potassium and Sodium	Need for supplementation very rare	Use in cases of exhaustion
Chromium	Exact amount required not known	May help diabetes, as it regulates blood sugar
Iron	Approximately 5 mg daily—exact amount required not known	Fights lead poisoning from commercial foods; builds immunity and energy. Iron oxide far less dangerous form than ferrous sulphate

Source: Adapted from Pat McKay, *Reigning Cats and Dogs,* pp.76–102; and "Your Complete Vitamin Guide for the Natural Pet," *Natural Pet Magazine,* Mar.–Apr. 1994, pp. 16–18, including additional suggestions from Dr. Nancy Scanlan.

Note: For in-depth discussion on individual supplements, I recommend Volhard and Brown's *The Holistic Guide for a Healthy Dog,* pp. 22–61.

INTERACTIONS	BEST FOOD SOURCE
Depleted by noise stress. Vitamin C needed to best utilize calcium/magnesium	Broccoli, dairy products, sardines, and bonemeal
Vegetable protein–based diets may dramatically increase requirement; phytic acid (in cereals) decreases availability.	Beef liver, chicken, oats, Swiss cheese, some nuts and seeds
Potassium depleted by cooking	Apple cider vinegar (1 teaspoon per pint of drinking water)
Depleted by white flour and white sugar	Calves' liver, vegetables, fruit
Too much dairy, eggs, yogurt block absorption	Citrus fruits, tomatoes, broccoli, cantaloupe, beef liver, poultry, beans

* Personal communication with Dr. Nancy Scanlan.

† Dr. Scanlan cautions that an excess in a growing puppy can cause signs that mimic rickets and not to add it as a separate supplement unless your veterinarian advises so.

†† Excess phosphorus can cause calcium deficiency. Excess calcium may contribute to bladder stones. Do not give more than recommended doses unless your veterinarian advises you to do so.

How to Be Your Dog's Supplement Detective

DIFFERENT AREAS OF the dog's body can give you clues to suspect deficiencies or possibly too much of a particular supplement. For example, if your dog has an eye or sinus infection, vitamin A may be needed topically. (I open a 5,000 IU capsule of vitamin A and dissolve it in 2 ounces of sterile saline solution and put a drop in each eye. It drains down through the sinus cavity to help inflamed sinuses.)

If your dog scratches his neck, you may be dealing with a vitamin F or essential fatty acid deficiency. Be sure that your animal is getting adequate essential fatty acids in his diet. Cold-pressed olive, canola, sunflower, salmon, borage, evening primrose, or black currant oil may be helpful.

For heart and lungs, we normally think of vitamin E_{10}, CoEnzyme Q_{10} and L-carnitine; for chest and lungs, vitamin C with bioflavonoids is valuable.

For the corner of the mouth, as well as umbilicus, consider vitamins from the vitamin B-complex group, and vitamin K, which is essential for blood clotting.

Vitamin D relates to proper bone growth.

For facial paralysis of the right side, potassium may be indicated, and sodium may be called for if there is a paralysis or stroke on the left side of the body.

Sulphur may be indicated for skin disorders, eczema and dermatitis, or skin discolorations. Taurine, one of the sulphur amino acids, along with zinc, is sometimes used to treat epilepsy. Sulphur deficiencies occur when the dog's diet is deficient in animal protein or after prolonged use of antibiotics, which deplete friendly bacteria in the intestinal tract.

Iodine typically prevents goiter and is necessary for a healthy thyroid gland. Deficiencies may manifest themselves in those symptoms common to hypo- or hyperthyroidism (specifically, weight gain, blackened skin, fatigue, itchy skin, sluggishness, patches of dry fur, thickened skin, immune suppression or feeling cold and having difficulty regulating body temperature, mammary tumors, deformities [such as thick tongue; short, broad head; wide nose; short bodies with heavy extremities], delayed loss of puppy teeth, shedding hair [alopoecia], and even timidity).

Calcium is critical throughout your dog's entire life. However, his third through fifth months are especially important because of his general growth and development of teeth. Too much and too little calcium apparently cause the same symptoms. Bonemeal is the best source because it provides phosphorus and magnesium in the correct ratio to the calcium. You will know you are dealing with a deficiency if your animal has porous or fragile bones, hip problems, muscle cramps, rickets, lameness, tooth decay, loss of teeth, gingivitis (which CoEnzyme Q_{10} also helps), irritability or aggression, kidney stone formation, calcification of soft tissues, toxemia in pregnancy, anxiety, muscle twitching, palpitations, or confusion. Too much or too little calcium and phosphorus can result in lameness, pain in the joints, too much extension in the carpal (wrist) joints, going down in the pasterns (ankles), and improper growth of the long bones.

Iron deficiencies would cause anemia, pale skin, fatigue, brittle nails, shortness of breath, red and inflamed tongue, low blood pressure, rheumatism in the back legs, dizziness, infertility, and rubbing his head on the right side near the eyes. Too much iron can cause gastrointestinal lesions.

Zinc is needed for proper growth and wound healing. Excess calcium can cause a zinc deficiency. Zinc affects the level of copper in the body, which, in turn, affects iron. Zinc is most effective if used along with copper, vitamin B complex, vitamin A, calcium, and phosphorus.

As you can see, supplements are a tricky business. That is why we in holistic health care are so adamant about fresh food diets. My best advice is to seek out a qualified veterinary practitioner or nutritionist. Perhaps have some blood work, urine analysis, and fecal testing done on your dog before attempting anything other than the fresh food with basic supplementation. You may contact Dr. Nancy Scanlan, Dr. Charles Loops, Dr. Russell Swift, and Dr. Robert J. Silver, as well as Dr. Kerry Brown (coauthor of *The Holistic Guide for a Healthy Dog* with Wendy Volhard—their book is a wonderful reference work that I keep handy when I need to research vitamin or mineral deficiencies).

Dr. Robert J. Silver of the Holistic Wellness Center (see "Resources") is an outspoken champion of holistic health care for animal companions. In his article "Neutraceuticals vs. Pharmaceuticals," Dr. Silver offers yet another aspect of supplementation.[36] He defines a neutraceutical as a food or part of a food that provides medical or health benefits, including the prevention and treatment of disease. Sometimes neutraceuticals are described as "designer" or "functional" foods. They can be dietary supplements, herbal products, processed foods such as cereals, soups, beverages, isolated nutrients, or genetically engineered foods. Essentially this definition covers just about everything except pharmaceuticals. A neutraceutical has most likely been extracted from a food, plant, or animal-based material, he explains.

Dr. Silver has found neutraceuticals to be of tremendous value in helping arthritis patients, and he feels that trauma, genetics, and poor-quality, highly processed, and chemically adulterated food (like commercial pet foods), as well as vaccinations and excessive and inappropriate use of antibiotics (I would add steroids to this list as well), play a role in arthritis. Each year, more and more powerful anti-inflammatory drugs are poured into people and their animals who suffer from arthritis, and many patients still do not receive much relief.

A recently conducted, double-blind, controlled study compared the effects of ibuprofen in human patients with a "chondroprotective" agent known as glucosamine sulfate. Glucosamine sulfate is a neutraceutical that actually aids the healing of joints. The result of the study using the chondroprotective agent demonstrates that after four weeks, 85 percent of the patients had more relief from their symptoms while taking glucosamine sulfate than did those taking ibuprofen. In fact, evidence suggests that glucosamine sulfate and its chondroprotective partner, chondroitin sulfate A, when given in adequate doses for a long enough period of time, can actually repair joint cartilage. There are no known toxic side effects. Glucosamine sulfate (in the form n-acetyl glucosamine) has also proved to be effective in treating inflammatory bowel disease.

Dr. Silver states that the human dose for glucosamine sulfate and chondroitin sulfate A is 500 mg three times daily. A large dog could be dosed at about 500 mg twice daily, a middle-sized dog at 250 mg twice daily, and a small dog at 250 mg per day. He warns that we must be patient because naturally assisting the body to heal itself takes more time than the "magic steroid bullets" doctors and veterinarians prescribe. Once you see benefits achieved with the chondroprotective agents, you may slowly reduce the dosage to find the minimum that is effective.

Dr. Nancy Scanlan suggests using a loading dosage of glucosamine sulfate for two to four weeks until you see improvement and then decrease it to an effective minimal dosage.[37] As always, your own holistic veterinarian will have a protocol that he or she is comfortable with.

Another neutraceutical known for its ability to stimulate the body's natural system of anti-inflammation is super oxide dismutase, a.k.a. SOD. It is derived from liver or from wheatgrass sprouts. Dr. Silver suggests administering 250–500 mg two or three times daily until you get the desired effect, then reducing the dosage to the smallest amount that is still effective. I use wheatgrass sprout supplements often (see "More About Supplements—Some Good, Some Bad").

Another supplement Dr. Scanlan suggests for dogs suffering with arthritic pain or muscle weakness in older dogs is phenylalanine (an amino acid).[38] She recommends a dose of about 500 mg for large dogs twice daily, 250 mg twice daily for medium dogs, and 250 mg once daily for small dogs. The dose can be cut in half when improvement is seen. Consult your holistic practitioner for his or her advice.

More About Supplements—Some Good, Some Bad

Vitamin C: I recommend the powdered form of vitamin C, as it is easy to use. Ester C, or sodium ascorbate, with bioflavonoids is less irritating to the gastrointestinal tract and is recommended when giving dosages of more than 3 grams a day. Daily amounts can be increased in weekly increments to avoid intestinal problems. (See "Resources" under Celeste Yarnall on how to obtain supplements recommended throughout this book.)

I often use a teaspoon of Bio-C formula, which is privately labeled for me by Best Friends. It provides 1,000 mg vitamin C with rose hips, 500 mg of bioflavonoid complex including rutin, and hesperidin. Give vitamin C and other water-soluble nutrients in frequent small doses, as they pass through the system in three to four hours. For this reason, putting Bio-C in food is an ideal way to administer it. I use 1 teaspoon per pound of raw meat for adult dogs. I also use Ester C with bioflavonoids when dosages of more than 3 grams are called for.

The primary function of vitamin C is to maintain collagen, a protein necessary for the proper formation and healing of connective tissue, ligaments, tendons, muscles, skin, and bones. Secondary functions include the formation of adrenaline (needed for stressful situations); protection of other vitamins from oxidation; formation of red blood cells; stimulation of interferon production; stimulation of the immune system, thus enabling the body to resist disease (including cancer); and inactivation of viruses and bacteria.

Found abundantly in the inner white pulp of citrus, bioflavonoids (vitamin P) are very important to the support of vitamin C. Rutin is part of the bioflavonoid complex, and it strengthens capillary walls. Hesperidin is a crystalline glycoside.

Bonemeal: I use bonemeal with fresh raw meat because the meat stimulates acid production in the digestive system and aids in calcium absorption. Mix $1^{1}/2$ to 2 tablespoons into every 2 pounds of meat. My Bonemeal supplement (see "Resources") contains less than 5 ppm of lead, and it includes, in balanced proportions, all the nutrients necessary for the proper assimilation of calcium. In fact, I feel this product is the only supplemental form of calcium that is complete and, therefore, safe for both dogs and cats.

MinerAll Plus: This is privately labeled for me by Best Friends. It is an excellent supplement for flea control and skin allergies. This powder is a unique blend of montmorillonite clay,[39] alfalfa, kelp, dandelion root, and garlic. Collectively, the ingredients in MinerAll Plus provide vitamins A, B complex, C, D, E, G, K, P, and U, as well as seventy-two trace minerals. Montmorillonite clay is a natural source of many trace minerals; alfalfa contains calcium, magnesium, potassium, phosphorus, silicon, and sodium; and dandelion root contains taraxacin, inulin, gluten, gum, and potash. These substances are useful for remedying chronic disorders of the kidneys and liver, as well as gallstones, anemia, and diabetes. Kelp contains iodine, iron, potassium, calcium, sodium, choline, sulfur, and silicon. Garlic contains protein, carbohydrates, calcium, iron, potassium, phosphorus, traces of sodium, and vitamins B_1, B_2, B_3, and C, as well as thirty-three sulfur compounds. It is also one of the best vegetable sources of selenium. Both selenium and vitamin E are antioxidants, which act to retard oxidation. I have combined Bio C and MinerAll Plus with bonemeal and lecithin in one product for convenience. I call it VM+Plus. Use 4 teaspoons for each pound of meat that you feed your dog. (See Celeste Yarnall in "Resources.")

Vitamin E: I add between 100 and 400 IU of high-quality vitamin E to the dog's food daily, like liquid vitamin E oil, which I keep refrigerated at all times.[40] (I prefer mixed tocopherols.) Vitamin E is known as the "fertility vitamin" and is of tremendous benefit in a breeding program. Dr. Nancy Scanlan suggests that you clear its use with your holistic veterinarian beforehand, especially if your dog has heart problems or diabetes.[41] He will need lower doses in these cases.

Essential Fatty Acids: Fatty acids, available in raw meat and uncooked oils, are essential to a dog's diet. I recommend high-quality, expeller-pressed, nitrogen-sealed oils. Never cook them; cooked fat clogs arteries. I include oils daily to promote luxurious coats.

You can make your own essential fatty acid mixture by combining 4 ounces of light olive oil, one 1-gram capsule of borage oil (containing 240 mg of GLA), 2 teaspoons (10 ml) salmon or cod liver oil (containing 1 gram of EPA), and 1,000 IU of vitamin E oil. Shake well and refrigerate immediately, as oils begin to oxidize the minute they are opened and may become rancid quickly. You may add 1 tablespoon of this oil mixture to each pound of raw meat or poultry.[42] I have my own product called EFA oil, which combines those ingredients. However, we have substituted grapeseed oil for light olive oil. (See "Resources.")

I rarely use flaxseed oil because it acts like a wet blanket for the enzymes that control the eventual flow of omega-6 essential fatty acids toward eicosanoids. In other words, it knocks out the production of good as well as bad eicosanoids.[43]

Herbs: From time to time, I use fresh herbs—but just a pinch for aroma and flavor. Sage, thyme, and marjoram, among other savory herbs, smell wonderful and are nice additions. I have also used a pinch of Sunrider Simply Herbs in my dogs' food now and then.[44] Red raspberry is known to be of benefit during pregnancy.

Acidophilus: This substance is most commonly produced by fermenting milk with lactobacilli (bacteria beneficial to digestion).

I keep vegetarian acidophilus (in either liquid or capsule form) in my refrigerator. If an animal has been on an antibiotic,[45] I recommend giving him acidophilus for a couple of weeks to a month afterward. Be sure to give the kind without lactose, because lactose can cause cramping, flatulence, or diarrhea in some dogs. The lactobacilli replace many of the friendly bacteria in the intestinal tract that are wiped out by the antibiotic. Supplemental friendly bacteria are referred to as *probiotics*. I also recommend enzymes (such as Dr. Swift's Florzyme) that contain friendly bacteria like acidophilus (good for the small intestine) and bifidobacteria (best for the large intestine). I currently use a probiotic called Florasource, which combines several friendly bacteria. I prepare my probiotic by mixing 1/8 teaspoon with 2 ounces of distilled water and syringe it in my animals' mouths thirty minutes before breakfast. I don't like the idea of adding it to raw meat since I add standardized extract of grapefruit as an antibacterial agent. These friendly bacteria might be destroyed in the process; besides, the probiotic's action seems to work best on an empty stomach.

Bee Products: Bee pollen, bee propolis, and royal jelly are excellent immune boosters. Bee propolis is the natural antibiotic the bees use to keep their hives free of bacteria. Combination products are available, but initially please be stingy with bee substances—they've been known to cause allergic reactions in sensitive individuals. I don't use them on a daily basis, but I have heard of good results. Try 1/4 teaspoon of bee pollen per pound of meat in your fresh food mixture and see how your dogs tolerate it. It's a good idea to clear its use with your animal nutritionist first; royal jelly, for example, can cause allergic reactions such as itchy skin.

Wheat Sprout Supplements: Biogenetics produces an impressive line of supplements (see "Resources"). Its Canine Balance and Nu-Pet wafers are antioxidant nutritional supplements containing a trademarked ingredient called Bioguard Sprouts, which fights free radicals. The use of antioxidants seems to improve the overall well-being and immune response of dogs. Bioguard includes vitamins C and E, beta-carotene, selenium, and beef liver, which provides B_{12} and other B-complex vitamins; it's blended with beef broth, which makes it palatable to dogs. You can crush the tablets with a mortar and pestle, putting the powder into the fresh food. However, most dogs love the tablets as a treat. Canine Balance, as the name implies, helps promote alertness, well-being, and composure in stressful situations such as boarding, training, showing, estrus, and illness. Bioguard Plus, which comes in both tablets and granules, is for people and animals. Introduce Bioguard Plus after two weeks on Bioguard.

Yeast: What about yeast? I don't include it in the fresh food recipe or as a supplement for my dogs. One reason is that it tends to cause or aggravate allergies. Alfred Plechner, D.V.M., lists yeast, yeast-containing foods, and brewer's yeast (given to animals for supposed flea protection) in his allergic "hit list."[46] Apparently, the DNA and RNA in yeast don't break down completely in the intestines and, when absorbed through the intestinal wall, may cause adverse autoimmune responses and weaken organs such as the liver and kidneys. If you're feeding your dog yeast and observe your dog itching and scratching excessively, with the appearance of patches of red skin, please discontinue use.

Yeast is a popular source of B vitamins in pet-food supplements because it's inexpensive! That's why it's in everything from vitamins to flea care. However, in high-quality human supplements, they advertise their products to be hypoallergenic and yeast-free. It's high quality B vitamins in supplements and garlic in the fresh raw food diet that keep fleas away!

Many other people in the holistic community do recommend yeast, including Richard Pitcairn, D.V.M., who suggests a mixture called Healthy Powder, and the Wysong Company, which puts yeast in its supplements. If you read labels, you'll find yeast in many other pet supplements.

Marina Zacharias offers the following cautions about yeast: "Brewer's yeast has been around for decades. Basically, it's a 'waste' product derived from the brewing industry. Although it did serve as a cheap ingredient for pet foods, it took the boys in the advertising department to come up with the idea that it's a great cure for (fill in the most common dog problem) flea, skin, and allergy problems. The problem I have with all this hype is a few facts that seem to have been ignored. Fact: Dogs can't digest it! Fact: Most dogs are actually allergic to it! A study done over six years ago on dogs with skin allergies proved that nine out of ten of them were allergic to yeast. Fact: Master herbalist Juliette de Bairacli Levy has been warning us against yeast for decades."[47]

Yeast is high in phosphorus, so it can cause a calcium deficiency by throwing off the calcium-phosporus balance within the body. All the big benefits you hear about this substance come from pet-food companies.

On the other hand, Michael Lemmon, D.V.M., advises that you refrain from using yeast if it obviously causes allergies or other problems such as skin or digestive disorders. Otherwise, he feels that yeast, in one or more of its forms, is good for animals, supplying high-quality proteins, B-complex vitamins, and trace minerals.[48]

Yeast comes in various other forms besides brewer's yeast, such as torula yeast, lactic acid yeast (available from Standard Process Laboratories, see "Resources"), and kefir, which is a milk product made from kefir grains cultured from milk-fermenting yeasts and bacteria. Kefir can be found in cheese and beverage form. I do not recommend Kombucha tea, which also contains a form of nutritional yeast, because it is made from black tea and white sugar. Zell oxygen yeast, according to Dr. Lemmon, may be used to help the body better utilize oxygen. Finally, BioStrath yeast (and its animal counterpart, AnimaStrath liquid yeast) combines yeast with sixteen herbs.

As always, consult your holistic practitioner, or conduct your own feeding trial and see what happens. From the results of my own experiments, I choose not to include yeast in my fresh food recipe. However, only you can be the judge as to your animal companion's tolerance.

Program: What about Program (lufenuron)? While we're on the subject of fleas and brewer's yeast, here's another highly touted product. I chose to follow the discussion of yeast with some information on Program rather than cover it in the "The Dangers of Conventional Care" because many people think of Program as a supplement. Marina Zacharias comes up with the best take on this drug yet: "Good grief! What are they going to come up with next? Ciby-Geigy has launched a massive promotional campaign on a new 'flea control' pill that they called 'Program.' Now you don't have to bother spraying poison on your carpets anymore. Just pop a poison pill into your animal once a month, and the animal will deliver the poison from its own blood directly to the flea!"[49]

The pill contains a chemical called lufenuron that prevents

flea eggs from hatching or larvae from developing. One must hope that every flea in your house and garden has taken a good bite out of your dog, ingested the poison blood, and laid infertile eggs. Only then will you have broken the cycle—no more flea problem. You see, Program is not a repellent like garlic. Your animal, who is no doubt allergic to flea bites, will still have to be bitten for the product to work.

You must continue to feed your dog this pill once a month, so that any new fleas that venture your animal's way can take that bite and suffer the same fate as the other guys.

Ciby-Geigy, the manufacturer, states in the brochure that Program is well accepted (there is a version for cats, too) and can be given to young, old, and pregnant animals. The brochure assures us that Program was given to nine beagles at ninety times the recommended dosage. Only six of the nine conceived—a conception rate of 67 percent. In the same test, eight beagles not on Program were bred, and 100 percent conceived.

Carol Scott Bardwick (Canine Cryobank, Inc.), a well-known reproduction specialist, has issued a "warning" bulletin on this product and its effects on both male and female reproductive systems. You also need to know that puppies born to dams on this drug on the ninety-time study had nasal discharge, respiratory congestion, dehydration/diarrhea, lethargy (sounds a bit like parvo, doesn't it?)—conditions that improved after the pups were weaned. What a coincidence! Evidently, the drug (lufenuron) concentrates in the dam's milk at a rate sixty times more than in the dam's blood.

Share this information with your veterinarian, and save your money. Use garlic; it's a lot safer!

What about fleas? In *Pet Talk,* a special supplement from *Love of Animals* magazine, Robert S. Goldstein, V.M.D., addresses this issue.[50] He asks his readers if they have noticed why some animals seem to be besieged with flea (and tick) infestation, spending all their time scratching, biting, and licking themselves raw. Dr. Goldstein suggests (as do I) that this is a wake-up call to their caregivers from Mother Nature herself. He states that something inside your dog or cat is not healthy. It is your opportunity to take action before a serious disease develops.

If our animal companions have strong, vital immune systems, pests find them less appetizing. Weak, sickly dogs and cats seem to attract fleas and ticks like a magnet attracts bits of iron. They are an easy target. It is impossible to eliminate all fleas and ticks with poisons, and Dr. Goldstein explains that because of these poisonous flea products, we now have today's "superflea"! This genetic mutation has actually adapted to today's poisons. Today's superflea and tick require higher doses of more potent insecticides and have longer life cycles than they did fifty years ago. They are no longer seasonal nuisances but can sustain themselves and their eggs all year long—even through the cold season. I am vehemently opposed to Program because it puts poison directly into an animal instead of on or around him. Dr. Goldstein suggests that if these poisonous substances continue to be prescribed and sold, we will poison ourselves long before we get rid of the fleas!

To treat flea problems, Dr. Goldstein suggests that the immune system of our animals be built up through nutrition and supplementation and that our yards and homes be treated with nontoxic methods to eliminate the problem. He provides a booklet on poison-free flea-proofing, which can be obtained along with his numerous other natural pet products and booklets by contacting him at *Love of Animals* (see "Resources").

I explain to my clients that flies don't buzz clean garbage cans. If you feed the fresh food diet, your dog will be clean and healthy inside, and pests will pick on some other poor animal. Note also that B vitamins repel fleas and ticks, as does garlic. My collie, Connie, is flea-free all year round thanks to the natural diet and supplementation.

You might also consider this tip passed on to us by Marina Zacharias: "A simple and elegant solution is to buy some regular old borax from the grocery store and sprinkle it lightly and thoroughly over all carpeted areas. Using a push broom, work it in well so that the borax is spread deep into the carpet fibers. Use a carpet sweeper or lightly vacuum the area to remove the surplus. This will prevent any risk of caking. The borax actually dehydrates the fleas' larvae and eggs, breaking the hatching cycle. As long as the carpet is not shampooed, this will control the fleas for a year or longer. There are companies (for example, Fleabusters) that use a similar process."[51] This is reported to be a safe, nonchemical method of protecting all in the household from the dangers of fleas. Dr. Scanlan warns to be careful since some dogs and people may be sensitive to borax. Inhaling it may cause lung problems.

You can make your own homemade insect repellent in a spray bottle. Combine 1 cup Avon Skin-So-Soft bath oil, 1 cup water, 1 teaspoon eucalyptus oil, and 2–3 tablespoons apple cider vinegar; mix thoroughly and spray on people, animals, holes on screens, carpets, inside cars, or on anything you don't want those little pests to land on.[52] Apparently the formula does not kill the bugs, but it makes whatever it covers highly distasteful to them. Be forewarned that it might make your dog's coat a little greasy. However, as a repellent, it sounds like it does a good job.

A safe way to treat yards for fleas (and several other pests) is beneficial nematodes. Beneficial nematodes are microscopic and attack these harmful creatures. Mix them with water and spray the selected area, or mix them into the soil. They are effective for approximately two years (although repeat treatments are recommended annually for maximum effectiveness). Beneficial nematodes are not harmful to humans, animals, or plants. They are, however, compatible with other beneficial insects.

Heartworm Plus: What about heartworm medication? I include it here because it is given regularly, and many folks think of these drugs as harmless supplements just because of the user-friendly way they are marketed. My role is not to challenge your veterinarian in dispensing this medication but merely to present facts not taught them in allopathic veterinary schools or by profit-minded pharmaceutical salespeople.

Heartworm is a risk in certain parts of the country. Dr. Scanlan says that the incidence of heartworm in California is less than 3 percent but advises to be careful to check for heartworm in the southern states and on the East Coast. Nevertheless, you should be aware of the ever increasing evidence that Ivermectin (the ingredient in Heartguard) has been linked to fertility problems, thyroid problems, and autoimmune disorders.

Dr. Jean Dodds was quoted in Marina Zacharias's newsletter: "For heartworm, I recommend using only the 'daily' form of medication as it is a totally different compound."[53]

Marina Zacharias tells us of one case reported in the Pacific Northwest a few years ago, after which local vets immediately jumped onto the latest "must have" drug that is pumped into countless animals as a precaution. Wouldn't it be great if the veterinary community could see how fresh-food-eating dogs resist parasites?

In her *Natural Rearing Newsletter*, Marina Zacharias reports that the president of Canine Cryobank, Carol S. Bardwick, D.V.M., saw in twelve years of her reproduction specialty practice a wide variety of cases involving the deleterious effects of Heartguard—and the animals' return to normal within sixty days after halting use.

Merck Pharmaceutical has data, apparently, only on rats and mice. Dr. Bardwick asked a Merck veterinarian in 1992 if any studies had ever been done on Ivermectin and canine reproduction. He retorted, "I'll get back to you." She is still waiting for an answer.

There is a homeopathic nosode recourse for heartworm, so check with your holistic veterinarian to see whether this is an option in your area.

Dr. Chambreau suggests that if you are currently using heartworm medication, or if your veterinarian has insisted upon its use, use the most basic product—not the ones that prevent intestinal parasites, which are rare in adult dogs and unlikely in naturally fed dogs anyway.[54] The nonchewables, she suggests, are better, again because they contain fewer chemicals. Most important, according to Dr. Chambreau, is to be sure that your dog is off the medication for at least a few months each year. She suggests that it be used only in the height of mosquito season and to pay attention to any differences your dog shows on and off the preventative. I personally have never given it to any of my collies and have never had a problem. However, I recognize that it can be a serious problem in susceptible dogs and in certain parts of the country, especially Florida.

Food Enzymes (Digestive Enzymes): I feel that enzymes are an important addition to the diet, especially if you suspect that your dog is not digesting his food thoroughly (check his stool for color and consistency; if abnormal, contact your holistic veterinarian or animal nutritionist). Freezing and refrigeration, even of the fresh food diet, may cause some enzyme loss. Enzymes are destroyed by cooking, and commercial pet foods are missing these vital substances (yet another reason to switch to the fresh food diet).

Dr. Russell Swift reports that food enzymes are beneficial to animals suffering from asthma, allergies, diarrhea, constipation, gastritis, colitis, obesity, poor weight gain, arthritis, liver and bladder problems, excessive shedding, and oily or dry coats, to name but a few ailments.[55]

Enzymes aren't exotic substances. They're mandatory for proper digestion and absorption of nutrients. If enzymes aren't present in adequate amounts in food, the body tries to make up the difference, increasing the risk of acute and chronic disease. By improving digestion and bowel function, enzymes relieve a large variety of physical symptoms.

I have had excellent results with Dr. Swift's enzyme formulations, both Florazyme LP, which contains liver and pancreas enzymes, and Florazyme EFA, an herbal formula. Dr. Swift and I have also created (under my own label) an excellent enzyme complex that is great for both dogs and cats. In addition to the basic Florazyme enzymes, it contains antioxidants, fructooligoosaccharides, gelatin, liver, and taurine. All Florazyme enzymes are highly active at body temperature and throughout a wide pH range, and they contain lactobacillus acidophilus, and lactobacillus bifidus. The Florazyme enzymes begin to aid digestion as soon as they are released in the act of chewing. I've found that approximately $1/4$ to $1/2$ teaspoon of Florazyme EFA, LP, or my Enzyme Supplement per cup of food at each meal is about right. You'll need to experiment, but follow the instructions on the label.

Digestive enzyme products I previously used in my fresh food contained pancreatic enzymes, papain, and aspergillus cultures. According to Dr. Swift, pancreas extracts, or pancreatin (marketed under the trade name Viokase) aren't the most effective enzymatic substances, because they function only in an alkaline environment. They do improve digestion in the intestinal tract, but since they're not designed to work in an acidic environment such as the stomach, they don't start the digestive process early enough to spare the pancreas overwork. Raw glandular pancreas extracts do help pancreatic function. Aspergillus fungal cultures are active throughout a wide pH range. Plant enzymes such as papain don't need environments warmer than body temperature to perform effectively.

Essiac: Marina Zacharias reports a fascinating story about an Ojibway medicine man who in 1892 offered to help an English woman with breast cancer.[56] The man gave her a recipe (which was ultimately named Essiac) containing eight herbs and told her to make a tea with it.

In 1922 Rene Caisse, R.N., was caring for this woman in a hospital where the woman was dying of natural old age. She had been free of cancer for thirty years. The woman gave Ms. Caisse the recipe in response to Rene's desire to help others. Two years later Rene used this recipe on her aunt who had terminal stomach cancer. Her aunt recovered and lived another twenty-one years.

Rene, a Western-trained nurse, did not simply accept the undocumented word passed down from the medicine man. Instead, she proceeded to experiment, vary the formula, and tried injecting it rather than drinking the tea. Rene Caisse named the product Essiac (Caisse spelled backward) and tried to isolate the active ingredients, refine, and perfect the ancient remedy with Charles Brusch, M.D., who became the personal physician to President Kennedy, was knighted by Pope Paul VI, and recieved the Post Gazette Humanitarian Award. Together they found that individually the herbs did not provide the same synergistic results as all eight did in the tea.

In 1977 Rene Caisse made an agreement with Resperin Corporation of Ontario, Canada, giving them a formula containing four herbs. In return, the corporation was supposed to open clinics across the country to treat terminally ill cancer patients, free of charge. The corporation never kept its bargain but trademarked the four-herb formula in Canada as Essiac. In the United States, the trademark is held by Mankind of Maryland.

In 1978 Rene Caisse died without ever making a penny in royalties. Dr. Brusch kept the original secret formula until he teamed up with the producer of the Canadian radio program *Staying Alive.* She and Dr. Brusch, whom she met during an interview on her show, reported in depth the Essiac story.

The eight-herb formula is now known as FlorEssence and contains the following herbs (however, the proportions remain proprietary to Flora, Inc.): burdock root, slippery elm bark, sheep sorrel, Turkish rhubarb, watercress, blessed thistle, red clover, and kelp. The formula is based on the original, and Marina Zacharias and Dr. Loops feel it has a place in our armament to help fight cancer.

Super Blue-Green Algae: Dr. Chambreau introduced me to Super Blue-Green Algae for animals. When her own fresh-food-eating cat was off her food a bit and suffering from a kind of lethargy, she offered this algae and the cat bounced right back.

Super Blue-Green Algae is a special strain that grows in the pristine, mineral-rich waters of upper Klamath Lake, high in the Cascade Mountains of Oregon. The lake is fed by streams in more than four thousand square miles of volcanically formed mountains. This algae is acclaimed for its wealth of vitamins, minerals, enzymes, amino acids, and chlorophyll, all in raw organic form. A noncellulose cell membrane makes its nutrients highly assimilable.[57]

The recommended dosage is $1/3$ teaspoon per pound of food, or $1/16$ to $1/8$ teaspoon per meal. However, as with all new substances, introduce it cautiously, beginning with just a pinch and increasing the dosage over a three-week period to ascertain your animal's tolerance. When using Super Blue-Green Algae, either omit your other mineral supplementation or use half the normal dosage along with a pinch of the algae. You may combine $1/2$ tablespoon of my MinerAll Plus and $1/4$ teaspoon of Super Blue-Green Algae for each pound of fresh raw food. Use bonemeal and Bio C (see recipe on pages 96–97.

Pycnogenol: Perhaps the most exciting food supplement I've come across is Pycnogenol, a special blend of a type of bioflavonoid called proanthocyanidin. This superantioxidant has many benefits.[58] It seems to enhance the effect of other antioxidants (such as vitamins A, C, and E and zinc) I use. Proanthocyanidin potentiates vitamin C, and some biochemists see evidence that Pycnogenol helps vitamin C enter cells. I certainly feel much better as a result of including it in my own health program, and I see increased vigor and immune response in my animals.

Maritime pine bark Pycnogenol and grapeseed extract (another source of proanthocyanidin) are beneficial to our dogs' health. I crush tablets of Pycnogenol and mix them into the dog's fresh food when I feel they need an extra antioxidant boost. Dr. Loops suggests 1–2 mg for each pound of body weight. Start with 1 mg per pound once daily, then increase to 1 mg per pound twice daily.

Colloidal Gold: I have no information at this time as to how gold, in this form, may be beneficial to dogs and cats. I include it for information purposes only. Don't administer colloidal gold to your dog without consulting first with your holistic practitioner.[60]

The use of gold in medicine is believed to have begun in Alexandria, Egypt, where a skilled group known as *alchemists* developed an elixir of liquid gold, which they professed had the ability to restore youth and perfect health. Paracelsus, who was one of the greatest known alchemists, founded the school of *iatrochemistry,* the chemistry of medicines, which was the forerunner of modern pharmacology. He developed medicines from metallic elements, including gold. Later, alchemy became more widespread, and gold was often used for its healing properties.

About 1857 English chemist Michael Faraday first prepared colloidal gold in a pure state. In the late nineteenth century, colloidal gold was commonly used in the United States as the basis of the cure for dipsomania (an uncontrollable craving for alcoholic beverages). Since then, traditional uses have included treatments for arthritis, burns, skin ulcers, and various types of punctures, as well as in certain nerve-end operations. The rural Chinese believe in the restorative powers of gold to this day; they cook their rice with a gold coin in the pot.

Colloidal gold can have a tremendous balancing and harmonizing effect on unstable mental/emotional states such as sorrow, fear, despair, anguish, frustration, melancholy, depression, and suicidal tendencies—ailments commonly associated with the heart—and even seasonal affective disorder (SAD). Reportedly gold directly affects the rhythmic, balancing, and healing activities of the heart and helps improve blood circulation.

The literature on gold suggests that it may be highly beneficial to the digestive system and to sluggish organs, especially the brain, and has been used to help rejuvenate the glands, stimulate the nerves, and release nervous pressure. Gold is supposed to help build strong natural defenses against disease and promote renewed vitality and longevity.

Aurum (Latin for "gold"), the Longevity Formulas, Inc. (LFI) version of colloidal gold, is an all-natural mineral supplement composed of minute particles of gold that have been electromagnetically charged and suspended in deionized water. It is flavorless and is reported to be nontoxic. LFI also has a colloidal trace mineral complex and a combination formula of copper, gold, and silver. Always consult your holistic veterinarian before introducing new therapies.

Oxygen (O$_2$): Oxygen, which all animals and plants need to survive, is obtained through respiration as well as by eating fresh raw fruits and vegetables (which contain hydrogen peroxide, converted to stabilized oxygen by the body). Stabilized oxygen comes in a powdered form that speeds digestion, facilitates removal of diseased and dying cells, and cleanses the system by oxidizing fecal matter without harming the mucous membranes or the lining of the intestines.

We can provide ourselves and our animal companions with supplemental oxygen, on a regular or occasional basis, just as we would with vitamins.[61] It has proved effective in the treatment of many serious animal illnesses. The brand I use is PuriZone by Best Friends. I have used somewhere between $1/16$ and $1/4$ teaspoon, depending on the animal's size and health, once daily for a few days.[62] Ascorbic acid (vitamin C) facilitates the action of O_2, so I add a pinch (about $1/16$ teaspoon) of Bio-C to $1/4$ teaspoon O_2 and about 1 cc distilled water. You may administer this orally (with an eye dropper or a syringe), or mix it into a tiny raw meatball or a little Beechnut chicken baby food as a treat. When O_2 is mixed with food or water, its action lasts only about twenty minutes, so be sure the mixture is consumed immediately.

If your animal has a creamy stool, which may look like anything from mashed potatoes to pea soup, it's time to cut back on the dosage (amount and frequency) of supplemental oxygen. Such a soft stool differs from diarrhea in that O_2 does not cause a loss of electrolytes, vital fluids, or nutrients. The stool probably becomes liquid to facilitate a deep cleansing of the lining of the colon. A stool looking like hard black balls is old fecal matter, which may have been in the colon for weeks, months, or even years (mucus and worms may be eliminated also). Check with your holistic practitioner prior to use.

DMG: Many experts recommend the supplemental use of DMG (N, N-Dimethylglycine) in our animals' diet. Extensive research in the United States has demonstrated that this nutrient may enhance health and well-being. Though DMG is not a vitamin or mineral and is not essential for the prevention of any deficiency, it does have an essential role in optimizing the metabolic workings of the body and in countering the consequences of stress. When used in conjunction with vitamins, minerals, and other cofactors, DMG neutralizes many of the wear-and-tear phenomena (including such degenerative diseases as arthritis, diabetes, heart disease, and even cancer) that are caused not by the lack of a specific nutrient but by the body's inability to cope with or adapt constructively to physical and/or mental stress.

DMG was first recognized as being a component of a metabolic pathway of the cell in 1941, but its true importance to optimum health and sustained physical output wasn't discovered until decades later. A normal, physiologically active substance found in such foods as cereal grains, seeds, and meats, it has a wide range of beneficial effects on the body:

- enhancing the immune response system, the body's natural defense mechanism against disease;[63]
- enhancing oxygen utilization and retarding the buildup of lactic acid in the muscles;
- reducing elevated cholesterol and triglyceride levels, and helping normalize high blood pressure;
- assisting detoxification of the body and improving the function of such organs as the liver, pancreas, and adrenals; and
- helping the body normalize blood glucose levels, and sustaining high energy levels and improved mental acuity.

J. W. Meduski, M.D., Ph.D., has evaluated DMG extensively and found it to be an extremely safe nutrient, even when fed at very high levels. Dr. Meduski has also shown that laboratory animals taking DMG may enhance their oxygen uptake ability when the environment is low in oxygen.[64]

I include DMG in my animals' regimen when they are stressed or ill. Many nutrition experts recommend administering DMG by dropper directly into the animal's mouth, but a few of my animal companions have thrown up when I used this method. When I mix it with their food, they don't even know it's there.

Dr. Chambreau suggests giving DMG only to sick animals, who may truly need such nutritional support, rather than administering it as a basic supplement. Dr. Loops usually recommends 125 mg twice daily under certain circumstances. Follow your own holistic practitioner's advice on the use of all supplements.

Standardized Extract of Grapefruit: Standardized extract of grapefruit, in its liquid concentrate form, is an essential product. *However, please exercise caution when using this extract. Never use it full strength! Keep it away from eyes and sensitive areas. If accidental contact occurs, flush with water for ten minutes. Irritation is temporary but may last for up to forty-eight hours.*

As previously mentioned, the citricidal action in standardized extract of grapefruit sterilizes meat (see "How to Prevent Contamination and Spoilage," page 118), ridding it of many harmful microscopic organisms.[65] It may also be used internally and topically, as follows:

All-purpose cleaner: Add 30-60 drops to a 32-ounce pump sprayer filled with water. Use on all surfaces where pets eat or where raw meat is handled.

Cutting board cleaner: Use as a spray or apply 10-20 drops to cutting board, and work into the surface with a wet sponge or dishcloth. Leave on for thirty minutes, then rinse with water. Keep animals away during this process.

Dish-cleaning additive: Add 15-30 drops to sink dishwashing water, to dishwasher detergent in automatic dishwasher, or to final rinse of either. You may add a few drops directly to dishwashing liquid.

Sink wash: Add 30 or more drops to a sink full of cold water and briefly soak vegetables, fruit, meat, or poultry.

Spray wash: Add 20 or more drops to a 32-ounce spray bottle of water. Spray on vegetables, fruit, meat, or poultry.

Shampoo: Add 1 drop to 1 ounce of shampoo then add 10 ounces of catalyst-altered water (CAW) (see "Pure Water and Catalyst-Altered Water," page 120) or distilled water. Shampoo as usual. Leave on for two minutes and rinse with water.

Skin treatment: Add 2 drops to 2 ounces of aloe vera juice or Willard Water, and apply topically three to four times daily. This is an excellent treatment for ringworm and other fungal skin problems. Also excellent for bite wounds.

Dental, ear, and nose wash: One drop in 2 ounces of purified water or aloe vera juice as a dental and gum swab. Apply with a cotton swab, gauze, or finger brush and massage gums. The same formula may be used to gently clean ears; use cotton to apply. If you use cotton swabs, be careful not to go past the outer ear, or you may cause inflammation or infection, or puncture the eardrum! Clean nostrils with a dilution of 1 drop standardized extract of grapefruit to 8 ounces of water or aloe vera juice, using a cotton swab or cotton ball to apply. Remember, keep away from eyes. Your holistic veterinarian may want you to administer it orally as a natural antibiotic. Check with him or her first as to how dilute this version should be.

Water purification (internal use): One drop in 8 ounces of purified water, poured into drinking bowl. If this is too strong, add more water. This also helps prevent *giardia lamblia* (a microscopic parasite that causes intestinal disease).

Chinese Herbal Patent Formulas

THERE ARE ALSO many Chinese herbal formulas and tonics (patent formulas) too numerous to mention. Their numbers fill entire volumes. Your holistic veterinarian or acupuncturist may suggest various formulas.

An excellent resource for the Chinese patent formulas is *Chinese Herbal Patent Formulas, A Practical Guide,* by Jake Fratkin. Unfortunately, it is designed for people, not our dogs. But many symptoms translate to both our canine and our feline friends. There is an index of products by symptom, an excellent glossary of traditional Chinese medical terms, and a practitioner's pharmacy-recommended patents. For Westerners' convenience, the Chinese characters on pages 308–19 carry a number code and are alphabetically arranged by English name. A handy spreadsheet on pages 282–94 cross-references herbal names as well. Acupuncturists can easily select a patent formula as an adjunctive therapy.

There are also several volumes available in English that explain the language and mechanisms of traditional Chinese medicine, which Fratkin's book points us to, including *Chinese*

Tonic Herbs, by Ron Teeguarden; *The Web That Has No Weaver,* by Ted Kaptchuk; and *The Essentials of Chinese Acupuncture,* by Foreign Language Press. You might also wish to add to your library *Love, Miracles and Animal Healing,* by Alan M. Schoen, D.V.M., and Pam Proctor. Schoen lists nine of his top Chinese herbal remedies with descriptions and case histories.

See "Resources" for distributors of Chinese herbal products.

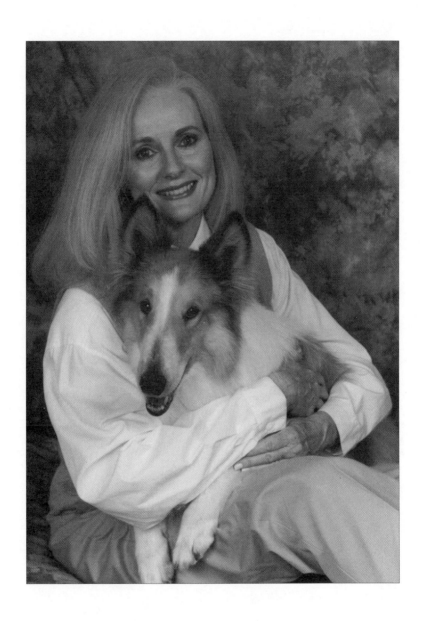

Chapter Five

Natural Remedies

DETOXIFICATION

AS YOU BEGIN to introduce natural healing substances and holistic therapies—such as herbs, supplements, homeopathy, nosodes, flower essences, acupuncture, and aromatherapy—into your dog's environment to remove the residue and effects of vaccines, anesthesia, cortisone, chemicals, and any other toxic substances, the animal will go through detoxification. In this natural part of the healing process, things often get worse before they get better; you experience a big step forward and then a small step backward, as health and balance are restored.

A cornerstone of holistic medicine is the emphasis on symptoms being the immune system's way of expressing weakness and crying out for help. Absorption and accumulation of toxins damage the immune system, which must then work harder to protect the body and keep it functioning normally. Eventually the immune system becomes overwhelmed, and various problems and symptoms develop that cause us to seek medical or veterinary treatment. In order to return the immune system to its normal healthy state, the toxins must first be removed. This is what detoxification is all about.

Dr. John Fudens and other holistic practitioners usually tailor their "detox" program to the individual animal. Through the use of all-natural therapies such as diet, supplements, homeopathy, herbs, and glandular extracts, the various toxins are released by the cells and are eliminated through the ears, eyes, skin, and respiratory and excretory systems. As a result, the symptoms that would normally be suppressed by conventional drugs and treatment return.

So don't be alarmed if the animal's symptoms worsen during detox. As long as his energy and vitality increase, the program is working. Whatever discharge or drainage you see is the result of the body cleansing itself and thus becoming healthier. For example, a dog with a skin condition is treated with cortisone, which only suppresses the symptom and harms the immune system. During detoxification, the residue of cortisone is removed from his system, and the skin rash returns. However, eventually the rash disappears, as the actual imbalance that originally caused it (such as improper diet) is corrected.

Sometimes additional holistic therapy is needed to rebuild the immune system and body, directing special attention to certain areas. But holistic therapy works very poorly or not at all in a badly contaminated body. So the detox program must come first, so that the animal can derive maximum benefit from further treatment.

As with all other healing therapies, this process must be done gently to avoid dehydration or undue stress. For example, detox that causes a softened stool (the consistency of mashed potatoes) is a gentle cleanse, whereas diarrhea (brown or yellow water) may dehydrate the patient. Stay in close touch with your practitioner so he or she can be sure that your dog's electrolytes and fluids stay balanced. If your dog suddenly stops eating and drinking a normal amount of water, call your holistic veterinarian or natural health practitioner as soon as possible. If you are in doubt about your dog's health, go to an emergency veterinary facility for fluid therapy; many animals die from dehydration and potassium loss.

But what if the dog is already suffering from something as serious as cancer? To most people, cancer is synonymous with death, but it's actually a symptom of our toxic modern lifestyle. Dr. Fudens has this to say about cancer:

[It is a] disease of the mind, emotions, and spirit . . . expressed on the physical body level . . . the way the spirit deals with its problems.

Carcinogens, stresses from virus, bacteria, pollutants, drugs, vaccinations, chemicals, radiation, and poor nutrition all play a part in creating the toxic and suppressed immune system that allows abnormal mutant cells to grow and organize into . . . cancers. But there also exists an ongoing aberrated negative force or energy in the family involving the pet and the person(s) the pet is bonded to. The negative force of energy is best described as a form of mental turmoil that leaves the person(s) paralyzed or helpless in controlling their lives, low self-esteem, anger, hostility, guilt, resentment toward life and others, lack of communication . . . feelings of mistrust and the lack of love and respect towards self and others. . . . Combined with the physical stresses and contaminants listed previously, our pet companions can very easily be overwhelmed . . . and thus a fertile breeding ground for cancer occurs.

It is their unhealthy, unwell attitude towards life, on all levels, that allows a cancerous process to develop. This negative force is stronger than surgery, drugs, and radiation, which is why, for the most part, these treatments do not work. Holistic therapies work by changing the negative energy or force into positive energy, allowing the immune system to repair and rebuild itself. This includes addressing the mental turmoil in the pet's environment to reduce that stress and strain. Animals . . . help heal us. They take away the negative energy or force, absorb it, neutralize it or become overwhelmed by it and get sick. They can show us how sick we truly are. Our pets are mirrors as to what is going on in and around us in this so-called modern society.[1]

Dr. Fudens recommends, as do all the holistic practitioners with whom I consult, that we start by changing the diet from commercial foods and any junk food or snacks to one with fresh, natural, and nutritious ingredients. Feeding the fresh food diet to your dog in the proper macronutrient combinations is the beginning of a full detoxification program that may also employ several natural remedies and therapies.

Please don't attempt to treat your animal without the guidance of a holistic veterinarian. The health of our animals is very precious, and we owe it to them to treat them with competent medical attention.[2]

HERBS

AS IS TRUE for so many of the healing therapies addressed in this book, herbs cannot be covered in depth here. What follows are just some of the highlights of this fascinating field. Herbal medicine is very powerful. As with homeopathy, I don't recommend self-diagnosis but rather working with a holistic veterinarian or an herbal practitioner.

Books I often use for reference include *The Complete Medicinal Herbal: A Practical Guide to the Healing Properties of Herbs with More Than 250 Remedies for Common Ailments,* by Penelope Ody;

Herbally Yours, by Penny Royal; *Today's Herbal Health,* by Louise Tenney; *The Complete Herbal Handbook for the Dog and Cat,* by Juliette de Bairacli Levy (see "Resources").[3] Penelope Ody provides a wonderful historical look at the use of herbs by the ancient Egyptians, Greeks, Romans, and Arab world. Influenced by ancient cultures, healing systems all over the world today embrace herbalism. The Indians embrace Ayurvedic medicine, which links the microcosm to the cosmos; they commonly include herbal remedies in their medical practices. Tibetans, whose medicine was under the control of the lamas and therefore closely linked to their religion, carefully coordinated the harvest of herbs to coincide with helpful astrological influences. Swiss alchemist Paracelsus subscribed to the doctrine of signatures, which used a plant's outward appearance as an indication of what it could cure (for instance, nutmeg and walnuts resemble the brain when they are cracked open, so they were thought to improve mental abilities).

The Chinese view disease as a sign of disharmony within the whole person. Herbs have been crucial to Chinese medical practitioners since about 2500 B.C. Many of their formulas go back thousands of years, handed down through the generations in herbal dynasties. The five elements in Chinese herbal medicine—wood, water, metal, earth, and fire—form a network of relationships. Each element represents a season, a taste, an emotion, a personality type, and parts of the body (for example, fire represents summer, bitter taste, joy, the heart, small intestine, tongue, and blood vessels). The forces of yang and yin (see Chapter 8), and *qi* (or *chi*) complement the basic model of the five elements. Yang and yin represent balance; and qi, vital energy.

Herbalists use the bark, berries, bulbs, flowers, fruit, gum, hips, hulls, leaves, roots, root bark, seeds, tops, and the whole plant—all according to tradition or recipe. It's important to remember that nearly all modern medicines are synthetic versions of the active ingredient of some herb. The salicylic acid in aspirin was isolated from white willow bark, cortisone from yucca, digitalis from foxglove, and Valium a synthesized version of valerian root.[3]

Herbs are often sold individually, but most work better in combination. There is a synergy that is created when they are combined. Most herbs shouldn't be given over long periods of time, no longer than two to three weeks, because the body seems to build up a tolerance and they cease to be effective. There are many herbs that do have nutritional value however, and are taken as supplements.

Administering Herbs

NOW LET'S EXAMINE the various ways to administer herbs. Remember, always use purified or spring water when preparing herbs.

Decoction: A tea made from roots and bark. Gently boil then simmer 1 tablespoon of cut herb or 1 teaspoon of powdered herb in 8 ounces of water for 15–20 minutes, then let stand for 5–10 minutes.

Infusion: A tea made from leaves or blossoms. Boil 8 ounces of water and remove from heat. Add 1 teaspoon of powdered herb, cover, and steep for ten minutes.[4]

Extract: A liquid solvent into which a principal ingredient of an herb has been dissolved. Herbs are put through a process of cold extraction—cold percolation of the herbs with suitable solvents for each herb, such as alcohol, water, grape brandy, or apple cider vinegar, singly or in combination—which causes the herbs to render their nutrients. Extracts come in liquid form, making them easy to assimilate. These formulations are excellent for dogs, as they may be further diluted in water when necessary.[5]

Tincture: An extraction of herbs in vinegar, alcohol, or, in some instances, vegetable glycerin or water.

Herbal oil: An extraction of herbs in an oil base.

Fomentation: A cloth soaked in a hot infusion or decoction, wrung out, and applied to an affected area.

Poultice: A moist, hot herb pack applied topically (more effective than a fomentation). When using fresh herbs, crush and bruise them. If they're powdered, mix with mineral water to form a thick paste. Spread on clean cloth and cover affected area. *Never reuse—always make a fresh one because poultices lose their potency.*

If you're a do-it-yourself kind of person, you can whip up many brews in your own kitchen. I don't pretend to be an herbalist but look to others whom I can trust to properly harvest and prepare food-grade and medicinal herbs.[6]

In addition to fresh herbs and grasses (see Chapter 4, "Nutrition"), I use extracts and tinctures, both internally and externally. I sometimes also employ *solarization* to prepare herbs, adding the contents of one herbal capsule to 2–4 ounces of water, placing it in a clear glass container outside in the sunshine for a few hours, and then strain the liquid through cheesecloth or a coffee filter, then dilute the mixture in water (1 drop to 1 ounce of water), and shake it. You may administer this dilution by eye dropper or mix it with a little food.

I've found the following mixture to be a powerful immune booster: 1 or 2 drops each of the herbal tinctures of echinacea (an herb prescribed for blood purification and as a detoxifier to increase resistance to infection) and goldenseal, 1 or 2 drops of Kyolic garlic, and a few drops of water. When I suspect an upper respiratory problem, I give a drop of this mixture in an eye dropper three to four times daily, at different intervals from the homeopathic remedy that I may be using. Animals Apawthecary, which makes glycerin-based herbal tinctures especially for dogs and cats, also makes an excellent mixture called Goldenseal/Echinacea. Their Allergy/Detox formula is also excellent, as is their Senior Blend and Tinkle Tonic (urinary formula). Good products are also available from Nature's Sunshine and Juliette de Bairacli Levy's NR Formulas (available from Marina Zacharias, see "Resources").

Herbal Combination Formulas

THE FOLLOWING SAMPLING of combination herbal formulas includes those most commonly used for various conditions that trouble dogs from time to time. These combinations have been suggested by several herbal experts but are not intended as medical advice. I also include a smattering of other alternatives, including homeopathy, diet suggestions, and supplements. Please consult your holistic practitioner prior to experimenting with any medicinal herbs. As always, proceed with caution. (See "Resources" for further information about brand-name supplements.)

You may find prepared combinations on the shelves of your health-food store; however, keep in mind that the dosage for dogs should be slightly lower than that suggested for infants or very young children. I generally begin by using one drop of an extract in 1 ounce of water. I combine the herbs in equal proportions unless my practitioner suggests otherwise. Check with your holistic veterinarian or herbal consultant prior to administering the substances listed.

For allergies, upper respiratory problems, or sinusitis, many herbalists combine:

   Goldenseal. Natural antibiotic-like herb for congested membranes. Reduces swelling, helps clean system.

   Lobelia. Stimulates, removes obstructions (acts as an expectorant), relieves spasms.

   Capsicum. Relieves congestion, disinfects, acts synergistically to increase power of other herbs.

   Parsley. Increases resistance to infection.

   Marshmallow. Helps remove mucus from lungs.

   Chaparral. Tones system.

   Burdock. Purifies blood.

   Helpful hints: Simplify diet (for example, for food allergies feed raw ground lamb, cooked barley flakes, zucchini); make changes weekly, one food at a time, and be certain to include vitamins A, B complex, and C with bioflavonoids (rutin and hesperidin), zinc, bonemeal for calcium (1 or 2 tablespoons per pound of meat) in each meal. Help build up pollen immunity by including Kyolic aged garlic and tiny amounts of bee pollen. Use trace mineral products such as montmorillonite clay, Super Blue-Green Algae, or spirulina to boost the overall immune response, and include alfalfa sprouts regularly. Consider adding lysine as a supplement if the herpes virus is suspected. Tea tree oil is also excellent diffused because it is antiseptic (see "Aromatherapy" for more about essential oils).

For lung problems:

   Comfrey. Soothes respiratory system.

   Fenugreek. Helps soften hardened mucus.

Helpful hints: Give vitamins A, B complex, C with bioflavonoids, D, and E in a high-potency multivitamin/mineral supplement including folic acid, which helps strengthen the lungs. Barley water helps relieve bronchial spasms. Offer lots of Kyolic garlic and honey (if your dogs enjoy it, blend in herbal teas served lukewarm). Foods high in potassium include dandelion greens, celery, string beans, and brussels sprouts; even melons are helpful. Run a warm-mist vaporizer with eucalyptus oil daily for two to three hours, but don't leave it unattended and make sure the air circulates freely. This treatment should be subtle, as dogs' sense of smell is much more sensitive than ours. If his eyes become irritated, discontinue the use of eucalyptus oil. Also, I find Nature's Sunshine homeopathic Asthma formula helpful. Diffusing the essential oil cinnamon may also be helpful to asthma sufferers.

For heart and circulation problems or fatigue, combine:

Hawthorn. Strengthens heart.

Capsicum. Facilitates the action of other herbs on the heart.

Garlic. Natural antibiotic and immune stimulant.

Helpful hints: Give cold-pressed oils (including EPA oils—fish oils, like salmon), barley, and oatmeal. Food-process zucchini, string beans, celery, carrots, and parsley; add liquid; strain and include with raw meat; and serve as a broth. Excellent for fasting days. One drop of Bulgarian rosewater may be added to drinking water for heart conditions. Consider discussing vitamin E and CoEnzyme Q_{10} with your holistic veterinarian as a supplement.

For digestive upsets, irritable colon, or diarrhea, combine:

Comfrey. Soothes lower bowel.

Marshmallow. Contains mucilage, which aids bowel.

Slippery elm. Soothes, draws out impurities, heals, acts as a buffer against irritation.

Ginger. Relieves gas, settles stomach.

Wild yam. Relaxes stomach muscles, acts as sedative on bowel.

Lobelia. Relaxant. Removes obstructions from bowel, heals.

Helpful hints: Vitamins A, E, and B complex, cold-pressed oils (including wheat germ oil), acidophilus, sweet potatoes, yogurt, comfrey, kelp, sprouts, and oatmeal are all good dietary choices. For diarrhea, have the dog fast for twenty-four hours to let his system rest and repair. Provide fresh purified water at all times; consider fluid therapy if dog becomes dehydrated. Administer fluids with an oral syringe or have your veterinarian administer subcutaneous fluids (my veterinarian taught me how to do this myself). I give Pedialyte, or mix it fifty-fifty with purified water. Return to solid food when diarrhea stops, but make it simple (boiled chicken and rice or oatmeal) for a day or so, then make the basic fresh food recipe (see page 96, in Chapter 4, "Nutrition"). For constipation, include aloe vera juice in fresh food diet (1 tablespoon per pound of food). Senna is also helpful for constipation. For fecal craving, bee pollen may be helpful.

For blood purifying, cleansing, eczema, ringworm, or cancer combine:

Pau d'arco. Natural antibiotic, antifungal.

Licorice. Natural expectorant. Supplies energy.

Red clover. Tonic.

Sarsaparilla. Cleanses, stimulates body defenses.

Cascara sagrada. Effective laxative.

Oregon grape. Tonic for all glands.

Chaparral. Cleanses deeply, fights bacteria.

Buckthorn. Calms gastrointestinal tract.

Prickly ash. Increases circulation.

Peach. Contains healing properties.

Stillingia. Removes toxic waste.

Helpful hints: Be sure food is fresh. Barley and oatmeal are excellent grains. Give sprouts and sprout supplements such as Biogenetics Bioguard or NuPet and Canine Balance twice daily. Full vitamin/mineral supplements, as well as Pycnogenol (1 mg per each pound of body weight daily). Lecithin, kelp, parsley, carrots, and celery, as well as lots of Kyolic garlic, chard, beet greens. It is imperative to work with a holistic practitioner for cancer cases. I recommend Dr. Charles Loops (see "Resources"). Consider the supplements vitamins E, C, CoEnzyme Q_{10}, A, beta-carotene (only for skin and internal problems), and FlorEssence (Essiac) for cancer and chronic disease.

For worms and other parasites:

Pumpkin seeds. Expel tapeworms.

Garlic. Makes the digestive tract inhospitable to parasites.

Black walnut. Oxygenates blood to kill parasites but can be extremely toxic.

Helpful hints: Once again, feed your dog the fresh food diet, including raw or cooked pumpkin (food-processed to a mulch), which will greatly help expel worms. Garlic is antibiotic in its effect, and fresh raw vegetables keep the colon healthy, creating an environment unfriendly to parasites. Be sure to keep your dog's environment free of fleas, through which dogs may contract tapeworms. A clean, healthy natural diet is the kind of preventative medicine I like best. Check with your holistic veterinarian regarding treatment for parasites. Dr. Richard Pitcairn has several natural ways to go about this, Juliette de Bairacli Levy's books offer herbal remedies, and Marina Zacharias carries an Anti-Parasite Remedy (see

"Resources"). Couch grass is also useful for worms, and papaya soothes the stomach after worm infestation. *Please contact your holistic veterinarian first and clear this course with him or her.*

For liver problems, combine:

Red beet. Nutritious for liver.

Dandelion. Stimulates liver.

Parsley. Cleans out toxic waste.

Horsetail. Builds, tones body.

Liverwort. Helps heal damaged liver.

Birch. Helps cleanse blood.

Lobelia. Removes obstructions from body.

Blessed thistle. General tonic to system.

Angelica. Helps eliminate toxins in liver and spleen.

Chamomile. Helps cleanse toxins from liver.

Gentian. Stimulates liver.

Goldenrod. Stimulates circulation.

Or instead combine:

Barberry. Causes bile to flow more freely.

Ginger. Stimulant.

Cramp bark. Good for congestion and hardening of liver.

Fennel. Helps move waste material out of body.

Peppermint. Cleans and strengthens entire body.

Wild yam. Good for hardening and blockages of liver.

Catnip. Strengthens liver and gallbladder.

Helpful hints: Give vitamins A, B complex (including B_6 and B_{12}), C, D, E, and K, as well as magnesium, zinc, sulphur, choline, inositol, methionine, and Pycnogenol. Vegetables—including cauliflower and collards with 1/2 teaspoon of nutmeg—are extremely important. Try dandelion tea mixed into food, along with watercress, alfalfa sprouts, and parsley. Avoid eggs, cream, butter, and all cooked oils and fats (cooked meat is greasy, so I recommend using only fresh raw meat and cold-pressed oils such as olive or canola; see Chapter 4, "Nutrition"). Consider glandular supplements and use naturally raised liver in small amounts in the fresh food diet.

For kidney, bladder, or urinary-tract problems, combine:

Goldenseal. Helps kidneys eliminate toxins.

Juniper. Antiseptic to kidneys.

Uva-ursi. Strengthens urinary tract.

Parsley. Nutritional to kidneys.

Ginger. Cleanses kidneys.

Marshmallow. Soothing to urinary tract.

Lobelia. Helps clear obstructions.

Helpful hints: Lecithin and vitamin E help purify kidneys. Some dogs enjoy melons, such as watermelon or cantaloupe, and even apples and grapes. Feed watercress, asparagus, celery, and parsley. Include zinc and high-potency vitamin and mineral supplements, antioxidants, and Pycnogenol. Cleavers may also be beneficial to the bladder. Adhere to the protein-to-carbohydrate ratio in the fresh food diet (page 96). Use an acidic form of vitamin C for bladder problems, and ester C for kidney problems.

For strengthening, stimulating, and cleansing the glands, combine:

Kelp. Contains iodine, which strengthens glands. *(Please check with your veterinarian regarding increasing any iodine, as certain thyroid conditions could be aggravated by an excess.)*

Dandelion. Stimulates glands, increases activity of liver.

Alfalfa. Increases glandular secretions.

Or instead combine:

Lobelia. Removes obstructions in system.

Mullein. Calms nerves.

Helpful hints: Glandular supplements are also helpful; check with a holistic veterinarian or nutritionist for specific suggestions. Feed raw meats and organ meats (liver, kidneys, heart—one to two parts organ to four to five parts muscle meat), alfalfa sprouts, avocado, broccoli, parsley, yams, raw nuts and nut butters (almond or peanut, but not walnut or flax—see Chapter 4, "Nutrition"), seeds (pumpkin, sunflower, sesame), oatmeal and barley, as well as high-potency vitamin and mineral supplements, including antioxidants, vitamin E, zinc, and Pycnogenol.

For thyroid and weight problems, combine:

Irish moss. Purifies, strengthens cellular structure.

Kelp. Promotes glandular health.

Parsley. Increases resistance.

Watercress. Acts as tonic.

Helpful hints: Give raw egg yolks (treated with standardized extract of grapefruit; for sterilization technique, see "How to Prevent Contamination and Spoilage" in Chapter 4, "Nutrition"). Iodine is a trace mineral known to be beneficial to the thyroid (but check with your holistic veterinarian because iodine can also aggravate certain thyroid conditions). Pumpkin and sunflower seeds, sprouts, yogurt, and kefir are helpful, too, but give yogurt only if your dog tolerates dairy products. Make sure your dog gets lots of exercise.

For Nervous disorders, combine:

Black cohosh. Relaxant.

Capsicum. Helps other herbs get to parts of body that need assistance.

Dill. Soothing to the stomach.

Valerian. Relaxes nerves.

Ginger. Soothes the stomach and also benefits travel sickness.

Hops. Contains B vitamins for nerves.

Rosemary. Benefits nervous disorders.

Passionflower. Combines well with valerian.

Chamomile. Calms and soothes.

Helpful Hints: Feed whole grains (for example, barley and oatmeal), which are rich in B vitamins, in small amounts. Fenugreek and chamomile tea are soothing. Brussels sprouts and cauliflower are excellent. Be sure to supplement diet regularly with trace minerals, such as AniMinerals; put a few drops in dog's water. Use Rescue Remedy (Calming Essence) by Bach (see "Flower Remedies," page 219).

For bone healing, combine:

Comfrey. Heals wounds, bones, entire system.

Goldenseal. Natural antibiotic with healing powers. Contains vitamins and minerals.

Slippery elm. Draws out impurities.

Aloe vera (unpreserved).[7] Natural detoxifier. Removes toxic matter from body, heals and protects.

Helpful hints: Kelp, broccoli, oatmeal, barley, vegetables high in calcium (such as kale and parsley), nuts and seeds (sunflower seeds and almonds are excellent) added to vegetable/grain mixture. Vitamins A, B complex, C with bioflavonoids, D, and E, bonemeal, and zinc all aid in healing bones. Also suggested for teeth and calcium deficiency are comfrey, horsetail, oat straw, and lobelia. Include Pycnogenol (from pine bark or grape seeds) daily.

For arthritis or inflammation of the joints:

Bromelain. Reduces swelling, inflammation.

Yucca. Precursor to synthetic cortisone.

Comfrey. Cleanses, purifies system.

Alfalfa. Contains alkaloid for pain, nutrients for body strength.

Black cohosh. Relieves pain, irritation, acid condition of blood.

Yarrow. Cleans blood, helps regulate liver.

Capsicum. Catalyst for other herbs.

Chaparral. Dissolves uric acid.

Devil's claw. Benefits rheumatism as well as arthritis.

Lobelia. Relaxant.

Burdock. Reduces swelling.

Centaury. Good for muscular rheumatism.

Helpful hints: Emphasize raw chicken and turkey in diet. The fiber in whole grains keeps dogs from getting constipated. Add chlorophyll extract to food or drinking water, just enough to turn the water light green. Use a pinch of fresh parsley in food. Include lots of sprouts; be sure wheatgrass is always available (for indoor dogs) to nibble on, or snip it and use it as a green vegetable in fresh food. Vitamin C is a must in each meal, at least one teaspoon of Bio-C (1,000 mg plus 500 mg of bioflavonoids), as well as a B-complex supplement in liquid or capsule form (see the sections on supplements in Chapter 4, "Nutrition"). For vitamin A, feed raw liver or cod liver oil occasionally. Consider a weekly fast (see Chapter 4) of raw meat broth and pure water. Be sure to exercise your dog and ask your practitioner about glucosamine sulfate as a supplement for control of inflammation, as well as shark cartilage. Vitmain E is extremely important, as is phenylalanine.

For skin and coat problems, combine:

Alfalfa. Contains trace minerals, which benefit skin and coat. It is also reported to be antifungal.

Aloe vera. Contains allantoin, which has healing properties. (I prefer a product by Mannatech called ManAloe. It is the isolated acemannon molecule that reportedly contains the healing action.)

Burdock. Good for burns and wounds.

Chaparral. For sores and wounds.

Goldenseal. Helps stop itching.

Helpful hints: The fresh food diet (see Chapter 4, "Nutrition") is the best approach to improving skin and coat. Cold-pressed oils, including wheat germ, cod liver oil, salmon oil, and borage oil, are excellent, as are evening primrose or black currant oil. Garlic taken internally helps heal all skin sores. Run a humidifier to moisten dry air. Bathe (therapeutic bath in gentle herbal shampoo mixed with aloe vera juice) and brush dog regularly. If your dog is very uncomfortable, spray aloe vera juice on him or dab the hot spots with cotton saturated with apple cider vinegar or aloe vera. Either one can be applied topically. Aloe gel heals burns. Try touch and massage therapy (see Chapter 6, "Hands-on Healing"). Try diluted Willard water as a spray. For bruising, *Arnica montana* and calendula are also beneficial. Horsetail ($1/2$ capsule per meal) may help restore hair. Dr. Scanlan suggests sulphur-based shampoo for greasy, scaly, crusty dandruff skin, and oatmeal-based shampoo for sensitive, itchy skin. Tea tree oil may be applied to small hot spots (not big ones).

For ear problems:

Diluted garlic oil from a capsule or mullein oil (1–2 drops) may be squeezed directly into the ears. Goldenseal and echinacea may be beneficial.

For eye problems, combine:

Goldenseal. Natural antibiotic.

Bayberry. High in vitamin C.

Eyebright. Strengthens immunity to eye complaints.

Helpful hints: Bathe eyes in sterile saline solution (or to 1 ounce of saline, add 1 drop eyebright). Also use homeopathic *Similasan,* Formula 1 for irritation and Formula 2 for allergies. Vegetables good for strengthening eyes are leeks, broccoli, cabbage, carrots, turnips, collards, and watercress. Pycnogenol has also proved helpful for eye conditions. My veterinary eye surgeon recommends dropping 1 drop of vitamin A oil (5,000 IU) in each eye twice daily. I dilute it in 1 ounce of sterile saline solution. I use 1 drop 2–3 times daily.

For birthing, pregnancy, estrus (heat cycles), combine:

Red raspberry. Strengthens uterus, regulates uterus during delivery, prevents hemorrhaging, reduces false labor pains.

Blessed thistle. Helps promote flow of milk, eliminates mucus congestion.

False unicorn. Strengthens ovaries, overall tonic for system, rich in trace minerals.

Black cohosh. Helps in uterine disorders.

Pennyroyal. Useful just before delivery (externally only).

Hops. Reduces problems associated with heat cycles, can reduce male sexual tension.

Helpful hints: Sprinkle a pinch of hops over food to reduce anxiety in both male and female breeding dogs. One tablespoon bonemeal per pound of meat. Do not feed aloe vera juice during first trimester of pregnancy because it can be too detoxifying. Include trace mineral complex and vitamin C (Ester C is easy on the gastrointestinal tract, as is sodium ascorbate) daily. Add a pinch of red raspberry to each meal in last trimester of pregnancy. Keep the homeopathic remedy *Caulophyllum* 30C–1M (homeopathic) on hand for difficult labor (administer 30C once weekly in last three weeks of pregnancy if your practitioner agrees). The homeopathic remedy *Urtica urens* 30C can help bring on milk, if needed. Female dogs usually love a little yogurt or kefir during pregnancy. Be sure all is ready for dam by the sixty-first day. Feed her as often as she wants, and give her lots of love and support. Try not to let her get too rambunctious prior to birthing. During labor, I give *Caulophyllum* 30C every fifteen to thirty minutes to keep contractions strong and then give one dose after the last puppy to help cleanse afterbirth. If 30C doesn't help, move up to four doses of 1M at one-hour intervals. I always clear this with Dr. Loops first. Also Marina Zacharias's homeopathic Pregnancy formula is invaluable, as is her Fading Puppy formula for both the mother and her pups.

For fasting, combine:

Raw meat broth and vegetable broth with a pinch each of one or more of the following herbs as seasonings:

Licorice. Good for strength and quick energy. Nourishes glands, inhibits growth of harmful viruses.

Hawthorn. Burns up excess fat, strengthens heart, helps insomnia, calms nervous system.

Fennel. Internal anesthetic. Relieves gas, cramps, and mucus accumulation.

Beet. Stimulates and cleans liver, strengthens system.

Helpful hints: Fasting is extremely cleansing but is not intended for the chronically ill, older dogs, or young puppies. Don't eat or cook in front of the dog—fast with him.[8] Provide pure water and broth at intervals throughout the day. Begin by feeding breakfast, substituting broth for dinner, then feeding a simple breakfast the following morning. (Broth may be fed by syringe.)

I have listed only some of the many herbs and combinations used in healing. Explore one of the books recommended or try some of the many preparations available at your health-food store. Talk to the salespeople—they're usually a wellspring of information—or join Nature's Sunshine as a distributor. There are regular meetings providing a wealth of advice. You may contact me for further information.

A word of warning: Medicinal herbs are exactly that—medicine. Please consult and work closely with a holistic veterinarian, someone who treats the whole animal. Before using any herb, remember that they are as powerful as any drug and that no one thing is good for everyone. Many of the associations listed in "Resources" will help you find practitioners in your area or those who will work with you by phone.

HOMEOPATHY

DR. DEEPAK CHOPRA defines "quantum healing" as the ability of one mode of consciousness (the mind) to spontaneously correct the mistakes of another (the body).[9] When in crisis, the body speaks through its symptomatic picture.

Allopathic, or conventional, medicine applies the Law of Opposites to the treatment of disease: the medicine is different from the disease. In other words, the medication prescribed by the doctor or veterinarian acts against the patient's symptoms (as indicated by such terms as anti-*inflammatory,* and so on). Allopathic drugs suppress symptoms, but in themselves they don't necessarily cure disease. The bodies of both humans and animals heal themselves.

Homeopathy takes the opposite approach, using remedies based on the Law of Similars. When used appropriately, homeopathy works with the body, not against it, promoting actual cure, not just suppressing symptoms. Symptoms are the banners of our immune system, manifestations of our attempt to heal ourselves, so we need to honor them, not rush to eradicate them. They are our windows to the internal process. Homeopathic remedies act in the same way as the natural defense reactions of the body—by stimulating the immune system so it can complete the job it was already trying to do. Homeopathy may also aid in ameliorating behavior problems.

For me, homeopathy is a wonderful method for treating both canine and feline imbalances because our companion animals are subtle creatures that live in the moment. When they don't feel well, they don't wish to be fussed with. Homeopathic remedies are easy to administer and give the body a gentle yet powerful nudge to help heal itself.

Most conventional veterinarians know nothing about homeopathy, but it truly cures most chronic diseases, whereas allopathic medicine provides only a quick, and often temporary, fix. Dr. Christina Chambreau finds that more and more people start with alternative therapy first and take the conventional approach as a last resort. She further suggests that you take your apparently healthy dog in for an evaluation by a holistic practitioner so that he or she gets evaluated before you are confronted with a health crisis with your dog.

If your dog has undergone long-term allopathic drug therapy, homeopathy may not work immediately; with persistence homeopathy may even help restore a dog's health when conventional veterinarians might recommend euthanasia. It's at such traumatic times that homeopathic veterinarians are asked to perform miracles, and many have done so. Very ill animals that are treated homeopathically may not be cured or even palliated, but the cure may make them feel better for a while so they die on their own, without any need for euthanasia. However, you don't have to wait until hope is all but lost—take your dog to a homeopathic veterinarian or arrange a telephone consultation now.

The History of Homeopathy

HOMEOPATHY WAS DEVELOPED by Samuel Hahnemann in the late eighteenth century. At that time people were treated with poisonous substances to "get the bad out of them" by making them vomit, have diarrhea, sweat, salivate, and bleed. Many died from such treatment.

Hahnemann felt that such practices were barbaric and stopped practicing medicine. While making a living translating books, he came across William Cullen's write-up on the action of *Cinchona officinalis,* the herb used to make quinine for treating malaria. Hahnemann disagreed with Cullen's conclusions and, to prove his point, took a small amount of the bark himself. He developed symptoms of malaria that lasted a few hours. Hahnemann repeated the experiment several times, always developing symptoms that went away by the next day. (He was a healthy man to start with, or this wouldn't have worked.)

From this research Hahnemann developed the Law of Similars, a concept that had been considered since ancient times by such men of science as Galen, Hippocrates, and especially Paracelsus. When an individual (human or animal) is made ill in a particular way by being exposed to a substance, that individual may also be cured by being treated with the same substance.

For example, bee venom *(Apis mellifica)* causes pinkish-red swelling in healthy individuals. Symptoms often appear suddenly, accompanied by itching and burning, and are relieved by applying cold water. At the same time, the person has no thirst, may be restless, and may feel better by not lying down. In homeopathic dilutions, bee venom improves or cures itchy, burning eruptions or swellings that come on suddenly, especially when the individual is less thirsty than usual.

The eruption doesn't have to have been caused by a bee sting for bee venom to be effective as a remedy. The eruption may have been caused by sunburn, hypersensitivity to food, vaccinations, or drugs. This remedy is also often prescribed for burning during urination and cystitis (bladder inflammation).

Hahnemann believed that the vital forces of the body respond to the energy of the remedy. The Theory of Vitalism—which states that our spirit (or soul) creates the physical substance of our bodies—predates our current biochemical understanding of life by thousands of years. Therapeutic touch and the spiritual aspects of disease and healing aren't new or foreign territory to even the most conservative doctors of internal medicine.

No one has yet been able to explain how homeopathy works, though Hahnemann did *provings* on humans for about 200 of the 2,000 existing remedies during his lifetime (fewer than 50 are generally given to dogs and cats). He gave each remedy to healthy people and meticulously recorded every change they underwent. Animal lovers will appreciate that Hahnemann did all his testing and research only on human subjects. Fortunately, homeopathic veterinarians have found that the symptoms in people correspond to symptoms in other animals, so our dogs and cats may now reap the benefits of this work.

How a Disease Runs Its Course

A HOMEOPATHIC CURE is obtained by giving the substance that produces symptoms in healthy individuals that are most similar to the patient's own symptoms. Since this therapy is based on an individual's total symptomatic picture, in order to use homeopathic remedies you must learn the characteristics for each remedy as well as observe carefully all the symptoms your dog is exhibiting, remember those he has exhibited in the past, and note his general characteristics. For example: First you sense an energy imbalance. Your dog seems to be getting sick; there aren't any symptoms, but you just know something's starting.

Then there are functional changes. For instance, he's frequently asking to pass urine, but there's no straining, and the urinalysis is normal. If the disturbance is treated homeopathically right away, even severe symptoms may be resolved quickly or avoided, although your conventional veterinarian may not be able to pinpoint the problem.[10]

If the disturbance remains untreated, you'll see inflammatory changes—the body trying its hardest to rebalance itself. At this stage the dog is sick—fever, redness, swellings, and the urinalysis shows white cells, red cells, and bacteria. Any conventional veterinarian will use some "anti" medications to treat a patient in this condition.

Finally, the body tries to ward off the problem by moving into pathology: thickened bladder wall; bladder stones; thick, hairless skin; distorted nails; fluid accumulation in abdomen or chest; thickened lung or bronchial tissues; and so on. Once this stage has been reached, it takes longer to effect a cure, and the dog must go back through the stages: inflammatory, functional, and energy imbalance. This is why it often looks as though the dog is getting worse before he gets better.

Working with Homeopathy

A CURE IN homeopathy involves more than just making the symptoms go away, which many kinds of treatments can do. Rather, it makes the symptoms go away and stay away permanently; the dog feels, and is, healthy in every respect (he has none of the symptoms of latent disease listed earlier). He may still get minor ailments, but he will recover from them with very little or no treatment. When a dog is given an appropriate remedy, you'll often see an immediate mental and emotional response of contentment, even though the final "physical" cure may take much longer. A rough rule of thumb is that it takes one month to heal for every year of illness.

It's important to understand that homeopathy is not herbal medicine. Rather, it utilizes medicines derived from plant, mineral, and animal sources. Just because a medicine is derived from plants doesn't mean it shouldn't be handled with caution. We must drop the stereotypical notion that if synthetic medicine is dangerous, natural medicine is mild. Since homeopathy is powerful enough to cure, it's also powerful enough to harm.

It's difficult for newcomers to fully grasp the idea that selecting a remedy in haste could cause an aggravation (make the condition worse), palliate the symptoms (cause the symptoms to return unchanged), or suppress them (cause the symptoms to go away, but make the animal feel worse overall or develop a more serious condition later). Allopathic medicine usually palliates or suppresses symptoms, but any modality can do any of the above.

It's always best to work with a homeopathic practitioner: selecting the right remedy in the right potency and knowing when to represcribe is not as easy as it might seem. I'm now able to treat simple things myself, but I always consult with my practitioner to be sure I'm on the right track before I administer a homeopathic remedy. You can't lose by deferring to those with more experience.

But beware—not every homeopath is competent. You must always take responsibility for observing what's happening to your animal companion. Later we'll discuss how to tell if your dog is responding well to a prescription. I recommend that you keep a journal, noting observations and remedies along with the date, time of day, and even weather conditions or related stress. The homeopath wants to know all current and past symptoms as well as all characteristics that make the individual unique. The homeopath asks about every body system and what makes each symptom better or worse. He or she looks for changes in the symptomatic picture and tries to discover a cause for the changes (for example, symptoms started after the dog's human companions divorced).

The smallest things are important in prescribing homeopathic remedies. How does your dog react to situations, people, other animals, noise, and other stimuli? Does he seek warmth under your covers or lie on top of the bed? Does he catch the breeze by the door or lie on the carpet or on cool, hard surfaces? How much water does he drink? Does he like dry, soft, or soupy foods? How does he interact with other animals in the house? Is he the boss or the low animal on the totem pole?

Once the homeopath has a complete picture, he or she

makes a list of characteristic symptoms (these are symptoms that aren't normally associated with the disease). For example, everyone with the flu feels tired and achy, but not everyone gets better from being consoled, worse from exposure to an open window, or better from having only cold drinks. These unique responses are what homeopaths look for.

Then the homeopath looks up the most important and distinctive symptoms (and this takes experienced judgment) in a *repertory* (such as by Kent, Kunzli, or Murphy, to name but a few of those most often used), which lists thousands of symptoms, along with recommended remedies. By cross-referencing the important symptoms, the homeopath comes up with the two to five of the best potential remedies. Then he or she studies a *materia medica* (a book containing in-depth descriptions of the remedies) to compare choices. Materia medica range from very small books (by Boericke, MacLeod, Day, and many others) in which the authors have put down their interpretation of the remedies, to multivolume versions (by authors such as Hering, Clarke, Allen, and Hahnemann) that list the specific symptoms that occurred in the provings. The more comprehensive materia medica are more useful in the treatment of animals.

Homeopathic References and Materials

I HAVE ON hand George Macleod's *Dogs: Homeopathic Remedies,* as well as his *A Veterinary Materia Medica and Clinical Repertory* with a materia medica of the nosodes; *The Homeopathic Treatment of Small Animals—Principles and Practice,* by Christopher E. Day; *The Science of Homeopathy,* by George Vithoulkas; Boericke's *Materia Medica with Repertory;* and repertories by Kunzli, Murphy, and Kent. *The Family Guide to*

Homeopathy, by Alain Horvilleur, M.D., helped me understand the role of homeopathy in the treatment of human problems. (See "Resources.")

Dr. Christina Chambreau cautions that the late Dr. Macleod's book is organized from an allopathic standpoint (that is, it advises on the best remedies to treat particular problems or diseases), so you'll need to discipline yourself to stand back and treat your individual animal and his symptoms as opposed to treating the disease (the way his book indicates). Potencies will need to be individualized. Your homeopathic practitioner can advise you on this. Christopher Day's approach is geared to the individual based on the symptom pictures, but he does list suggested remedies for specific conditions. Be sure to read the first half of the book and not just the disease section.

Dr. Pitcairn has many tapes on homeopathy, which are available through his office, and there are tapes available through the annual conferences of the American Holistic Veterinary Medical Association (AHVMA) and the National Center for Homeopathy (NCH). Look through the publications list in "Resources" for more suggested reading.

Dr. Chambreau teaches a wonderful veterinary homeopathy course and has made a video, *Homeopathic First Aid for Pets,* in which she explains six remedies for simple problems. She reminds us, however, that it's best to create health by preventative homeopathic care. Moreover, homeopathy may not help your dog if you continue to vaccinate and feed him commercial pet food (see Chapter 4, "Nutrition").

Homeopathics can be difficult to find in the United States, unlike in Europe, where homeopathic pharmacies seem to outnumber conventional drugstores. But more and more places (even regular pharmacies) are beginning to carry homeopathic remedies, as the alternative health care movement sweeps the country. Some homeopaths advise using homeopathic combination remedies with caution because a remedy in the combination may actually aggravate the problem. However, I use them when there isn't time to select the perfect remedy—for example, in an emergency. I personally have had success, when all else failed, with several combination remedies.[11] There are homeopathic kits for home use, containing remedies for common symptoms.

See "Resources" for more information about books, tapes, courses, and supplies.[12]

Cure, Palliation, and Suppression

THERE ARE FOUR possible outcomes of any treatment—complete cure, partial cure, palliation, and suppression—whether you use allopathic medicine, homeopathy, herbs, acupuncture, or any other intervention.

The body's energy field immediately starts to react to the medicine of a curative homeopathic remedy (which is why it's best to give single doses even of the lower potencies). At first you see the primary response (the drug response), which may be that the animal starts to feel better overall and/or there is a lessening of the symptoms, or perhaps you can't discern any changes but you get a sense that, energetically, things are better.

Then, three to five days later if the dog has been sick for a while or has been treated inappropriately over the years—or it may be within only minutes to hours with more superficial or newly contracted diseases—you see a reaction, possibly the current symptoms get worse or older symptoms return. This is a good sign—the body is starting to heal itself. One clue that this is a good aggravation—and not just a response to a wrong remedy—is a feeling that the dog is better (even with the symptoms)—you're picking up on his improving energy.

At this point, wait and don't use another homeopathic remedy. You can make your dog more comfortable with other gentle treatments, such as massage, herbs, flower remedies, and Reiki, but not homeopathy and acupuncture or conventional medicines. (Although I have had to resort to traditional medicine along with homeopathy with certain upper respiratory or gastrointestinal disturbances.) You need to follow the advice of your veterinarian: these problems can be very stubborn indeed, so please don't feel like a failure. Certain herbs, such as mint and other strongly aromatic substances, can counteract homeopathy. Check with your homeopath for any contraindications of other substances you may consider using. Your homeopath may simply tell you to wait and see whether the body stops reacting to the remedy's "push." If the symptoms get worse again, then the animal may have been antidoted by that specific substance.

Finally, the symptoms slowly start to abate. Again, the length of time needed for a cure is proportional to the depth of an illness and the amount of inappropriate prior treatment (whether allopathic, homeopathic, herbal, or some other kind). Cures take time and patience, often requiring several remedies over years' time. It's best to start with the parents and then treat the offspring deeply. Finally, in three or four generations (with fresh food and no vaccines, of course), you'll have very healthy dogs who rarely ever need treating. (If you're not a breeder, this may not be welcome news, but keep the faith. Things usually get better using natural remedies, especially homeopathic ones.)

The second outcome is toward a cure, but not all the way there yet.

The third outcome, a very common one, is that the symptoms go away almost immediately (even if they've been present or recurring for years), which makes us happy because the dog has, for instance, stopped itching or stopped crying when urinating. But then the symptoms come back. So we think, Okay, let's give another dose of that remedy or herb or drug—and again the symptoms go away. But then they return, so we try another remedy or drug. And so on and so on. This is palliation, the need to keep giving something to keep the symptoms away. The dog just keeps getting sicker, on the deeper, energetic level. Work with your homeopathic practitioner to avoid palliation or change to another holistic therapy such as acupuncture. Dr. Nancy Scanlan feels that under the right circumstances, acupuncture and homeopathy can be used together. Classical homeopaths disagree. The jury is still out on the subject. She feels the benefits of acupuncture are just as curative as homeopathy (see "Acupuncture" in Chapter 6, "Hands-on Healing"). Dr. Loops feels that homeopathy and acupuncture can antidote each other and that interpreting the case homeopathically becomes more complicated when acupuncture is used.

The fourth outcome is suppression. Again the symptoms go away immediately. They may not reappear, or they may come back even worse! But the dog is less friendly or more aggressive, or a few months later he comes down with hepatitis or another more serious disease. The symptoms are gone, but the dog is sick at a deeper level. It's like plugging the outlet of a volcano: it gets hotter and hotter inside until it explodes at a deeper, more dangerous level.

Allopathic medicine is very good at palliating and suppressing. Homeopathy and other natural therapies may cure (complete or partial), palliate, or suppress, so you must be the judge of how your dog is responding. If you feel that symptoms are going away too fast (as mentioned, a minimum of one month is needed for each year of disease) or recurring too often, talk to your homeopath. If he or she can't convince you that your dog is moving toward a cure, get a second opinion.

Dr. Chambreau shared the following case with me:

Quimby was brought to me when he was seven years old. He is a boxer who had lived with his family since he was fourteen weeks old. When he was three years old, he developed a problem whereby he would have to be carried around for twenty-four hours after he had exercised too long. The conventional veterinarian first diagnosed hip dysplasia and said that, short of surgery, there was nothing to be done to cure the problem. One year later, a second veterinarian diagnosed a cruciate problem in one knee and calcium deposits in both knees. The dog was on prednisone occasionally, lame if taken on walks that were too long or if he played too hard in the backyard. He had been taking ascriptin twice a day every five to six days when at his worst. He was stiff every day. The veterinarian recommended surgery for the knee but warned that because of the calcium deposits, surgery would still leave him stiff. He sat squarely but on the right side. Hypothyroidism was also diagnosed at that time, and he was taking the drug soloxine. He had a history of demodectic mange, licking his feet, occasional ear infections, and skin allergies for which he had taken shots, to no avail. He seemed to have a fear of metal bowls, tin foil, rain, baths, shouting, and fast-moving objects. Quimby, an affectionate dog, loved being outside when it was cold or even cool. His stools could be changeable from soft to firm. For a big dog, he did not drink a lot. Within one month after the first homeopathic remedy, the dog was running around like his old self with more spunk and energy. He was a little more thirsty and less bothered by the heat. He was still sore and lame, but less so. Within one year, he was completely sound and has remained so. During those first two years of treatment, he was better in many ways but developed incontinence for two months, ground his teeth for one month, and a sneezed a lot for a while. He re-experienced many of his old symptoms for short periods of time. He is now thirteen years old, has not been vaccinated, and is fed a raw meat, fresh food diet. He has occasional problems (every six to twelve months) that respond to short therapy, and strangers think he is a four-year-old boxer.[13]

Homeopathy is tailored specifically to each individual. If one remedy doesn't produce the cure after an appropriate period, your homeopathic practitioner may try another. Often an aggravation occurs (the crisis point of the disease), which is extremely trying, of course, for both us and the animal. Patience is the key. We're so used to the quick fix we get from drugs. We must learn to trust that our bodies have the ability to heal themselves if we will only work with them.

Again, a word of caution. I don't advocate amateur diagnosis. You should always consult a responsible veterinary practitioner. Many symptoms require immediate attention by a qualified emergency veterinarian. You have every right to explain to an allopathic veterinarian that you're working with a homeopathic veterinary practitioner who needs to be consulted prior to (or as soon as possible after) any drug therapy or medical procedure.

Dr. Chambreau feels that emergency allopathic care is fine as long as you call your holistic practitioner as soon as possible. If your dog develops a life-threatening asthma attack on Saturday, steroids may be lifesaving, a reasonable intervention until you can reach your homeopath on Monday. But it could be a problem if you panic during a healing crisis with a dog already under homeopathic care, and get allopathic treatment or give a homeopathic remedy on your own. It is difficult to know what requires emergency treatment and what is an acceptable level of crisis reaction. Only you with the help of your holistic veterinarian can make that decision. I have found that all too often, traditional veterinarians recommend euthanasia when animals appear to be suffering. The healing process or acute phase is not pleasant, but if the animal can get through it, he may heal himself with homeopathic assistance.

Many caring conventional veterinarians welcome your search for another way to heal your dog. Others may be threatened by new approaches or find them inappropriate. Just be honest and, if you can, enroll them as partners in healing. Dr. Chambreau suggests telling your allopathic veterinarian that you value and need his or her expertise in examination and diagnosis but don't want him or her to administer drugs or vaccinations. Dr. Chambreau doesn't recommend using homeopathic remedies along with allopathic drugs but feels that all other therapies in this book may be used compatibly until you find a homeopathic practitioner.[14]

Dr. Russell Swift sees a growing consensus that most allopathic/antipathic drugs do not interfere with the homeopathic remedy if it is the *simillimum* (curative medicine). He also has been told that suppression with homeopathic remedies is unusual unless a remedy is given frequently and in fairly high potency.

I feel that when necessary, perform emergency medicine or surgery and then restore balance—using acidophilus, B complex, other supplements, or perhaps intravenous fluids for severe dehydration, to build the animal back up and get him ready for holistic help. Such procedures are complementary medicine and should never be deemed detrimental to a holistic program. All we can do is the best we can at any given time. And if drugs need to be used, so be it. Your holistic practitioner will soon be able to clear their effects, but get the animal out of danger first. The point is to use everything we have in order to heal—as long as the method does no harm and saves the animal's life!

How Homeopathic Remedies Are Prepared and How They Work

ORIGINALLY, THOUGH Dr. Samuel Hahnemann gave small amounts of his remedies in their crude form, his patients got very sick before they were cured. He decided to dilute the remedies in order to see if they'd be gentler in their action. Indeed, the dilutions worked just as curatively but didn't cause such severe aggravations. Homeopaths following Hahnemann diluted the remedies further, finding appropriate levels for each case. James Kent taught that the *simillimum* is the right remedy at the right potency. This is the concept of the minimal dose.

Today homeopathic remedies are prepared according to specific guidelines found in the *Homeopathic Pharmacopoeia of the United States,* which follow the instructions given by Hahnemann in his book *The Organon.*[15] If possible, an alcoholic tincture is made (some substances are not soluble in alcohol and are prepared differently). The process is known as *trituration.* One grain of the element and 100 grains of milk sugar are ground together. After three dilutions, it is usually possible to carry out successive dilutions with water and alcohol marking the commencement of liquid potency. Dilution and *succussion* (shaking) of the tincture then produce a *potentized* homeopathic remedy.

The following notation is used to indicate the level of dilution: 1 drop of the mother tincture diluted with 9 drops of alcohol (or other solvent) creates a potency of 1X (as in the Roman numeral for ten). Similarly, 1 drop of the mother tincture diluted with 99 drops of alcohol creates a potency of 1C (as in the Roman numeral for 100). You will also hear of 1M potencies (1 drop of a 1C dilution + 99 drops = 2C; do this 1,000 times [serially dilute] and you have 1M). Potencies range from 1C to CM (100,000C). (There is also a category of potencies referred to as LM, which are prepared and administered according to Hahnemann's *Organon*.)

By the time a potency of 12C is reached, the dilution is beyond Avogadro's number (6.023×10^{23}), which in physical chemistry means that not one molecule of the original substance remains in the dilution; therefore, nothing poisonous or toxic is left, no matter what the remedy has been made from. For instance, the nosode Lyssin,[16] which holistic veterinarians recommend giving after rabies vaccinations, is made from rabid dog saliva, but a 30C dose is even more dilute than a 12C, so it contains not even a single molecule of the toxic saliva. Think of the remedy as containing the energy of the original substance imprinted on the molecules of the alcohol mixture.

It's important to know that, paradoxically, the more dilute the remedy, the more powerful it is. At the lower potencies you're dealing with a dilute solution of the physical substance, but as the potency increases, so does the energy of that substance. Thus, potencies lower than 30C can be given one to three times a day for a week or so. Higher potencies should be given only once (except in emergencies), and then the dog needs to be given time to react—perhaps a week, or maybe six to twelve months. The remedy is repeated only when there is no change in symptoms for a few days to a few weeks, depending on the severity of the symptoms.

Homeopathic remedies are made from a wide variety of substances, from innocuous herbs such as chamomile to known poisons such as hemlock. But even the most toxic substance is safe to ingest in submolecular dilution. Poison ivy, agaricus, aloe, leopard's bane, arsenic, nightshade, blister beetle, oyster shell, Spanish fly, lava from Hekla in Iceland, coral snake, flint, club moss, sulphur, cranberry, salt, aurum, rue, cuttlefish ink, tissue from dogs with distemper, and tissue from tubercular lungs are among the many sources of these remedies.

Cell Salts (The Twelve Tissue Salts of Schuessler)

CELL SALTS ARE among the homeopathic remedies listed in materia medica. Wilhelm Heinrich Schuessler, a nineteenth-century physician, physiological chemist, and physicist, saw that when the cells of the body were reduced to their basic elements, there were twelve integral salts. Each of the twelve cell salts serves to stimulate the body in a certain way. He deduced that illness reflected an imbalance of these twelve cell salts. He felt balance could be restored to the body using only these twelve remedies from among hundreds of homeopathics:

Calcarea flourica (calcium fluoride)
Calcarea phosphorica (calcium phosphate)
Calcarea sulfurica (calcium sulfate)
Ferrum phosphoricum (iron phosphate)
Kali muriaticum (potassium chloride)
Kali phosphoricum (potassium phosphate)
Kali sulfuricum (potassium sulfate)
Magnesium phosphoricum (magnesium phosphate)

Natrum muriaticum (sodium chloride)
Natrum phosphoricum (sodium phosphate)
Natrum sulfuricum (sodium sulfate)
Silicea (silica)[17]

Hyland's Homeopathic makes a combination of all twelve cell salts (called Bioplasma), compounded according to the biochemical theory of Dr. Schuessler. I have found it useful as an overall tonic to help build up the constitution of animals that suffer from chronic or acute problems. Two tablets three times daily on an empty stomach is the usual dosage.

How to Select a Potency and Administer a Homeopathic Remedy

THE CHALLENGE FACING homeopaths is not only to select the appropriate remedy but also to determine the optimum potency from a wide range of possibilities. H. G. Wolff, D.V.M., recommends that you keep a homeopathic kit on hand (see "Resources") for emergencies (6X dosage).[18] When a different potency is required, purchase it from a homeopathic pharmacy either in person or by mail, if a prescription isn't required (see "Resources").

Dr. Wolff warns that just reading a book does not make you a homeopathic practitioner. Homeopathy is more complex than you may think at first. So don't take chances with your precious animal companion's life. Join a homeopathy study group, in which you can get support from your lay peers; if there isn't one in your area, consider starting one yourself. And always, either in person or on the phone, work with a practitioner well versed in small-animal homeopathy to select the right remedy, potency, and schedule of administration.

Homeopathics stimulate the immune response; if symptoms

disappear, there is no need to repeat the remedy. Your dog's curling up and taking a nap after his dosage is a good sign that the correct remedy has been chosen, says Dr. Wolff. When the illness is acute, you may administer two or three doses a day for several days; some remedies may be administered every hour for up to five or six hours.

Remedies are available in pellets, tablets, and granules. The dosage is the same for humans as for animals; the size of the animal isn't important:

1 dose=1 tablet or 5–10 granules (tiny, poppylike seeds) or 3 pellets (#20 or #35)

The potency selected and how frequently it's given is of primary importance. If your dog doesn't swallow a complete dose (for example, exactly 3 pellets), don't worry, he'll still get the benefit of the medicine. All vials of homeopathic remedies indicate a condition or symptom and recommended quantity and frequency. This is a requirement of the Food and Drug Administration (FDA), not an absolute, so work with your homeopath to determine the proper potency and schedule of dosage. Also note that the symptoms suggested are only one or two of the "too-numerous-to-mention" possibilities.

Marina Zacharias adds: "To defend the right to practice homeopathy in this country, a homeopath named Dr. Clayton founded the FDA."[19] It seems that the FDA was developed in 1938 in America as an institution to protect homeopathy. The first page of the FDA's enabling legislation refers to the existence of homeopathic pharmacoepia in the United States and how a homeopathic pharmaceutical can be used with a patent in America. But the FDA today seems to work against homeopathy.

The FDA requires that an expiration date appear on all pharmaceutical containers even though homeopathic remedies don't seem to lose their effectiveness unless they're stored improperly. So please don't throw away remedies when they "expire." Remedies even a hundred years old have been used successfully! In fact, Samuel Hahnemann's original remedies that are 180 years old are still used (albeit rarely) successfully. Just make sure to store your remedies in a special corner far from sunlight, heat, microwaves, and disinfectants. Strongly aromatic substances, such as perfumes, camphor, chamomile, mint, tea tree oil, coffee, garlic, and even powerful herbs such as goldenseal and echinacea may also neutralize the effects of homeopathics and even antidote a homeopathic action if included in your dog's food.

As much as possible, try to avoid touching the remedy with your hands, as you may have the residue of chlorine (from tap water) or other strong substances on your skin, which will deactivate the remedy. Or you yourself may be susceptible to the remedy and accidentally absorb it.

Dr. Chambreau recommends that you not push pellets down your dog's throat. Instead, crush the pellet, tablet, or granules in a folded index card, then open the dog's mouth just enough to pour the powder into the flap at the side of his mouth, or on the tongue, using the folded card as a funnel. (Homeopathic remedies are administered orally because the mouth contains such a large number of nerve endings.[20] However, some companies prepare injectable homeopathics.)

It's best that the dog not have a taste of food in his mouth when you administer a remedy, so if giving only one dose, before bedtime might be best. I usually give my animals their dosage upon arising, on an empty stomach (thirty minutes before a meal or one hour after is the general rule). Your practitioner may suggest that certain remedies be administered at specific times of the day for greater effectiveness (see page 218).

If necessary, the remedy may be given in milk or cream, since lactose (milk sugar) is the medium of the pellets, tablets, and granules. If you can't get your dog to take the remedy any other way, it's okay as a last resort to mix it with some baby food chicken or raw hamburger. This isn't ideal, but it's better than not administering the dosage. But if the remedy then doesn't work, you're left wondering whether it was the wrong remedy or whether it was inactivated by the food.

I find it easier to dissolve the remedy in water and administer it orally with an eye dropper. Add the prescribed number of pellets or tablets to 1 ounce of distilled water in a sterile amber dosage bottle. Shake the bottle vigorously for 1–2 minutes, or until the remedy has dissolved completely.

For external use in treating eye inflammations and conjunctivitis, tinctures such as calendula (marigold) or euphrasia (eyebright) are often recommended. They should never be used undiluted. To make your own eye bath, start with 1 drop of tincture in 1 ounce of boiled or distilled water, or sterile saline solution (unpreserved), in a sterile dropper bottle; if this mixture is too strong, dilute it even further.

Shake or tap the bottle against your hand several times (this is called succussion) when diluting tinctures in water or saline. I use 10 seconds as my guideline. Remember to be very cautious about anything you administer to the eyes; it must be sterile.

I especially like euphrasia as an eyedrop; mix 1 drop into 1 ounce of sterile saline solution. I use this to cleanse the nasal passages as well, as it helps dogs suffering with nasal and sinus conditions smell their food or broth.

The homeopathic *Similisan* formulas are excellent as eye-drops as well (Formula 1 for red and irritated eyes, Formula 2 for allergies).

The following materia medica and minirepertory are for general purposes and information only. I don't advocate working without the guidance of an experienced homeopathic veterinary practitioner. Remember that every remedy listed here may be used for many different conditions—again, homeopathy treats the whole individual, not the problem. Each being presents a different picture, so if your dog has an abscess, you'll need help from an expert to find the proper remedy. For example, if *Carbo vegetabilis, Aconite,* or *Hepar sulphuris calcareum* fits the patient's total symptomatic picture, it'll treat an abscess better than, say, *Silicea,* which doesn't fit the picture, even though *Silicea* is another remedy used for abscesses. See how tricky this is?

Materia Medica

THE FOLLOWING, in my experience, are excellent remedies to have on hand for emergencies or for convenience when tele-consulting with your homeopathic veterinary practitioner. Each remedy is listed by its full Latin name, although each also has an abbreviated name (for instance, *Aconitum napellus* is commonly referred to as *Aconite; Cinchona officinalis* is known as *China,* as it is the source of quinine).

I prefer the lower potencies (6X to 30C) and recommend starting low (6X) for chronic disease and working up from there; acute disease may require higher potencies. Always consult your practitioner before administering remedies. Note that I also recommend decreasing the dosage with improvement. During an acute stage or crisis, you may need to repeat the dosage. When a condition is chronic, sometimes one dose is sufficient.

Aconitum napellus. For early stages of feverish conditions of sudden onset associated with chills: high temperature, dry skin, anxiety, intense thirst, agitation. Ailments due to fear or fright. Prior to surgery; also used for shock. Dosage: 3 pellets every one to two hours; decrease frequency with improvement.

Allium cepa. For what appears to be a head cold or upper respiratory infection with acrid, watery nasal discharge, mildly tearing eyes, and sneezing. Symptoms producing laryngeal discomfort; dog may even sound hoarse. Dosage: 3 pellets every one to two hours; decrease frequency with improvement.

Alumina. For conditions affecting mucous membranes. Constipation with inertia of the rectum. Dryness (skin, nose, cough, and so on) is characteristic of this remedy. Dosage: 3 pellets twice a day.

Antimonium crudum. Has strong action on stomach and skin, producing symptoms that are aggravated by heat. Also for nausea and vomiting after excess intake of food, with white tongue. Dosage: 3 pellets three times a day.

Antimonium tartaricum. For respiratory discomfort and excess mucus. There could be a rattling in the chest and/or shortness of breath, and an accumulation of mucus in the chest, associated with little expectoration and a desire for frequent sips of cold water. Could also show lack of thirst. Eyes may be covered with mucus in pneumonic stages. Dosage: 3 pellets two times a day.

Apis mellifica. For stings and bites that usually feel better with cold applications. Also for irritated skin or tissue that's pinkish and puffy but looks whitish when pressed. A guiding symptom is intolerance of heat around eyes and ankles. Also useful for throat conditions in which the tissues seem full of water (edema). For stings and bites, remove stinger and wash well. Dosage: three pellets every half hour for six doses.

Argentum nitricum. For eye conditions. Produces irritating effect on mucous membranes and free-flowing mucopuruent discharge. Dosage: 3 pellets three times a day; decrease frequency with improvement.

Arnica montana. Helps relieve discomfort of mild trauma (accidental injuries). Reduces shock and helps control bleeding. Helps relieve bruising. Excellent after surgery or delivery of puppies. Dosage: 3 pellets immediately, then 3 pellets every half hour; decrease frequency with improvement. See also "Creams and Ointments," page 215.

Arsenicum album. For gastric disturbances, diarrhea, and vomiting, or if bad food is the expected cause. Animal is anxious, restless, feels weak and cold, and has a strong desire for small amounts of water. Good remedy for colibacillosis or coccidiosis, upper respiratory problems, and pneumonia if symptoms become worse toward midnight. Dosage: 3 pellets two or three times a day.

Baptisia tinctoria. For low-grade fevers and muscular lethargy. Secretions are offensive, and gums become ulcerated and discolored. Tonsils are red, and stool tends to be dysenteric. Dosage: 3 pellets every hour; decrease frequency with improvement.

Belladonna. For feverish inflammatory conditions that appear violently, and in which symptoms progress rapidly. Condition causes a state of excitement and active congestion. Animal has a full, bounding pulse and dilated pupils, cannot tolerate bright light, and experiences painful swallowing. Dosage: 3 pellets every two hours; decrease frequency with improvement.

Bryonia. For upper respiratory symptoms and pleurisy. Rheumatism of the joints with inflammation. Animal is worse from movement, wants to lie still. Dosage: 3 pellets three times a day.

Cantharis. For severe rash with intense itching of skin. Cystitis with blood. Dosage: 3 pellets two to four times a day.

Carbo vegetabilis. For lack of resistance to infection and/or conditions that develop slowly with a general lack of vitality. Coldness of body surface; this remedy may help raise a below-normal temperature. Dosage: 3 pellets one time and check temperature.

Caulophyllum. For difficulties at parturition and uterus disability, which may be accompanied by fever and thirst. Tendency to retain afterbirth with accompanying bleeding. May revive labor contractions and has been used in place of Pituitrin injections. Especially helpful in establishing normal pregnancy in those who have had miscarriages. Dosage: 3 pellets for three or four doses.

Chamomilla. For teething and accompanying gum irritation, pain, mild fever, and diarrhea. Condition improved by motion. Dosage: 3 pellets three times a day.

Cinchona officinalis. For conditions characterized by draining fluids, associated with a general weakness, bleeding, and diarrhea. Dosage: 3 pellets every ten minutes for bleeding and after each bowel movement for diarrhea; decrease frequency with improvement.

Cocculus indicus. Mainly for motion or travel sickness with tendency to vomiting. Dosage: For travel sickness: 3 pellets one hour before trip and then every hour as needed; decrease frequency with improvement. For general malaise from travel, 3 pellets in the evening once you've arrived at your destination.

Colocynthis. When diarrhea is yellowish and forcibly expelled. Aggravation occurs after eating or drinking. Dosage: 3 pellets at time of discomfort.

Cuprum metallicum. For occasional sudden severe cramps. Muscles contract and show twitching. Also for fits and convulsions that take an epileptic form. Head is drawn to one side. Dosage: 3 pellets every hour; decrease frequency with improvement.

Euphrasia officinalis. Mild inflammation of eyes and tearing. Principally, conjunctivitis and corneal ulcerations. Dosage: 3 pellets three to four times a day. As an eyedrop: 1 drop of mother tincture in 1 ounce sterile saline solution. One drop in each eye three or four times daily.

Ferrum phosphoricum. This cell salt, like *Aconitum,* may be used in early stages of fever, throat inflammations, and pulmonary congestion. Also if hemorrhages are present. Dosage: 3 pellets three or four times a day.

Gelsemium sempervirens. For conditions that produce weakness and muscle tremors. Dosage: 3 pellets four times a day; decrease frequency with improvement.

Hepar sulphuris calcareum. For conditions showing extreme sensitivity to touch, indicating acute pain. Also for upper respiratory problems with purulent discharge. Dosage: 3 pellets three or four times a day; decrease frequency with improvement.

Hypericum perforatum. For lacerated wounds with damage

to nerve endings. To give relief from pain caused by injury to spine. Injured part usually feels worse if moved. Dosage: 3 pellets every hour; decrease frequency with improvement.

Ignatia amara. For animal that seems unhappy, which could be result of either excitement or emotions (fright, grief, disappointment). Also for indigestion or motion sickness. Dosage: 3 pellets in the morning; decrease frequency with improvement.

Ipecacuanha. For persistent vomiting or diarrhea usually caused by diet. Dosage: 3 pellets every fifteen minutes; decrease frequency with improvement.

Kali bichromicum. For runny nose, discomfort, and pressure at base of nose. Nasal discharge is yellow-green and viscous and may form a crust. Sinusitis, presence of thick, sticky, stringy mucus. Could be useful in bronchopneumonia. Dosage: 3 pellets four times a day.

Ledum palustre. To give relief from pain caused by minor puncture wounds from sharp, pointed instruments such as teeth, claws, or bee stings. Excellent following surgery or for insect bites. Affected parts are generally cold to the touch and feel better after cold applications. Dosage: 3 pellets every fifteen minutes; decrease frequency with improvement. See also "Creams and Ointments," page 215.

Lycopodium clavatum. For flatulence with distension of abdomen under navel, gastric symptoms that increase in the evening (4:00 P.M.–8:00 P.M.), and right-sided symptoms. Dosage: 3 pellets once a day for three days.

Magnesia phosphorica. For cramps, such as uterine spasms, and leg and foot cramps; acts on muscles that cramp or go into spasm; effective for symptoms that are improved by heat, pressure, massage, and exertion. Dosage: 3 pellets every fifteen minutes; decrease frequency with improvement.

Mercurius solubilis. For spongy, sore gums; sore throat; mild fever; thirst; shivering; and excess salivation associated with a cold, thick, coated tongue. May be useful in acute stomatitis (inflammation of gums). Dosage: 3 pellets every hour; decrease frequency with improvement.

Nux vomica. For intestinal discomfort, abdominal pain, diarrhea, indigestion, travel sickness, congestion. Stools are usually hard. Dosage: 3 pellets every hour; decrease frequency with improvement.

Phosphorus. One of the most important remedies in homeopathy. For dry, hard, racking cough with fever that develops rather quickly from a cold settling in the chest. Has an effect on eye conditions. Animal craves cold food and water. Also for nosebleeds. Dosage: 3 pellets at time of bleeding; don't repeat. For other indications, 3 pellets three times daily.

Pulsatilla. Recommended when there is a creamy, bland, thick, yellow nasal or vaginal discharge. Animal is better with cool air, cold food, and water. Dosage: 3 pellets three times daily.

Pyrogenium. For fever with weak, thready pulse. Dosage: 3 pellets (200C potency) one time or as directed.

Rhus toxicodendron. Pains from joint conditions such as rheumatism, neuritis, and achy flulike symptoms that are worse when animal is inactive and much better when active. Cold applications make symptoms worse; heat or warm compresses make them better. Also for skin eruptions looking like eczema or herpes, and so forth. Dosage: 3 pellets every six hours until symptoms improve.

Ruta graveolens. Facilitates labor by increasing tone of uterus, and for injury characterized by a sore area near where the tendon is attached to the bone. Excellent following the use of *Arnica* for the muscles. Also used to assist rectal prolapses. Most symptoms are worse when animal is lying down. Dosage: 3 pellets three times a day or until improvement.

Silicea. For acne, fibrous growths, minor skin eruptions and abscesses, and chronic sinusitis. Also for certain cases of renal insufficiency and bone disorders. Dosage: 3 pellets two times a day until improvement.

Spongia tosta. Thyroid gland becomes enlarged. Lymph system also involved. Used as a heart remedy. Dosage: 3 pellets every six hours.

Staphysagria. Postoperative remedy, reduces trauma and helps heal wounds. Dosage: 3 pellets following trauma.

Sulphur. Has a wide range of action, among them skin conditions such as ringworm★ and mange. Also aids action of other remedies. Dosage: 3 pellets the first day symptoms appear; decrease with improvement or cessation of symptoms.

Symphytum. Hastens union of bone in fractures. Helps relieve pain and promotes healing of injured tissues, especially those injured by a blunt object. May be used with *Arnica.* Also used for symptoms relating to the eyes. Dosage: 3 pellets three or four times a day.

Thuja. Used (along with *Sulphur*) to clear the effects of vaccinations. Dr. Pitcairn has recommended this treatment prior to administering nosodes to clear vaccinations. Dosage: 6X *Sulphur* two times daily for seven days; 6X *Thuja* two times daily for seven days. Repeat for an additional fourteen days.

Urtica urens. Used in urinary tract problems. Helps dams to increase milk supply and to dry it up later on. Dosage: To bring milk in, 3 pellets (30C) three times a day. To dry up milk supply, 3 pellets (6X) three times a day.

★Bacillinum has also been found to be effective for ringworm. Dosage: Two doses of 200C each administered one week apart.

Ustillago maydis. For alopecia and dry coat. The remedy has an affinity for the genital organs of both sexes. Dosage: 200C 3 pellets one time.

Veratrum album. Vomiting associated with painful, watery diarrhea and cramps alternating with extreme exhaustion and cold sweats. Chills extend from head to feet, limbs are cold. Also used in cases of collapse. Animal craves cold water, which is then vomited. Dosage: 3 pellets two to four times a day.

Also keep on hand:

Mother Tincture

Calendula officinalis tincture. For mild burns, insect bites, and superficial skin irritations. Dosage: a few drops in wet compress two or three times a day.

Creams and Ointments

Arnica montana cream. Stimulates healing of wounds and bruises, also for spasms. Dosage: two or three applications a day.

Calendula officinalis cream. For mild burns, insect bites, and superficial skin irritations. Dosage: two or three applications a day.

Ledum palustre ointment. For punctures, bites, and stings. Dosage: three or four applications a day.

Warning: As with any drug, when your dog is pregnant or nursing, seek the advice of a holistic veterinarian before using any of these remedies. If symptoms persist or worsen for more than three days, consult your practitioner. Keep these and all medications out of the reach of children and animals.

CHRONOBIOLOGY

WHAT IS CHRONOBIOLOGY? It is a theory of time and rhythm. It involves the study of the interaction of time among

MINIREPERTORY
(ORGANIZED BY SYMPTOM)

Note: Please consult a homeopathic practitioner prior to administering remedies.

Abdominal distension associated with gas	Carbo vegetabilis
Abscesses	Silicea
Anxiety	Aconitum napellus
Bee sting	Apis mellifica
Bleeding gums	Phosphorus
Boils	Hepar sulphuris calcareum
Boils (grouped, recurring, red)	Sulphur
Bruising	Arnica montana
Burns (mild and dry)	Calendula tincture/cream
Colds (of the head with acrid, watery discharge and tearing)	Allium cepa
Colds (high temperature of sudden onset, strong thirst)	Aconitum napellus
Colds (sudden onset with redness and rapid pulse)	Belladonna
Constipation	Alumina
Cough (croupy, early stages)	Hepar sulphuris calcareum
Cough (dry, hacking, croupy)	Spongia tosta
Cough (dry, hard with fever)	Phosphorus
Diarrhea (with cadaverous smell)	Arsenicum album
Diarrhea (dietary indiscretion)	Ipecacuanha
Eruptions (recurring, burning, itching)	Sulphur
Exhaustion (emotional cause)	Ignatia amara
Eyes (inflammation, tearing)	Euphrasia officinalis
Fever (sudden onset with rapid pulse)	Belladonna

Flatulence (bloating under the navel, worse in evening)	Lycopodium clavatum
Gas	Carbo vegetabilis
Gastric upset	Pulsatilla
Grief	Ignatia amara
Indigestion	Nux vomica
Indigestion (with gas)	Carbo vegetabilis
Injury (sore area located where tendon connects to bone)	Ruta graveolens
Insect bites	Ledum palustre
Insect bites (improved by cold)	Apis mellifica
Insect bites (topical applications)	Calendula tincture/cream or Ledum ointment
Kidneys, pain over (with depression and vaginal discharge)	Helonias
Leg cramps (improved by heat, massage, pressure, exertion)	Magnesia phosphorica
Leg cramps (sudden, severe)	Cuprum metallicum
Milk, deficient	Urtica urens (30C) (lower dosage [6X] dries up milk)
Motion sickness	Ignatia amara or Cocculus indicus
Nasal discharge (bland, yellow, creamy)	Pulsatilla
Nasal discharge (yellow-green, viscous)	Kali bichromicum
Nausea	Ipecacuanha
Nervousness before an event (such as dog show)	Gelsemium sempervirens or Aconite
Pregnancy (stimulate uterus)	Caulophyllum
Puncture wounds (superficial)	Ledum palustre
Pyometra (bland, creamy yellow vaginal discharge)	Pulsatilla

Rash (dry, scaly skin)	Arsenicum album
Rheumatism (joints)	Bryonia
Runny nose	Kali bichromicum
Sinusitis (thick, sticky)	Kali bichromicum
Skin rash (sudden onset)	Arsenicum album
Sprain	Arnica montana
Strain (overexertion)	Arnica montana or Rhus toxicodendron
Surgery	Arnica montana alternated with Hypericum
Teething	Chamomilla
Throat (sore)	Belladonna
Trauma (general, minor)	Arnica montana
Vaccinosis	Thuja or Sulphur
Vaginal discharge (yellow, creamy, bland)	Pulsatilla
Vomiting (nausea/indigestion caused by diet)	Ipecacuanha or Nux vomica

the various body systems (that is, nerve, hormone, and metabolism). At any time of day, our body's energy ebbs or flows like the tides of the sea. If these times can be charted, then various remedies can be targeted at certain organs, with greater effectiveness. Researchers at Stanford University[21] are currently studying the concepts of chronobiology on people.

False/negative responses may also occur in diagnostic procedures when carried out at the wrong time of day. Wendy Volhard and Kerry Brown D.V.M. state that this concept has been effectively used in properly diagnosing heartworm. They also suggest that any diagnostic work be done when the energy is in the appropriate organ:

liver between 1:00 and 3:00 A.M.,

lungs between 3:00 and 5:00 A.M.,

large intestine between 5:00 and 7:00 A.M.,

stomach between 7:00 and 9:00 A.M.,

spleen between 9:00 and 11:00 A.M.,

heart between 1:00 A.M. and 1:00 P.M.,

small intestine between 1:00 and 3:00 P.M.,

bladder between 3:00 and 5:00 P.M.,

kidneys between 5:00 and 7:00 P.M.,

heart constrictor between 7:00 and 9:00 P.M.,

triple heater between 9:00 and 11:00 P.M.,

and gallbladder between 11:00 P.M. and 1:00 A.M.[22]

If a remedy (or for that matter, a drug) is necessary for a particular organ, you would dose the animal at the appropriate time.

FLOWER REMEDIES

UNLIKE DANGEROUS antidepressants and tranquilizers, which only mask emotional distress, flower remedies act as gentle catalysts to alleviate underlying causes of stress and to restore emotional balance. Reportedly, flower remedies are benign and may therefore be safely prescribed for humans, animals, and even plants. The subtlety of this therapy makes it especially well suited to the profound emotional nature of our animal companions.

Note that flower essences are not herbal remedies. Herbs possess powerful medicinal qualities and should not be dealt with lightly (see "Herbs," page 168). Herbal extracts may indeed be made from flowers (such as chamomile and goldenseal), but flower essences are merely the life force collected from the energy field, or aura, of plants.[23]

To make these remedies, the flowers of wild plants, bushes, and trees are picked at dawn—at the height of their vitality—

submerged in water, and solarized (exposed to sunlight) for a few hours (see below for how to make your own). The resulting liquid is diluted and strengthened several times.[24]

The History of Flower Remedies

THE CONCEPT OF flower essences dates back to the ancient alchemists, who felt that the morning dew was sacred. They used an early form of flower therapy in their healing practices. Flower remedies have been used for centuries in India and China, in Australia by Aborigines, and in Europe as far back as the sixteenth century by the master physician and alchemist Paracelsus.

But the first formal research and development of flower essences is attributed to Dr. Edward Bach (1886–1936), an acclaimed British physician, bacteriologist, and homeopath. While practicing medicine, Dr. Bach had observed that his patients' state of mind was directly related to their physical ills. In 1930 he gave up his lucrative medical practice and research so he could dedicate his life to studying the relationship between the mind and the onset and progression of disease. He noticed that inharmonious states of mind such as fear, loneliness, depression, hopelessness, and boredom not only inhibited our natural ability to heal ourselves but were actually the primary cause of disease itself. He believed the only way to truly cure illness was to address its underlying emotional causes, a view diametrically opposed to that of traditional medicine, which treats symptoms.

After many years of researching the healing properties of flowering plants, Dr. Bach developed thirty-eight natural remedies to alleviate every negative emotional state he could identify.

He also created the combination formula Rescue Remedy (Calming Essence), intended for emergency situations. Today these remedies are world renowned for their effectiveness.[25]

The Flower Remedies Handbook: Emotional Healing and Growth with Bach and Other Flower Essences, by Donna Cunningham, describes several other prominent sources for flower remedies, including Flower Essence Services (FES). Working with North American species, FES has created more than seventy well-documented essences, and many more are being developed.[26]

Dr. Christina Chambreau highly recommends the flower essences produced by Molly Sheehan's Green Hope Farm. Sheehan's Emergency Trauma Solution may be taken in situations of sudden trauma (just like Rescue Remedy), and she claims this remedy was even used to help keep the electrical system of the farm from shutting down.

Recognizing the importance of animals in our lives, Sheehan has also developed Animal Emergency Care, a fine-tuned version of the original emergency formula.[27] Ellon USA (an American company that distributes flower remedies) receives correspondence reporting wonderful results when flower remedies are administered to cats, dogs, birds, tropical fish, horses, cattle, snakes, and even African rhinoceroses and elephants. Some people include flower remedies in the water they use on their special plants.

No one can dispute the genius of Dr. Bach's pioneering contribution; his work has touched the lives of countless health practitioners and individuals throughout the world. However, though many of his followers believe his thirty-eight remedies are the only viable ones, other pioneers continue to expand the repertory, offering us a vast array to choose from.

How to Use Flower Essences

AS YOU EXPLORE the flower remedies, it's important to remember Dr. Bach's belief that negative thoughts and feelings poison the system, bringing about ill health and unhappiness and hindering treatment and recovery. Every one experiences negativity from time to time, but some of us are better able to deal with it and thus bring our systems and minds back into harmony. Flower essences help us achieve a healthful balance.

The Flower Remedies Handbook, by Donna Cunningham, includes affirmations to be spoken aloud when using flower remedies. We animal lovers may speak these words while administering the remedies to our animal companions. Being the highly sensitive creatures they are, they react even to subtle changes in their environment, including the moods of their human companions. Since our animal friends often suffer from the same stresses that affect us, I usually take the same remedy I give my pets, saying, "I accept my feelings and deal with them openly," or whatever seems appropriate.

Especially when obvious medical problems are ruled out as the cause, flower remedies assist the animals suffering from the ill effects of stress, which we all know leads to disease. In fact, many behavioral problems are a sign of physical illness. So check with your holistic veterinarian, who may recommend a complete workup, including but not limited to a fecal (stool) test and complete blood panel, in order to rule out (or, if necessary, treat) any pathological problems.

Bach flower remedies may be used to complement treatment recommended by your holistic practitioner, as they seem to act as a catalyst for healing. Many homeopaths recommend their use since they don't, as herbal formulas sometimes do, interfere with homeopathic treatment. But other practitioners believe differently, so it's best to ask. You may wish to contact a certified flower essence consultant for a personalized program.[28]

Administering flower remedies couldn't be easier. Vigorously shake the dosage bottle vertically, in increments of eight shakes (twenty-four is a good number) to energize the remedy. Then simply add a few drops of the concentrate to the animal's drinking water (2 drops of remedy per ounce of purified or spring water). With Rescue Remedy, mix 2–4 drops of the concentrate into the food, or place 2 drops on the tip of the nose or ears (so they'll lick it off) or administer it orally, but dilute it with spring water first.[29] You may fill a spray bottle and atomize the air with appropriate remedies, too.

Ideally, flower remedies are given four times a day. In cases of extreme stress, they may be given as often as every half hour—and Rescue Remedy may be administered every five to eight minutes in times of crisis until you see improvement. If there is no improvement or symptoms worsen, seek advice from your holistic veterinarian.

You may use up to a maximum of six remedies, including Rescue Remedy (even though it's a combination, it counts as one when mixed with others). Make up and store the combinations you deem appropriate for your dog; I use 1-ounce amber dosage bottles with glass droppers.[30] With these combinations I usually administer half a dropper's worth at a time, orally. Afterward, be sure to rinse the dropper in warm water because the dropper may have touched the animal's tongue, and you don't want to risk contaminating the remainder of the formula.

When the remedies are given in food or water, there's no need to worry about their effect on your other animals. If another animal (or human, for that matter) doesn't need the remedy, it will have no effect, so all your animals may share the same bowls freely. To ensure potency, always prepare the remedy-enhanced food or water daily. To preserve flower essences, keep the bottle in the refrigerator or mix an ounce of remedy with a teaspoon of vegetable glycerin.

Before you begin using flower remedies, look at yourself and your animal companions as objectively as possible. It's important to know which of their behaviors are normal. Many times we human beings accuse animals of being spiteful or vindictive when they behave in ways we don't like, but this is often only our own inability to understand animal behavior. For instance, it's natural for puppies to bite when teething; it's not a sign of mean-spiritedness. But since such natural behavior isn't acceptable to us, we must find gentle ways to discourage it—or rather, to channel the animal's normal behavior into acceptable outlets with positive reinforcement (see "Nonverbal Communication" in Chapter 2, "Interacting with Your Dog"). This way a young animal soon learns to play with toys instead. The flower remedies Chestnut Bud and Walnut can help this transition.

You can obtain a self-help guide to flower remedies (designed for human use) through Ellon USA (see "Resources"). As you read the descriptions for each essence that follow, compare the behaviors listed with those of your dog, and then read the canine interpretations below.[31] You'll soon get the hang of it.

See what combinations you come up with both for yourself and for your animal companions. Use a little poetic license as you interpret the descriptions and explore other flower essence companies, which are making major breakthroughs in this exciting field. I especially like Healing Herbs' emergency formula,[32] called 5 Flowers, and use it often in my own custom formulations.

The Flower Remedies and Their Uses with Dogs

Agrimony. For animals suffering from skin irritations, wild dogs that cannot adjust to captivity, and restlessness at night when you'd rather the dog slept.

Aspen. For the shy dog who startles easily at any sound, even nonthreatening ones (if this condition was brought about by trauma or abuse in the past, use Star of Bethlehem; when in doubt, use both). Give Aspen during intense storms or after earthquakes, or to a kenneled or sheltered animal who senses impending harm. Aspen may actually help reveal to your dog what he's actually afraid of, so he can learn to deal with his own fear.

Beech. For dogs with little tolerance for other animals or certain people. Effective with Walnut to assist in keeping peace between two animals who are always fighting. For the dog who is intolerant of a new relationship in the house. For the dog who always seems irritated. Also good for picky eaters.

Centaury. For the quiet, submissive dog who doesn't stand up for himself, allows himself to be abused by a cat, a child, or another dog. Increases will to live when fighting an illness or during the hard delivery of a puppy.

Cerato. For flighty, inattentive animals. Valuable during shows or training sessions, when dog's ability to be undistracted and to relate to your requests is required. Excellent for anxiety and related problems, such as canine eating disorders, especially during pregnancy.

Cherry Plum (one of the ingredients in Rescue Remedy). For the dog who loses control, becomes wild, angry, and vicious when provoked. In competition situations, when the dog is stressed by strange people, the smell of other dogs, and unfamiliar noises. For the dog who doesn't travel well. For retaining control during heat cycles and/or mating (for both sexes); good for pregnant dams who seem unusually stressed. In situations where the dog could lose bladder and/or bowel control. Also for the dog who constantly chews himself or chases his own tail. For allergies to grasses, and to help dogs stay away from biting at stitches after surgery.

Chestnut Bud. Used to break bad habits, or during training sessions, to increase memory retention and a keen sense of awareness. Helps dogs learn lessons necessary for us to coexist.

Chicory. For the extremely affectionate dog, who may be possessive and jealous, wanting always to be near you, to be held, petted, and fussed over. For the mother dog who is overly possessive with her litter, especially when it's time for her pups to leave home. For the dog who thinks he owns the house or tries to get attention in negative ways.

Clematis (one of the ingredients in Rescue Remedy). When the dog appears stunned or experiences unusual, prolonged patterns of sleep, beyond the typical nap. To help while regaining consciousness following surgery or an accident. In conjunction with Rescue Remedy, helps newborn pups wake up and breathe. Give them one drop every few minutes on tips of ears or nose.

Crab Apple. This remedy is especially cleansing during or after any illness, rash, open wound, worming, or flea infestation. Used to detoxify and heal. For dog with a poor self-image, one who cowers during shows, or the dog who was previously abused or abandoned.

Elm. For the dog who must change location, go to the groomer, or be subjected to too many people at a time (a show or guests and relatives).

Gentian. For setbacks of any kind (for example, when the dog gets worse before he gets better during the course of an illness, arthritis symptoms, rehabilitation from surgery, the ill effects of a stillborn puppy). Helps to give dogs an inner fortitude to deal with whatever comes their way.

Gorse. For apathy, depression, and despair, when the dog refuses to eat or to improve. When battling cancer, a critical injury, or surgery.

Heather. For the center-of-attention dog, the dog who annoys or is a pest, or the dog who cries when left alone. For the dog left at a kennel or in a shelter, wanting attention from everyone.

Holly. For the dog showing signs of temper. When there's a need for more love. Especially good for abused or neglected dogs who need to be quarantined, or rescued dogs at the shelter or the veterinarian's office. Helps nourish the heart and releases jealousy and anger.

Honeysuckle. Helps dogs stop sulking after change or loss of loved one. For the dog who has been chased by a cat, a child, or another dog. After a long birthing experience; for the mother caring for her young after a cesarean section. For the dog who has lost too much blood or whose vital signs are low. Before selling a dog or puppy or when moving to a new home. Also for when the dog must be hospitalized or placed in a kennel.

Hornbeam. For fatigue. A strengthening remedy, helpful in assisting the runt of the litter or building up any sickly animal.

Impatiens (one of the ingredients in Rescue Remedy). For the dog who gets agitated by too much excitement or gets overly anxious at mealtimes or before a dog show. Also for the dog in pain.

Larch. For dogs low in the dog hierarchy of the household, or the runt of the litter. Also for the dog with low self-esteem. Increases confidence before a show, so he can hold his head high.

Mimulus. For fear of particular things or circumstances, such as thunderstorms, vacuum cleaners, trips to the veterinarian, or visits by small children. Also for deep fears, such as fear of starving, strangers, abandonment. When fear turns to terror, use Rock Rose or Rescue Remedy. For illnesses that don't respond to treatment, such as postinfluenza.

Mustard. For the depressed dog, complicated by hormonal changes (such as puppy coming into heat for the first time, or the stud discovering girls). During pregnancy if depression is noticeable, or if the dog is cantankerous during heat. Use on cranky older dogs who like to be alone and get obnoxious when approached.

Oak. For last weeks of pregnancy, when the dog feels overburdened. For long chronic illness, especially if the dog begins to struggle. To rebuild strength after harsh living conditions, starvation, or abuse. For loss of elimination functions and/or loss of control of limbs or muscles.

Olive. For exhaustion following a long ordeal or long-term pain. For elderly dogs who become exhausted easily. For the dog plagued by stressed adrenals or allergies. For caged dogs who exhaust themselves to get out.

Pine. For the dog given away or left behind. In competition, for the dog who never makes it to the finals though he's show quality. For the dog who looks guilty whenever his human companion is upset, even though it wasn't the dog's fault.

Red Chestnut. For the dog who constantly watches out the window when his human companion is late coming home. For the mother worrying over her pups.

Rescue Remedy (a.k.a. Calming Essence—a combination of Star of Bethlehem, Rock Rose, Impatiens, Clematis, and Cherry Plum). For any kind of trauma. Be sure to take it yourself; if you're calmer, it helps your dog. In the case of an accident, see your veterinarian immediately; however, Rescue Remedy can help you through the trauma of getting the dog to the veterinarian's office. Used on pregnant dams, on car trips, for boarding, during long absences from home, before and after surgery, or whenever the dog experiences unusual stress. Also, it can stop a seizure very quickly. Often used as a last resort, with remarkable results. I always reach for it first. I use Rescue Remedy or 5 Flowers Remedy during travel to and from shows and often just before going to the ring for judging.

Rock Rose (one of the ingredients in Rescue Remedy). For dogs who experience panic or terror. After an accident, injury, or other terrifying event.

Rock Water. For increased joint flexibility. For picky, inflexible eaters.

Scleranthus. For the dog with equilibrium problems or

neurological confusion, as in some kinds of seizures, with complications to one side of the body (such as with stroke or partial paralysis).

Star of Bethlehem (one of the ingredients in Rescue Remedy). For all trauma. Loss of loved one, after injury or abuse, birthing difficulties, intense heat or cold. Use to comfort those left behind in a kennel. For the ill or injured dog who must be hospitalized and is deprived of his human companion's comfort.

Sweet Chestnut. For the high-strung dog, at his wit's end. For the dog forced to remain in a tiny kennel or carrier. To prevent burnout in show dogs, or anytime the dog needs endurance or energy.

Vervain. For intense, hyperactive, or for the very high strung dog.

Vine. For the "boss dog," who thinks he's in charge ("top dog"), the strong-willed dog. To boost the self-esteem of the "underdog."

Walnut. Helpful through any changes, including weaning and heat cycles. Eases adjustment to houseguests, holidays, or a new home. Protects against pollutants and pollens from grasses. For the very sensitive dog who is easily disturbed.

Water Violet. For grief, loneliness, and lack of joy.

White Chestnut. For constant and persistent unwanted thoughts such as worries that prevent peace of mind and disrupt concentration. Good remedy to use for focus in dog training sessions.

Wild Oat. For the bored dog who doesn't feel useful anymore, the dog retired from shows, movies, or TV. For competitions, where the dog needs to have a strong desire to win.

Wild Rose. To remain happy and content when you bring

home a new animal. For the older, grouchy dog, or the dog placed in a cage during a dog show.

Willow. For resentment—the dog who ignores you when you come home because you left him alone all day, or the show dog who punishes you by urinating where he shouldn't (check for health problems, too, with this behavior) for not taking him to shows anymore or not paying attention to him, or the dog who chews up your favorite shoe.

Flower remedies often work well in combination. Use your intuition to come up with mixtures that are right for your dog. Here are a few ideas: Aspen, Star of Bethlehem, and Larch may be used singly or in combination with shelter or stray animals who have been abused or neglected; Aspen and Larch for fear and mistrust; Star of Bethlehem for grief and trauma. Try combining Red Clover, a great calmer for group hysteria (such as at dog shows), with Rescue Remedy or 5 Flowers. If travel is traumatic for your dog, with accompanying motion sickness, withhold food and water for at least one hour before departure, and give Rescue Remedy (or 5 Flowers) and/or Scleranthus. Use Crab Apple, Olive, and Rescue Remedy together or separately for dogs with respiratory problems. They're also good to use after spaying, neutering, or during and after bouts of fever.

The Australian Bush Flower Essences (see "Resources") include a wonderful remedy called Kapok Bush that supports those who get easily discouraged and give up. Borage, by FES, gives us cheer and courage in facing up to challenges—healing ourselves and assisting the healing of our companion animals is indeed challenging.

Consultant Yolanda LaCombe recommends several of the healing herbs and FES remedies for dogs, among them Mariposa

Lily for the motherly dog who needs to mellow out, Queen Anne's Lace for dogs who have experienced trauma to the head (you may suspect abuse in their past), Manzanita for anorexic dogs, and Red Clover for calming in tense situations.

I've started carrying my flower reference books with me to shows, as I'm always being asked what makes my animals so centered and able to handle this unusual stress.[33] If you consider that each animal is an individual made of the same "stuff" we are, it isn't any wonder that when we observe their personalities and traits, we can prescribe flower essences for them as easily as we can for ourselves.

How to Make Your Own Flower Essences

IN *NATURAL HEALING for Dogs and Cats,* Diane Stein explains how easy it is to become a do-it-yourself maker of flower essences.[34] You'll need a clear glass bowl, free of design, which can hold up to 12 ounces of water. Stein suggests using distilled or spring water; I prefer spring water when making flower essences as well as gem elixirs (see "Crystals and Healing" in Chapter 7, "Other Healing Approaches"). You'll also need stainless-steel tweezers, several amber glass dropper bottles sterilized in boiling water, a glass funnel, some labels for the bottles, and brandy (to use as a preservative).

Place the bowl outside on the soil or grass, next to the flowers. Fill the bowl with spring water. Pick blossoms or petals from the healthiest plants; use the tweezers, not your fingers, for picking so you don't contaminate the essence with whatever may be on your hands. Cover the surface of the water with the flowers or petals. Organically raised flowers or wildflowers are best; don't use flowers that have been treated with chemical pesticides.

Pick only one kind of flower at a time; it's okay to select from different plants and colors, just stick with a single species (such as only roses) in your bowl. If you can obtain only a single flower, this is fine, too.

Leave the water and flowers in the sunshine for three hours. If you begin in the early morning, while the dew is still on the petals, you may need to solarize longer. Spring and summer are the best seasons; pick a cloud-free day for best results.

Fill the sterile dosage bottles halfway with brandy. With tweezers (again, no fingers, please; you may also use a leaf from the same plant or even a crystal) remove the flowers and any debris from the water. Add the water to the bottles containing the brandy, filling them to the neck, sealing, and labeling them. It's a good idea to include the date. You may even label them with the phase of the moon or astrological sign under which they were prepared.[35]

If you're making more than one flower essence, wash your hands before proceeding to the next flower. In fact, it's a good idea to wash your hands before preparing or administering any treatment. Try to use unscented soap, as aromatic materials may interfere with the potency of flower essences and homeopathics.

You now have a mother tincture. Potentize your essences by succussing (shaking) or hitting the bottle against the heel of your hand in increments of eight shakes or taps.

For everyday use, add 2 drops of the mother tincture to another dropper bottle filled with equal amounts of spring water and brandy. Another way to dilute the remedy is to mix 1 ounce spring water, 2 drops potentized flower essence, and 1 teaspoon brandy; or substitute 1 teaspoon vegetable glycerin for the brandy if you wish to avoid the alcohol altogether.

Now you may use your homemade essences just as you would those you buy at the health-food store.

Nature and the Higher Self

FOR A LESSON in communing with the nature spirits, or devas, I recommend reading *Behaving As If the God in All Life Mattered,* by Machaelle Small Wright, one of my favorite authors; her *Flower Essences* and *Nature Healing Conings for Animals* are also excellent resources. One of Wright's Perelandra Essences is comfrey, which is used to repair soul damage occurring in the current or a past life.[36]

Wright and other spiritual writers have awakened in me a confidence that each one of us is blessed with an ability to contact our higher selves. This higher self can in turn be in touch with another person's or animal's higher self, and thus be a party to healing. I've found that even if I feed the perfect diet, select an array of herbal and homeopathic remedies, use every kind of supplement imaginable, and even pray for an animal friend to be healed, unless I release myself to the laws of nature, healing will be thwarted every step of the way.

AROMATHERAPY

WHAT IS AROMATHERAPY? It is the skilled use of essential oils to heal, nurture, and care for the body, mind, and spirit.

Scent is a powerful component of holistic health care. The subtle use of aromatherapy can enhance all healing therapies, especially those for dogs, whose sense of smell is so much more complex and acute than our own. Their olfactory ability is the result of evolution: their acute senses allowed dogs to survive predators and other dangers in the wilderness.

The history of humans' use of scent dates back to the ancient Egyptians. Symbolic representations of incense appear on the walls of Egyptian tombs and temples, author Scott Cunningham recounts in *Magical Aromatherapy*. The Egyptians had such a high regard for scent that they traded valuable commodities such as gold for fragrant substances and used them in medicine, food preparation and presentation, and the rituals of religion, magic, and even their journeys to the afterlife.

The Greeks anointed their deceased with essential oils, burned incense on altars, and lavished their bodies with expensive fragrances. They also believed that the fresh scents from living plants maintained physical health, and they built their homes so that rooms would open out onto herb gardens surrounded by flowering plants. They inhaled specific perfumes to heal various ailments, such as quince or white violet for stomach upsets, grape leaves to help clear their head, and roses to relieve headaches. Hippocrates, the father of medicine, stated, "The way to health is to have an aromatic bath and scented massage every day."

The American Indians, through centuries of trial and error, developed uses for fragrant plant materials in every aspect of their daily lives, from food, medicine, and tools to personal adornment and toys.

The Hawaiians have traditionally used fragrances (especially scented coconut oil, maile, *hala,* and *pukiawe*) that were burned by the kahuna, or witch doctor, who chanted and prayed while they fumed.

Aromatherapy stimulates the immune system and promotes healing. Typically, essential oils, the distilled or expressed product of aromatic plant materials, are used for this purpose. These aromatic essences have many desirable qualities—ranging from antibacterial and antiviral to antispasmodic and other properties that help ease daily aches and pains and assist in recovery from injuries, accidents, and other mishaps. They also provide quick relief in emergency situations.

Some essences are reported to have diuretic properties (promoting the production and excretion of urine), are vasodilators or vasoconstrictors (widening or narrowing blood vessels, respectively), and act on the adrenals, ovaries, and thyroid. Others aid in digestion or are beneficial in treating infection, modifying immune response, and balancing moods and emotions, according to Kurt Schnaubelt, director of the Pacific Institute of Aromatherapy.[37] Essential oils are also invaluable in the day-to-day grooming needs of your animal companion from head to toe.

Scott Cunningham describes the use of scent in three different forms:[38]

Fresh plants contain large amounts of energy in their flowers, twigs, and leaves. Grow your own or buy them at health-food stores, farmers' markets, and/or organic nurseries.[39] If you plant your own garden, please observe organic principles, and never let the dogs sniff plants sprayed with synthetic pesticides.

Dried herbs are ideal because if they have been harvested, dried, and stored properly, the essential oils haven't evaporated. Check local herb shops for a lovely variety or peruse the shelves of your health-food store for both herbs and spices.[40]

Essential oils are volatile aromatic substances that naturally occur within specific plants, such as rose and garlic, giving them their pungent odor. Distilled or expressed essential oils can be purchased at most health-food stores.[41] Essential oils can help our animals because they contain properties that sedate, calm, and soothe.

The essential oils most frequently used in animal care are eucalyptus, tea tree, lavender, citronella, rosemary, pennyroyal, cedarwood, chamomile, cinnamon, tangerine, patchouli, mint, lemon, terebinth, thyme, and sage. They may be used to mask odors; help with exhaustion, fatigue, birthing, and weight loss; treat anemia, anorexia, abscesses, coryza (common cold), fractures, sprains, and poisoning; and control fleas and other pests, among other conditions.

There are three points of caution regarding essential oils.

First, you need to recognize the difference between fragrance oils and essential oils. For example, calendula oil is not an essential oil. Calendula can be sold as a tincture or an infused oil, made by steeping calendula flowers in oil. Sweet Pea oil is not an essential oil. Mimosa, though it may produce an essential oil, is mixed with chemical solvents for use in the perfume industry. Even then it is too expensive for our use, and the solvents would be toxic to our companion animals. Apple oil is a fragrance oil; apple does not produce an essential oil. The same goes for melon, water lily, lilac, hyacinth, and gardenia (they are produced chemically by scientists in a lab). They do smell lovely and are enjoyable in that sense, but they do not have therapeutic value.

Second, we need to use the best quality essential oils. My personal aromatherapist, Marla Wilson (see "Resources") recommends these suppliers: Oshadi, Isha, John Steele, Laboratory of Flowers, Tisserand, and Aroma Vera.

Third, essential oils can be very dangerous if used directly on the skin. Never take them internally because the oils contain chemicals that could cause such allergic reactions as seizures, burns, and, in some cases, death. Once I spilled a drop of cinnamon oil on my dining room table, and it ate a hole in the wood finish. I consult with Marla now to learn about any special safeguards before I experiment with a new essential oil.

Some *hydrosols*[42] (a whole floral water–steamed distillation of plant materials with all the essential oils intact), such as those sponsored by aromatherapist Jeanne Rose and those available through reputable essential oil suppliers such as Oshadi, Isha, White Rose of Provence, and Palmetto (see "Resources"), are organic and could be taken internally under certain conditions in small dilutions (consult with a trained veterinary aromatherapist first). You want to be sure you are getting a true hydrosol with no additives. Check the label first; if your supplier doesn't know, try another supplier.

Note that Scott Cunningham's books contain references to many synthetic oils and incense. For our purposes, do not use such oils, because they do not possess medicinal properties.

Essential Oils for Your Dog

JOAN CLARK AND her colleagues at AromaPet feel that "aromatherapy is a new paradigm for the care and nurturing of our animals as we usher in a new vision of health and fitness, not only for ourselves but for the animals that are a part of our lives. Every stage of our pet's life can be enhanced with aromatherapy. From birth to death, essential oils make each transition more memorable and sacred."

It's only natural that our companion animals be part of this new, holistic vision in the twenty-first century.

Aromatherapy is valuable in holistic veterinary care. For example, for animals suffering from an upper respiratory condition, Joanne Stefanatos, D.V.M., mixes equal parts eucalyptus oil (a well-known respiratory stimulant) and diluted catalyst-altered water (CAW; see "Pure Water," in Chapter 4, "Nutrition") and places this solution in the infuser cup of a vaporizer. Patients inhale the fumes for the first twenty-four to forty-eight hours of their stay at her hospital, after which they can usually breathe better, smell their food, and begin eating (so they are permitted to leave the hospital). Dr. Stefanatos suggests continuing the therapy at home. I use a diffuser or a nebulizer.

For the same purpose, Nelly Grosjean, author of *Veterinary Aromatherapy*, suggests using the following blend of essential oils in an aromatic diffuser: 20 ml eucalyptus, 10 ml pine, 5 ml tea tree, and 2 ml thyme; she also feels eucalyptus is fine on its own.[43]

Don't forget to dilute the eucalyptus oil in water if you use a vaporizer, since used straight it may irritate your dog's sensitive eyes. Some vaporizers warn not to add anything to the water because oils may cause damage to the unit. You may use your diffuser or nebulizer along with your vaporizer to get the benefits from the humidity as well as the scent. My humidifier has a little cup in which I add a few drops of essential oil to a small amount of water.

Dr. Stefanatos uses oil of lemon to sedate a fever. For tonification she suggests rosemary, peppermint, sage, or thyme. Essential oils of sage and lavender can be used to stimulate a diuretic response; Dr. Stefanatos suggests administering them in a nebulizer or diffuser for two to eight hours. For gastrointestinal problems, she uses basil, chamomile, thyme, and peppermint. Oil of bane helps speed restoration of health after many diseases have run their course.

For excessive heat cycling, false pregnancy, and swollen mammary glands, oil of sage is recommended. Dr. Stefanatos believes oil of cloves may prevent the need for a cesarean section. For heat as well as asthma problems, she prescribes oil of cinnamon at bedtime. I also use it in a diffuser for diarrhea.

For abscesses, Grosjean suggests a poultice of cabbage leaves (crush large outer layers first) or of clay, followed by cleaning with compresses and several drops of lavender. She also recommends clay poultices to promote the healing of wounds,[44] and sprinkling mint leaves or lavender seed into the dog's bed for flea problems.

You may buy or assemble little bags of herbs, dried flowers, fruits, seeds, pods, and so on, and lace them now and then with essential oils. Try the following oils and combinations to assist in a variety of circumstances:

- To enhance beauty: *catnip, rose*
- For comfort: *lavender*
- For courage: *yarrow*
- To relieve depression: *jasmine, lavender, marjoram, tangerine*
- For stilling emotions: *costmary*
- For happiness: *apple, neroli, orange*
- For healing: *clove, coriander, cypress, eucalyptus, myrrh, niaouli, palmarosa, pine, sandalwood, spearmint*
- For maintaining health: *eucalyptus, garlic, lavender, lemon, pine, tea tree*
- For longevity: *rosemary*
- For love: *carnation, jasmine, rose (and many more)*
- To improve memory and impart wisdom: *sage*
- For peace: *chamomile, rose*
- For physical energy: *cinnamon, lemon, nutmeg*
- For sleep and calming: *chamomile, jasmine, lavender*
- For training sessions: *lavender*

Dr. Nancy Scanlan is certified in aromatherapy (besides her other callings) and offers the following list of essential oils for various common complaints:

- Arthritis: *black pepper, garlic, juniper, lemon, thyme*
- Asthma: *cajeput, eucalyptus, lavender, marjoram, peppermint, pine, rosemary, thyme*
- Barking and chewing: *chamomile, geranium, lavender, marjoram, sandalwood*
- Cystitis: *eucalyptus, lavender, pine, thyme*
- Dandruff: *cedarwood, geranium, juniper, lavender, lemon, rosemary*
- Diarrhea: *chamomile, cinnamon, clove, geranium, ginger, nutmeg, savory*
- Flatulence: *chamomile, ginger, lemon, peppermint, rosemary, tarragon*
- Gingivitis: *lemon, sage*
- Respiratory infection: *black pepper, eucalyptus, lavender, lemon, peppermint, pine, rosemary, sage, sandalwood, thyme*
- Skin infections: *chamomile, geranium, juniper, lavender, sage*

My friends at AromaPet (see "Resources") offer an aromatherapy pet pharmacy—an essential oil pet-care line that consists of the following products already blended for our convenience (which takes the guesswork out of it for me!):

Fennel Fever. A combination of peppermint, spearmint, rosemary, and ginger to help with fever and chills caused by various conditions.

Ginger-Vitus. A perky oral hygiene blend of cinnamon, lemon, tea tree, peppermint, and more to help keep the gums and teeth healthy as well as assist with halitosis.

Helycriscum Hot Spots. A soothing antiseptic and anti-inflammatory blend to help alleviate itchy, red, raw, and inflamed conditions.

Juniper Joints. A blend of birch, juniper, peppermint, tarragon, pepper, and thyme to help with arthritic conditions, muscular aches and pains, and aging. Base oil of arnica, St. John's wort, calendula, and sweet almond.

Lavender Blues. A soothing and supportive synergy of lavender, marjoram, and tangerine to help with depression, grief, sadness, or any difficult change.

Lemon Boo Boo. An antiseptic blend of lemongrass, tea tree, eucalyptus, and lemon to help with cuts, scratches, wounds, and cleansing of skin injuries.

Mellow Out Marjoram. A blend of lavender, marjoram, ho wood, and patchouli to assist with stress, hyperactivity, and change.

Mugwort. An antifungal antiseptic blend for warts, nail care, and skin lesions.

Peppermint Peppy. A zesty, uplifting blend of peppermint, spearmint, lime, birch, and eucalyptus that helps with low energy, fatigue, and aging.

Ravensara Rub. A respiratory blend with oils of ravensara, eucalyptus, peppermint, and niaouli to assist with any conditions relating to the respiratory system.

Rosemary Flush. A stimulating blend of rosemary, grapefruit, cypress, lemon, and fennel to assist with detoxification, circulation, weight gain, and release of fluids.

Tarragon Tummy. A blend of tarragon, peppermint, fennel, and marjoram to help with digestive ailments, flatulence and nausea.

Weeping Cypress. A tonic of cypress, cedarwood, lavender, palmarosa, marjoram, and patchouli for skin conditions which tend to drain.

AromaPet has also created a travel kit to take to dog shows or just for on the road. It consists of lavender, tea trea, peppermint, rosemary, eucalyptus, birch, lemon, marjoram, jojoba, St. John's wort, arnica, calendula, sweet almond, and grapeseed.

Guidelines for Using Essential Oils

JOAN CLARK, OF AromaPet, recommends: "Animals are scent sensitive and, therefore, a little goes a long way. Animals need only small dosages of the oils to see results. If the condition is severe, you may use a larger dosage. Begin with less and build up. Depending on the size of the animal, and the energy/emotional level of the animal, you will determine the dosage."[45] Before applying essential oils, contact AromaPet for further details (see "Resources"). Prepare these blends in a 1-ounce amber glass bottle.

Large dogs. Up to 3 percent of the blend. A 1-ounce blend would contain 27 drops of essential oil in a carrier like sweet almond oil.

Medium dogs. 2 percent of the blend. A 1-ounce blend would contain 18 drops of essential oil in a carrier.

Small dogs. 1 percent of the blend. A 1-ounce blend would contain 9 drops of essential oils in a carrier.

I like to use essential oils daily in my diffuser, and Nelly Grosjean recommends the use of the aromatic diffuser not only to help us benefit from the fragrance of essential oils but also to protect against microbes and pollution. She feels that the regular use of the diffuser regenerates, cleanses, ionizes, enriches, and revitalizes the air we breathe.[46] This particular practice is widely used in France, where Ms. Grosjean resides.

Another means of distributing scent is to bring distilled or purified water to a boil in a nonmetallic pot, pour the water into large heatproof bowl, and add a few drops of an essential oil or fresh herb while you visualize pictures (such as your dog restored to glowing health or in harmony with your family).

Whatever form of aromatherapy you use, remember to practice nonverbal communication through visualization and affirmations as you and your animal inhale the aroma; according to Scott Cunningham, this is the key to the power of aromatherapy.[47] Focus on positive images, as they are the best form of communication (see "Nonverbal Communication" in Chapter 2, "Interacting with Your Dog").

Never use synthetic scents. Like synthetic food (canned and dry) and synthetic vitamins and minerals, synthetic oils are missing "life energy," so they should never be used in veterinary aromatherapy. The "real stuff" comes from living things and thus has a direct link with the earth, a subtle energy that can't be duplicated in a laboratory. The energies of these plant materials merge with our own and those of our dogs to support healing. For example, genuine rose oil envelops us in scent and guides us through a field of flowers, just like the aroma of fresh roses. A synthetic rose oil contains nothing living; it would probably give you a headache and repel your dog.

Essential oils should always be sold in dark bottles. Citrus oils can deteriorate easily and become too terpene rich to be used on animals. Be careful with them.

Keep essential oils away from strong light, heat, air, and moisture. Never let any living thing drink them. Watch for allergic reactions, and be sure dogs, cats, and children don't have direct access to the oils. And take care with your choice of houseplants, as some are poisonous to dogs and cats, who may nibble on them if the scent is attractive. See the brief discusion on poisonous plants (page 56).

Chapter Six

Hands-on Healing

A NUMBER OF hands-on therapeutic interventions normally associated with human healing are also beneficial to dogs. Any therapy you choose is usually welcomed if you approach your companion animal with honor and respect. Consult your holistic veterinarian before embarking on any course of treatment and remember that the foundation for these treatments is the fresh food diet. Optimum results cannot be achieved if your dog's diet is overlooked. For further information about any of the treatments described in this chapter, see "Resources."

CHIROPRACTIC

FOR AT LEAST a hundred years, humankind has been helped by chiropractic therapy, even though the profession has been maligned and discriminated against by the American Medical Association (AMA), many of whose member physicians believe alternative therapies are practiced by "quacks" and are not based on scientific principles. Since alternative health care is perceived as a threat to allopathic doctors' income, it's in their best financial interests, along with those of the pharmaceutical companies, to discourage us from seeking alternatives. Most physicians and veterinarians opposed to chiropractic have no direct experience with it.

The basic principle of chiropractic, whether for people or for animals, is to work with the peripheral nerves at the root level, which is where the nerves exit between vertebrae. The nerves are very sensitive to pressure there, and the spine can get sprained just like any other joint. A misalignment, or *subluxation,* between two vertebrae puts pressure on the nerve root, thus interfering with its function. This pinched nerve is usually accompanied by pain but may also cause a functional problem.

Chiropractic Treatment for Your Dog

CHIROPRACTIC IS ANOTHER method that treats the whole being. Dr. Christina Chambreau maintains that this modality is one of the best ways to help an animal being treated homeopathically. Applying chiropractic to dogs is not such a strange idea: they have many of the same musculoskeletal problems we do. A chiropractor trained in animal anatomy can work effectively to restore healthy functioning to your animal companions.

Sharon Willoughby, D.V.M., enrolled in chiropractic school and learned that when a dog's vertebrae (the bones that protect the spinal cord) are out of alignment, they keep the spinal cord from sending certain nerve impulses to the rest of the body. When some of the vital parts of the dog's body get cut off from these impulses, the dog can become ill. He can be in intense pain. He can have difficulty moving. The chiropractor works to realign the vertebrae by applying gentle force to the spine, tail, knees, shoulders, and other areas of the body. When a dog's vertebrae are out of alignment, the joint caps stretch. The surrounding muscles may go into a spasm. This can be very painful.

If you notice that your dog persistently chews at a spot, perhaps on his chest or back, he may be trying to tell you something about his physical state. You may think you're dealing with an attitude problem, but when dogs hurt, they have a very limited means of communicating their pain.

Chiropractic can treat certain internal disorders as well. Dr. Willoughby cautions that chiropractic is most helpful when an internal disorder has just begun. In advanced cases, it's usually not as effective. Chiropractic isn't the correct treatment for fractures, infectious diseases, abscesses, or blocked urinary tracts. It's best to have a veterinarian examine the animal before you try chiropractic therapy. Often X rays are needed to determine whether there's a fracture or some other reason the animal should not be adjusted by a chiropractor.

Veterinary schools don't teach chiropractic, and chiropractic schools teach how to work on people, not animals. So in 1989 Dr. Willoughby founded the American Veterinary Chiropractic Association (AVCA). A hundred-hour course in animal chiropractic is available to both veterinarians and chiropractors. After certification, practitioners may take postgraduate courses. In 1991 twenty AVCA-certified practitioners were accredited in the United States, with another forty working toward accreditation.

Because chiropractic is a very sophisticated science, find a practitioner who is AVCA-certified and trained. An unqualified practitioner may inadvertently do great harm to the animal's skeletal system. A thrust at the wrong angle could injure the joints permanently.

Prior to making an adjustment, the chiropractor needs to observe how the animal stands, moves his head, walks, and turns, as well as how he behaves or reacts, in order to determine where soreness occurs. Sometimes the practitioner must work on parts of the body that are already painful to the touch. Dr. Willoughby teaches her clients how to massage animal companions at home between visits, so the animal will be more relaxed during the next treatment and she can more easily make her adjustments.

Network Chiropractic

CREATED BY Donald Epstein, D.C., in New York, network chiropractic pulls together the various approaches to this modality. I was first introduced to it by Mark Haverkos, D.V.M., who spent six years with the Hopi as their veterinarian. In addition to network chiropractic, he also practices homeopathy, acupuncture, and herbal medicine. In 1993 he demonstrated his network chiropractic techniques at the American Holistic Veterinary Medical Association (AHVMA) conference.

As we become aware of our body, according to Dr. Haverkos, we begin to realize that all its parts are related, that they're all part of a single system. Rather than viewing a body as something that needs to be fixed (a view held by conventional medicine), network chiropractic aims to remind all the particles of the body that they're relatives and deserve a loving relationship with one another.

Dr. Haverkos learned from the Hopi that everything happens for a reason. Animals do the best they can to adapt to whatever conditions prevail, and their current physical state reflects these conditions. Just as the Hopi know that less is more, so do practitioners of network chiropractic. They don't need a heavy hand, but simply a specific intent, so the body can make positive use of the energy offered.

If a chiropractor tries to force the spine into "normal" alignment (the problem with traditional chiropractic), it will quickly revert to misalignment. Network chiropractic seeks to discover why the bones are aligned the way they are, and then it seeks to release some of the chaos that caused the misalignment so the body can move on to another level.

Dr. Haverkos asks animals' permission to work on them before he begins, rather than imposing himself. This request need not be in words, which aren't our highest form of interaction (see "Nonverbal Communication" in Chapter 2, "Interacting with Your Dog"). When beginning a treatment, Dr. Haverkos feels himself "resonating" energetically and spiritually with his patient. He can actually sense, in his own body, what he does to the animal.

Certain manipulations provoke particular emotional responses. Though we think of animals as being present in the moment, their spines may tell a different story. For example, an abused animal (perhaps one rescued from a shelter) may have been dishonored by a human being, and thus, on an energetic level, he may be stuck in the past. During a network treatment, emotions associated with such mistreatment may come up and be released. Dogs respond very quickly to this kind of therapy.

Dr. Haverkos does nearly all his adjustments on standing animals. As he feels down the spine, he asks the animals how they feel, whether they feel heat or a sticking sensation, for example. He palpates the musculature and asks himself, "Does it feel smooth or rubbery?" He advises practitioners not to think too much but rather just to feel.

Even if you can't find a network chiropractor, you can learn to "resonate" with your animal to facilitate his well-being. Gently feel your dog's muscle tone. Watch the way he moves and how he looks at you as you go over his body. Watch him breathe—his breathing should have a nice, rhythmic flow. If it catches somewhere, there's a blockage, a residue from the past. Trust your senses. Such observation may give you insight into his homeopathic type and so may lead to the appropriate remedy. Or you may feel he needs acupuncture or some other intervention.

ACUPUNCTURE

ACUPUNCTURE, A TECHNIQUE that stimulates specific points in the body to rectify imbalances, originated some 3500 years ago in China.[1] According to legend, thousands of years ago someone noticed that lame warhorses, when wounded by arrows in certain spots, would stop limping. (Another legend tells a similar tale about humans.) The same spots were stimulated in other lame horses, who also stopped limping.

After the energy pathways of the body were discovered and mapped, it was concluded that any disruption of the energy flow, qi (or chi), caused disease. Placing small needles along exact points on these energy pathways was found to enhance the flow of qi and promote a state of health. So, in essence, acupuncture is simply another means to help the body heal itself. Originally, stone needles were used. Today acupuncturists may choose from among metal needles, heat, pressure, massage, electrical stimulation, injections, magnets, gold beads, lasers, or any combination of the above.

Human and veterinary acupuncture began separately, using different charts. The human charts show a system of interconnected pathways (meridians and collaterals) through which flows the energy of the body. Hundreds of acupuncture points are spread throughout these pathways. Identification of animal meridians was less complete, and their points were usually given different names, even when their location and function seemed identical to human ones. Charts were developed primarily for farm animals, especially horses, chickens, pigs, and water buffalo. Today in China, though cats and dogs are treated with acupuncture, the emphasis is still on farm animals.[2]

Impressed by research and clinical results, the American Veterinary Medical Association sanctioned further study of acupuncture as a valid method of treatment in 1989. Many holistic veterinarians now embrace this technique in their practice. To become a certified veterinary acupuncturist, a practitioner must complete a four-month-long training course accredited by the International Veterinary Acupuncture Society (see "Resources"), pass an oral and written exam, and submit a complete report of a successful acupuncture case.

Dr. Richard Pitcairn, who is primarily a homeopath, speaks positively about acupuncture and Eastern medicine. He tells us that the Chinese advocate the holistic approach as a means of preventing disease. They resort to acupuncture and herbs when their preferred methods—meditation, exercise, diet, and massage—have proved insufficient. Although acupuncture, like Western medicine, may be used to treat symptoms alone, the best approach is to correct the underlying imbalances that created the conditions fostering specific diseases. Therefore, most contemporary acupuncturists emphasize a total approach to health.

"The basic theory behind this comprehensive system," says Dr. Pitcairn, "is that the fundamental energy fields that compose the body (as well as all aspects of the universe) manifest two poles which are actually expressions of one whole."[3] The Chinese refer to these poles as *yin* and *yang*. They are opposites, not looked upon as good or evil. (Yang is masculine and active, and yin is feminine and passive.) For good health, we need to achieve a proper balance between these two extremes.

As John Ihor Basko, D.V.M., reaches deeper levels of mastery with acupuncture, he often discovers that the more you know, the more you don't know. "Oriental medicine comes from [the insight] that ultimately we don't know how the body works, and nature cannot be explained by the mind. You can't always go by the recipe." Sometimes Dr. Basko gets a hunch to put a needle in a certain point without knowing why, then later he will read about it and discover how it was appropriate. Ultimately, any improvement seems to be due to a rebalancing of the entire body and mind.[4]

Acupuncture and Your Dog

AS WITH HOMEOPATHY, it's important to glean as much information about the dog's general habits, attitude, background, and family life before commencing treatment. The placement of the needles may be determined according to such factors as the personality and characteristics of the dog, the time of day the problem occurs, and the kind of weather that makes it worse.

During the physical exam, the anatomy of the dog is examined, as are acupuncture points along the backbone. A specific point may be tender or painful when a dog has a problem with certain organs or the meridians associated with that point. Some veterinary acupuncturists, including Dr. Nancy Scanlan, use traditional tests such as blood panels, X rays, and stool tests to help them assess the animal's condition.

Animal acupuncture is used to treat arthritis, spinal and disc problems, kidney disorders, metabolic imbalances, aging disorders, cataracts, asthma, and allergic dermatitis. It can be helpful in unblocking obstructed urethras in unneutered males and may be used during surgical emergencies for shock and respiratory arrest, in treating infertility, and to build immune response. Have your acupuncturist show you how to needle the emergency rescue point; nonbreathing puppies and kittens can sometimes be resuscitated this way.

Acupuncture has also been used in place of an anesthetic; studies have shown that endorphins and enkephalins (the body's natural pain relievers) are released when certain acupuncture points are stimulated. However, restraining an animal anesthetized by this means is problematic because it does not make him sleepy.

Relief of ailments often comes after only one acupuncture treatment, but it usually takes at least three visits before dramatic results are seen. The most difficult thing about acupuncture, as with homeopathy, is that some animals may get worse before they get better. But once they weather the crisis, their improvement may be quite dramatic and enduring. Says Diane Stein, "In veterinary use, the method is described as giving successful cures in seventy to seventy-five percent of animal cases, many of them listed as incurable by standard veterinary medicine."[5]

You may wonder how your dog will tolerate acupuncture. Many holistic veterinarians report that dogs and cats who resist treatment on the first session often prove extremely cooperative in subsequent visits. Many times the animal lets the practitioner know where it hurts and then relaxes throughout the treatment. If your dog resists acupuncture, please don't force him to be "needled." Try just one point and come back another day. Dr. Scanlan wrote an article in *Natural Pet Magazine*[6] about acupuncture that states the case well for this treatment:

Acupuncture is performed by stimulating specific points on the body, usually by using needles. They can also be stimulated with a small current, massage, heat, injections, implants, or other methods. These points have the ability to alter various conditions in the body in order to achieve a desired effect. Acupuncture has been used successfully for nearly 5,000 years on animals as well as humans. As a matter of fact, it is still the treatment of choice for one-quarter of the world's population for many problems. It is now being utilized by an increasing number of veterinarians for various conditions. It is not a cure-all but, where indicated, it works well.

Dr. Scanlan continues,

Some people look askance on acupuncture. The idea that needles can do anything but cause pain is hard to imagine, and the choice of acupuncture points looks like voodoo to some. When I found out that anyone can find an acupuncture point by measuring the electrical resistance of the skin, I realized that there might be some foundation to what I thought was superstition. Acupuncture points have a lower electrical resistance than do other points on the body. The resistance is further changed when there is a problem in the area of the body that the point corresponds to. There are instruments called "point finders," which are just ohm meters, measuring electrical resistance. These are used to find and treat acupuncture points.

Another problem that people have in understanding acupuncture is how a point on the hand can have anything to do with something as far away as the heart. Western medicine has already recognized the phenomenon of referred pain, in which a problem in an organ is felt as pain somewhere else. Most people are aware that during a heart attack, people often feel pain starting in their shoulder and traveling down the left arm. When cattle have a problem in the reticulum (one of their four stomachs), they feel it as pain in their breastbone area. Acupuncture points work in a similar way, often showing unusual sensitivity when a corresponding organ is damaged or diseased.

There has been legitimate research by physicians and veterinarians in the United States, Canada, and Western Europe as well as in Asian countries, that has shown specific effects obtained by stimulating specific points. These effects include:

- increase of circulation to an area
- decrease of inflammation
- release of endorphins (body's natural painkillers)
- relief of muscle spasms
- stimulation of the body's immune system
- release of hormones
- release of various substances in the brain and spinal cord

Because of this research, and because of the beneficial results achieved many times over by veterinary acupuncturists, the American Veterinary Medical Association has recognized acupuncture as a valid treatment for animals, when performed by properly trained professionals.

Acupuncture works especially well for conditions involving nerves, muscles, bones, and joints. Arthritis is one of the most common conditions treated by acupuncture in my practice. Animals that come to me usually have been through all other available treatments, and nothing else is working like it used to. The choice is acupuncture or euthanasia. With acupuncture, about 80 percent of these animals respond well enough that they have an additional year of quality life, sometimes longer, before age catches up with them again. These animals may need continuous treatments as often as once a week to once a month.

Guido was an aptly-named German shepherd cross who came to me for treatment of arthritis in his lower back, along with neck and shoulder pain. His owner warned me that Guido didn't like veterinarians, and I spent the first visit hanging on to the scruff of his neck so he couldn't bite me. I placed needles as we circled around each other, him lunging for me, and me lunging for acupuncture points. On his second visit, he sat in front of me, begging with his eyes, as if I were holding a special tidbit. On the third visit, he sat on my feet with his back toward me so I couldn't get away without doing something to that back. He has been that way ever since.

Another group of animals with arthritis come to me because their owners don't want to use cortisone any longer. This group is usually a little younger and healthier, and about 90 percent will show improvement. In about two-thirds of these cases, the improvement varies from satisfactory to excellent. In one-third there is not as much improvement, and owners may prefer to use other treatments instead of or along with acupuncture. The amount of improvement does not correspond to the animal's response to other drugs, so the only way to know whether it will work for your pet is to try it. Once this group starts improvement, additional treatment is usually required at intervals anywhere from once a month to once a year.

Mugs, the boxer, started coming to me because his guardian's livelihood had been saved by acupuncture. His guardian was a professional bowler who hurt his back, and whose doctor told him he couldn't bowl for at least six months, and maybe forever. With acupuncture he started bowling within weeks, and with occasional "tune-ups" he has had no problems for years. Mugs has hip problems and a bad back. At first he needed weekly sessions, but now I see him about every six months, when he lets his owners know he needs help.

Acupuncture is also used for nerve damage, disc disease, long-term injuries, lameness, some skin problems, and other long-term illnesses. Any problem that overwhelms an animal quickly, such as parvovirus in dogs, needs to be taken care of much more quickly. In these cases, it may not be safe to wait for acupuncture.

When you take an animal in for acupuncture treatment, he will be examined as usual, and a complete record of his problem will be obtained. You may be asked questions that other veterinarians don't often ask, such as whether he seeks heat or cold, seems to want company or wants to be alone, and other things that may not make sense to you. Traditional Chinese medicine is involved with the whole animal, not just the leg (or back or wherever the main problem is), and sometimes these other questions can make a difference.

Dr. Scanlan offers the following story[7] to illustrate the benefits of acupuncture for our animal companions and the necessity of treating the whole animal, not just the body:

One of my patients was brought to me because she was following her owners around and didn't want to let them out of her sight. Utah didn't want to go outside, and when she did, she went out just long enough to go to the bathroom and then immediately want back in the house. She always had been attached to her owners, but she had gotten to the point where they felt obliged to stay home for the dog's peace of mind. She was a Doberman, a little too big to carry around or take easily on car rides.

I X-rayed Utah and found arthritis of one hip. I treated her with acupuncture for the hip problem, and she was slightly improved one week later but still followed her owners everywhere. I then stimulated some very strong yang points to treat the clinging behavior (an excess yin characteristic). The next week I found a very yang dog (opposite of yin) who was boisterous and wanted to be outside all the time, avoiding her owners. Once she got through this stage and things were back in balance, she was back to her old self. In addition, a lick granuloma (a nonhealing sore that dogs create by constant licking) that she had had for seven years healed up and never came back.

Most often, acupuncture is accomplished by inserting needles into the acupuncture points. The needles used are smaller in diameter than anything normally used to give injections. Once in place, they are not painful, and most animals relax or even fall asleep during treatment. Other methods may be used also—which can be troublesome for some animals—including electrically stimulating a point, injecting a solution into a point, heating the point, massaging the point, and implanting gold beads at the point (this is usually done under an anesthetic).

The owners of three of my patients tell me I'm the only veterinarian they don't try to bite. Others may still be nervous about coming, but with each treatment, they're less nervous, not worse. One dog whom I see at the same time every week brings his leash to his owners and gets excited every week before it's time to visit the doctor.

I wish more conventional veterinarians were open to referring their patients to alternative practitioners when their own methods fail. Many use steroids to rescue animals from acute or life-threatening episodes, but the practice gets out of hand when they prescribe these powerful drugs routinely for chronic conditions. Steroids are known to lead to the loss of normal function in the adrenal glands, which regulate so many body processes essential for a long and healthy life. Furthermore, these substances don't cure; they merely get rid of symptoms. However, animals that have long suffered with chronic disease, such as arthritis, often get safe relief through acupuncture, especially if nutrition and other holistic treatments are included in the healing regimen.

I personally have had great results with acupuncture for my own health problems from time to time and find it to be a wonderful experience. My practitioner uses aromatherapy along with the acupuncture treatment, and for me this is a lovely addition. Perhaps veterinary acupuncturists could employ this mode of healing, too.

Some Common Acupressure Treatments for Your Dog

ALAN M. SCHOEN, D.V.M. (author of *Love, Miracles, and Animal Healing*), wrote an informative piece on acupuncture and acupressure wherein he states that you should always consult a veterinary acupuncturist to deal with serious illness, but he also offers the layperson some simple acupressure techniques to do at home.[8] He recommends that you study six critical acupoints to relieve temporary distress and give the animal some relief in times of crisis. There are two emergency points and four master points known to have generalized beneficial effects on the body; they can also be helpful for particular diseases.

First, it is important, according to Dr. Schoen, to use the tip of your index finger or thumb to apply pressure to the specific acupoint. Press firmly but gently. If you get a "flinching" reaction, or the animal cries out, you're probably pressing too hard.

Second, for relaxation, rub in a circular motion counterclockwise over the acupoint. To stimulate, rub clockwise.

Dr. Schoen uses human descriptions of acupoints such as knee, elbow, hand, or foot and suggests we visualize the dog standing up on tiptoes on his hind legs like a human.

This method of treatment does not negate the need for emergency veterinary care, which should, of course, be sought immediately.

Acupoint #1 is known as the emergency point for cardiac arrest, Governing Vessel 26, or GV26. This point is centered just below the nose and above the upper lip. Animal guardians may give a series of sharp jabs to this point for cardiac arrest or shock. Dr. Schoen suggests the finger or a needle to stimulate the fight-or-flight surge of adrenaline (also called epinephrine). If this is done early on, the chances are good that the animal will recover.

However, never stimulate this point in this manner on a conscious animal or you risk getting bitten. You may perform this procedure on newborn pups (if they are having difficulty breathing or, for that matter, are not breathing at all).

Acupoint #2 is the emergency point for asthma attacks. It is what the Chinese refer to as Lung 7, or LU7. It is located on the inside of the front paw just above the wrist bone. Not all animals respond to this, so emergency procedures may be called for immediately. Dr. Schoen tells us that "in a pinch, having an alternative like LU7 might save you and your pet hours of anguish."

Acupoint #3 is the master point for an upset stomach or other gastrointestinal complaint. It is located just below the knee on the outside of the shinbone in a depression where the muscle of the lower leg joins the knee. Dr. Schoen recommends exerting pressure at Stomach 36, or ST36, with your fingertips to help relieve gastrointestinal problems. The Chinese have a special name for this very special spot, "Walk Three Miles," presumably because of the increased energy received once this point is stimulated.

Acupoint #4 is the master point for head- and neckache. The acupoint is known as Large Intestine 4, or LI4, and is located on the hand (front paw) near the point where the thumb and index finger meet. I use this often on myself. It is also known as a "longevity" point because it increases microcirculation, contributing to a longer, healthier life (according to Chinese tradition). Stimulating this acupoint may soothe a painful neck, front legs, or shoulders. It also helps nasal congestion, diarrhea, or constipation. Try it on yourself for headaches.

Dr. Schoen warns that some animals don't like their paws fussed with, so be respectful. If your dog gets aggressive when his toes are touched, you probably want to avoid massaging them.

It's always advisable to have a veterinary diagnosis prior to administering acupressure. If your animal is undergoing acupuncture, clear this procedure with your practitioner first.

Acupoint #5 is the master point for the immune system, allergies, and metabolic imbalance. This acupoint is known as Large Intestine 11, or LI11, and is located on the outside of the elbow joint where the biceps join the forearm. The Chinese refer to this point as *qu chi* or "Pond-in-the-Curve" because it is located in the curve in the elbow. When this point is stimulated with pressure, pain in the shoulder and elbow can be reduced. This is a critical spot for arthritis discomfort.

Acupoint #6 is the master point for endocrine disorder. Spleen 6, or SP6, can work wonders for menstrual cramps in humans. However, when this point, on the inside of the foot on the rear legs just to the front and above the heel, is stimulated on animals, it can be of benefit to diabetes sufferers as well as those with other endocrine disturbances.

Dr. Schoen advises that acupressure is not a substitute for needle treatment, which goes deeper and provides a stronger stimulation, but he does not discount the potent healing possibilities of acupressure—not to mention the loving connection we can make with our animal companions through this practice.

ACUPOINT CHART

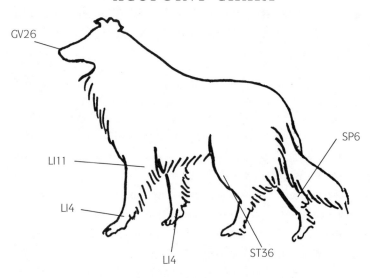

GV26

LI11

LI4

LI4

SP6

ST36

THERAPEUTIC TOUCH

THERAPEUTIC TOUCH (T-TOUCH) therapy, a method devised by Linda Tellington-Jones, is a type of nonverbal communication through cellular memory. The practitioner speaks to the cellular intelligence in her hands, which in turn speaks to the cells in the body. When working on animals, simply placing our hands on the body and moving them in a circular manner creates a kind of kinesthetic (sensory) interspecies communication. Tellington-Jones addresses the issues surrounding Therapeutic Touch in her books, articles, and videotapes (see "Resources").

Many holistic veterinarians employ Therapeutic Touch to calm and soothe their patients prior to therapy. Circular touch (generally clockwise) is done gently all over the body and sends the caregiver valuable information concerning the dog's state of well-being. Moreover, the circular method provides the animal with all four types of brain waves (alpha, theta, beta, and delta). Dr. Chambreau feels that this therapy supports animals under homeopathic treatment, and she has heard of excellent results through the use of this treatment for behavioral problems as well as severe physical problems. Tellington-Jones cannot explain scientifically how Therapeutic Touch works; nevertheless, it does.

Tellington-Jones initially studied the Feldenkrais method, which opens new neurological pathways to the brain through the use of nonhabitual movements.[9] Tellington-Jones then developed her own techniques based on Feldenkrais's work, beginning with the concept that every cell in the body knows its function. Using the circular movement, when done with respect, increases the speed of healing at the cellular level.

Animals may actually be born with habitual holding patterns, but even the most resistant animals respond to this technique and learn to release their stuck energy. Tellington-Jones has even been successful in changing an animal's self-image and increasing his self-confidence.

Allow your hands to find their own way as they communicate with the cells of your animal companion. Try to tune in to his breathing and his response to your touch. You may find your own breathing falls into sync with your dog's. The caregiver need not do anything more than concentrate on making the circles and on sensing the animal's response. And, as always, approach your dog with respect.

I imagine the face of a clock as I touch my animal. The spot where you begin is six o'clock. Gently push the skin clockwise all the way around, past six, and finish at nine. At nine o'clock, I pause and begin again in another spot. It's important to maintain a constant pressure and close the circles. I use my middle three fingers and make 1¼ circles at each spot, then I move on and repeat the procedure. I rest my thumb and pinkie against the animal's body to steady my hand.

At the beginning of each session, the speed of your circles should be about one per second. As you feel your dog entering a state of bodily listening, slow down to one circle every two seconds. Don't do the same area twice, and don't connect three circles in a row (which we all tend to do initially). Remember to lift your fingers as you close each circle and begin again. You may also use your left hand. Tellington-Jones has found her right hand to be more effective, but she has trained herself to use both hands.

Tellington-Jones calls this massage method circular touch. It generates an energetic release, what she calls the "clouded leopard touch." The circular motion seems to imprint on the animal's cells more than simple petting or stroking, which although loving and beneficial, doesn't seem to activate the cellular awareness in the same way.

Tellington-Jones also makes little butterfly motions, a kind of touch-and-lift maneuver. Remember, nothing is gained through force. This healing technique enables people and animals to release fear and replace it with trust. Experiment to find the optimal pressure; it may vary from very light, with just one finger, to somewhat heavier, using the entire hand. Be gentler, of course, in areas where the animal feels pain. You shouldn't get tired doing this; it should benefit you as much as it does your animal companion. Stroke your animal's ears. Many of us do this instinctively. Like most major breakthroughs, this technique is so simple that you may be doing it without even knowing you're healing. However, it becomes even more effective when you do it intentionally. Let your fingers lead you, but don't forget the ears. It's often the best place to start. Work the area of the muzzle and move inside the mouth (working the gums calms the fight-or-flight mechanism). Also work the hindquarters and neck. Do short sessions (fifteen minutes is fine) on a daily basis.

When using Therapeutic Touch, we become focused and grounded and thus focus and ground our animals, rather than just offering a few absentminded strokes. When we are fully present, our animal companions allow us to connect with them in a profound way, so much deeper than with words. Touch is basic to both our species and theirs, and may even extend life.

A Therapeutic Touch video for dogs is available (see "Resources"), and courses are offered frequently around the country.

REIKI—UNIVERSAL LIFE FORCE ENERGY

PROFOUND HEALING IS possible through the power of touch. The Reiki practitioner, an initiated individual, channels energy in the form of a pure white light to heal the sick. Reiki originated in Tibet thousands of years ago, and its history may be traced through India, Egypt, Ephesus, Greece, Rome, China, and Japan to the United States.

Reiki differs from Therapeutic Touch in that it isn't dependent on the energy clarity or healing ability of the practitioner, who only serves as a conduit for the flow of pure white light. Thus, no negative energy may be absorbed by the healer or transferred from the healer to the subject. In Therapeutic Touch the intensity and effectiveness of the healing varies with the state of the healer; moreover, the healer needs protection from negative forces and energies and should center and focus meditatively when working.

But the Reiki initiation involves a series of four "attunements," which activate and set the energy path in the individual; this energy path remains active for life. It runs from the crown chakra of the individual through his or her chakra system and ultimately to his or her hands (for a detailed explanation of chakras, see "The Aura and Chakras of a Dog," p. 273). Whenever an initiated individual touches anything alive, the Reiki energy automatically flows through his or her hands, with no effort or expenditure of energy on his or her part.

Three levels are available. First-degree Reiki activates the healing energy so that it flows when anything is physically touched. Second-degree Reiki activates the energy so that it flows when certain symbols are activated by the Reiki practitioner, who can activate healing at a distance, without physically being present; the practice of second-degree Reiki heightens the power of the energy tenfold. Third-degree Reiki activates the healing energy that sets the Reiki pathways in another individual, allowing the Reiki master to initiate others.

The Reiki method may be used on plants, animals, people (from babies to elders), even on mechanical things such as cars and computers. It has been shown to be effective in treating anything from mild imbalances to life-threatening illnesses. You may learn more about this modality by reading *The Reiki Handbook: A Manual for Students and Therapists of the Usui Shiko Ryoho System of Healing* or by contacting Eleanor Haspel-Portner, Ph.D. (see "Resources").

Dr. Portner, also a psychologist and an accomplished astrologer, felt that I'd be able to make good use of this healing therapy in my work with animals. During my initiation, one of her own cats became very vocal, jumped into my lap, and nudged me. I saw in my mind's eye (or through my third eye) a pyramid with a white light coming up and out through the top of my head, and then great bursts of purple, magenta, and rose. My body went from cold to warm, and my hands felt energized. That evening I read the material Dr. Portner had given me and practiced on one of my kittens, which had injured her ankle slightly by jumping down from the cat tree. Within a day she was healed.

Dr. Portner told me the story of her introduction to Reiki. After the first attunement, she was instructed to do the first four Reiki positions on herself at home that night. When she awoke the next morning, she noted that she could see without her glasses (she has severe myopia). After the second attunement, her perfect vision lasted even longer.

Dr. Portner (by then a Reiki master) and her family worked on their cat Tippy, who had a malignant tumor, from a distance while he was in surgery and in the days following. Much to the surgeon's surprise, Tippy recovered with amazing speed and without any negative effects. At another time Dr. Portner's elderly cat Noble was near death and was being given fluids by his veterinarians. The family did round-the-clock Reiki on him, sustaining him until they could find a veterinarian able to intervene. Within twenty-four hours, he was stable and proceeded to recover.

In recent times, many factions have developed in the Reiki organization. Be careful in your choice of practitioners, since not all individuals who claim to teach Reiki have the keys to do the attunements, and some people who claim to teach Reiki don't even realize that a specific attunement process is required to set the energy path. If you have a desire to learn Reiki firsthand, check holistic publications for lectures or seminars near you.

MASSAGE THERAPY

ANIMAL MASSAGE TECHNIQUES are described in both *The Magic of Massage,* by Ouida West (one section), and *The Healing Touch,* by Michael Fox (the entire book). Fox suggests the following sequence: feet and paws, legs, abdomen (when pregnant animals are in labor, I use the same effleurage movement of little butterfly circles on the belly that I learned in my own Lamaze natural childbirth classes), torso, spine, and neck, head, and ears. Since touch seems to be such an important conduit in the human/animal bond, it's no wonder that it can be an important healing element.

SUMMING UP TOUCH

TOUCH THERAPY OF any kind is also an excellent way to help us get closer and strengthen the bonds with our animal companions. But never force an animal to accept any hands-on work (see also Chapter 7, "Other Healing Approaches")—let him tell you how much is okay with him, and for how long.

Here's what many touch therapists recommend. Hold your hands, if your dog will allow it, on any one of the seven chakras or on a painful spot. See if you can let positive healing energy flow from you through your right hand into your dog, and let any negative or painful energy flow from the dog into your left hand. (If you are more comfortable using the opposite hands, this is fine, too.) Then—and this is very important for your self-care as a healer—shake your hands to release any negative energy from your body. Let the dog rest comfortably and use this healing in his own way.

Chapter Seven

Other Healing Approaches

VETERINARY ENERGY MEDICINE

A CHANGE IN energy precedes a change in structure. Dr. Joanne Stefanatos believes that as we understand more and more about the workings of the body, medicine will be increasingly energy based, instead of relying on drugs and surgery.[1] Robert Becker, M.D., and Strom Nordenstrom have demonstrated that electrons flow through the body in complex circuits at the cellular level and that in many disease conditions the flow of electrons changes. Likewise, Kirlian photography presents evidence that a halo, or aura, of energy surrounds every living thing and that disruptions in this aura may be associated with various disorders.

An electroacupuncture biofeedback instrument can detect pathological dysfunctions in animals before any physical conditions or symptoms arise. Using such technology, veterinarians in the future will be able to recognize potential danger signs, pinpointing and eliminating disease-producing toxins from the body long before they can become destructive. Most agree that when this form of medicine is readily available, we'll look back on invasive procedures such as surgery and vaccinations as if they were from the Dark Ages. Until then, our only alternative is to think constantly about prevention.

Below are described some of the modalities that apply principles of energy to healing. See "Resources" for further information about these techniques. As always, consult your holistic veterinarian before implementing any therapy.

Light and Color Healing

THE HISTORY OF light and color healing is both extensive and impressive. Records found in the Pyramids revealed that the Egyptians used colors to heal with great success. The Rosicrucian Society has used color therapy since the fifteenth century. Edward D. Babbitt, author of *The Principles of Light and Color*, told of the many values of color healing nearly a century ago; noted spiritualist Edgar Cayce also wrote of its benefits. More than two dozen significant twentieth-century works have expounded on this therapy.

Einstein proved that light is an electromagnetic phenomenon and that color is a manifestation of the vibration of light waves at distinct and measurable frequencies; each color has its own frequency. White light contains all colors, as seen in a rainbow or prism. The primary colors of white light are red, blue, and green; the secondary colors are yellow (a combination of red and green), cyan (green and blue), and magenta (red and blue). See Chapter 8, "Astromedicine for Your Dog," for the correlation of colors to the sun signs of the zodiac.

The colors of an aura vary depending on the condition of the being. A vitamin and mineral deficiency, for example, would affect the aura colors. Vitamins themselves possess color:

vitamin A is yellow, B vitamins are orange and red, vitamin C is lemon yellow, vitamin D is violet, vitamin E is scarlet and magenta, and vitamin K is indigo. In addition, each *chakra,* or energy center, in the body has its own frequency, color, and harmonic note. Cats and dogs, like humans, have seven chakras, each of which corresponds to a color.

Dr. Stefanatos refers to light as waveforms or pockets of energy cells (*photons,* particles that travel at the speed of light). Light carries information; sunlight carries all the wavelengths of the color spectrum, including infrared and ultraviolet (UVA) light, which are not visible to the human eye. The sun's rays are absorbed by the aura of the body and, through the chakras, penetrate the body itself. At the cellular level, DNA traps light within the water molecules of an organism. Thus, sunlight resonates within the body to create glowing health.[2]

Though many practitioners may not be aware of it, all healing systems depend upon the body's chemical reaction, which produces color and brings about a change in body function. Stanley Burroughs, author of *Healing for the Age of Enlightenment,* tells us that a human burn victim or someone running a high fever has a surplus of red, which relates to the element hydrogen. When a blue light (related to oxygen) is projected, the two elements combine, producing water—in this case perspiration. Thus, blue is apparently cooling; it lowers the fever and cools the burn.[3] However, when color is integrated into the body through medications (generally allopathic), there's a danger of side effects in functions such as digestion, ingestion, and oxidation.

How can you use color therapy at home with your animal? Dr. Stefanatos suggests that you surround him with color in the form of bedding, blankets, collars (you might even use colored kerchiefs for whimsy, if he'll tolerate it), or harnesses. Through color, you can introduce energy that assists in the elimination of waste and congestion. Color, many healers feel, can also repair damage done by illness and injury.

By wrapping a jug of water in red plastic wrap and leaving it in the sunshine for about twelve hours, you can create energized water, which Dr. Stefanatos says boosts the immune system and acts as a blood builder. Other colors produce different effects. Green-energized water stabilizes; yellow treats constipation problems. Note that the water doesn't actually become colored; it is merely energized by color.

Dr. Stefanatos uses colored utility lights to treat her animal patients, clipping the appropriately colored light onto the animal's cage and turning it on it as often as she deems necessary. She uses only Dura Test Vita lightbulbs at her hospital, because they provide the full spectrum of visible light along with UVA rays; these bulbs may be purchased, along with a compatible holder, at hardware stores and some health-food stores.

If your dog has a painful area, use the color green on the area for ten minutes, followed by the color red, which stimulates the immune system and decreases pain. You can use pieces of colored fabric to make a kind of color compress.

For stress, Dr. Stefanatos suggests using blue, which stimulates the pituitary gland and decreases anxiety, over the sixth chakra (at the brow, or third eye). A cool color, blue also reduces nerve paralysis and may be used to treat mange, eye problems, or an itchy rash (hot spots). Blue light also helps dogs to sleep.

I provide color therapy for my animal companions by making their beds the appropriate colors. A wonderful seamstress, my mother, Helene Yarnall, makes colored slipcovers for the beds, which I change as needed. She also designs the exhibition-cage curtains for my show cats, selecting colors that both soothe the animals and show them off.

As you can see, color is important to our well-being and healing, as well as to that of our animals. In addition to being beneficial, color therapy has no harmful side effects.

THE AURA AND CHAKRAS OF A DOG

THE AURA IS made up of four bodies (see page 275): the physical body (and, just above it, the etheric double), the emotional body, the mental body (two layers—higher and lower), and the spiritual body (three layers—higher, middle, and lower). Dr. Stefanatos explains that the chakras are aligned along a spiral column in the etheric double, and energy is absorbed from the surrounding air and brought through the chakras into the physical body.

The ancient clairvoyants saw the seven major chakras as spinning wheels of light (*chakra* means "wheel" in Sanskrit). The various spiritual schools have different ways of identifying the chakras, but a widely accepted version delineates seven major chakras, beginning with the first, or root, chakra located at the base of the spine and moving up the body to the seventh, or crown, chakra located a few inches above the top of the head. (There are also five minor chakras, at the hands and feet/paws and the hollow at the base of the skull, where the brain meets the spine.) A color is associated with each chakra.

First chakra (root/base of spine): Red stimulates the immune system by building up the blood and detoxifying it. This color fights tumors, has an antiviral effect, and relates to the reproductive system and the procreative imperative to survive. Dogs with compromised immune systems should be surrounded by the color red as much as possible.

Second chakra (qi/below navel): Orange is an appetite stimulant and a lung builder. It depresses the parathyroid glands and stimulates the thyroid as well as the mammary glands in the production of milk. The qi emanates from this chakra.

Third chakra (solar plexus): Yellow stimulates the gastrointestinal system and helps keep hormones in balance. It's also beneficial for the liver, gallbladder, and kidneys, as well as for diabetes and hard chronic tumors. The fight-or-flight mechanism originates here.

Fourth chakra (heart): Green stabilizes energy and is a bronchiodilator. It helps treat infections. Many believe that love emanates from the heart chakra.

Fifth chakra (throat): Turquoise (blue/green) aids in healing third-degree burns, scratches, sores, and infections. It reduces fevers that respond quickly when used in conjunction with holistic remedies. Turquoise soothes irritations, inflammations, and itching. It helps induce sleep and should follow green in treating infections. It is known as the chakra of self-expression.

Sixth chakra (third eye/brow): Indigo worn around the neck helps stabilize the thyroid if an animal has a hyperthyroid condition. The brow chakra is best known for providing living things with intuition and instinct.

Seventh chakra (crown/above head): Violet increases the white blood cell count, stimulates the spleen, and is a color for high spiritual attainment in humans.

A DOG'S AURA

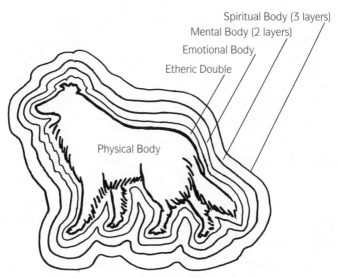

Spiritual Body (3 layers)
Mental Body (2 layers)
Emotional Body
Etheric Double
Physical Body

The etheric double is the nearest nonphysical level.

THE MAJOR CHAKRAS AND THEIR COLORS

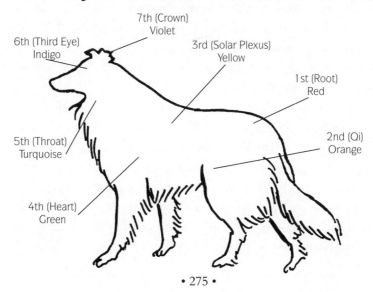

7th (Crown)
Violet

6th (Third Eye)
Indigo

3rd (Solar Plexus)
Yellow

1st (Root)
Red

5th (Throat)
Turquoise

2nd (Qi)
Orange

4th (Heart)
Green

CRYSTALS AND HEALING

MANY OF US have browsed through crystal shops at one time or another. But what are crystals? Basically, they're solidified substances created when water combines with an element under certain conditions of pressure, temperature, and energy.

Sand (silicon) combined with water forms quartz (silicon dioxide). Quartz amplifies, transforms, stores, focuses, and transfers energy. This crystal has the ability to vibrate at precise rates, making it invaluable in the manufacture of modern timepieces. When quartz is squeezed, it generates electricity. Alternating electrical currents cause quartz to swell and shrink, an action that when done rapidly becomes oscillation. Quartz vibrates at specific rates depending on what shapes it's cut into, and it transforms electricity into waves that can be broadcast (such as radio and television signals). A bit of quartz crystal in a microcircuit increases an electrical signal; this is how microphones and all audiovisual equipment evolved.

Quartz is also used to transmit information within computers, thin slices storing large amounts of data in memory. Quartz focuses energy in lasers and helps astronomers measure distances in seconds. It can burn through a steel wall as readily as it assists in delicate eye surgery.

Dael Walker, author of *The Crystal Book,* explains that crystals have *piezoelectric* properties[4] (that is, they can produce a small electric current when applied with mechanical stress). Since the body is electromagnetic, it responds to crystal therapy. The physical body exists only by virtue of energy; we get energy from food, water, air, and the earth itself. Crystals don't interact directly with the physical body but rather with the fundamental energy system that creates and supports the body, and connects that energy system with the mind and emotions. When used in conjunction with the mind, crystals can create functional changes that manifest themselves in the physical body.

Healing can be viewed as getting energy back into the cells of the ailing being when something has been blocking energy flow. When energy is brought back, new and healthy cells form, and the patient becomes well. Pain is a signal from the cells to the brain that something is wrong in the body. When painkillers coat the nerve pathways, blocking communication from the cells, the brain doesn't receive the distress signal and, therefore, doesn't know anything's wrong. So it doesn't send the necessary healing energy to the cells, and the condition worsens.

Unlike painkillers, crystals actually feed energy to the cells, which can then repair themselves and turn off the pain signal once it isn't needed anymore. Quartz crystals oscillate at the same frequency as the RNA and DNA in human beings and animals, according to Dr. Stefanatos, because their geometric structure is the same.

The Shapes and Sizes of Crystals

TUMBLED OR POLISHED stones seem to open up and increase energy.

Crystal balls disperse energy in all directions. Egg-shaped stones are excellent for scanning auras; just point the small end toward the body. Some practitioners use the egg shape in acupressure.

Collect several crystals in different sizes and shapes. Listen to your heart as you select them. But please don't use your own crystals on your dog—get special crystals for use on other beings.

Varieties of Healing Crystals

IT'S IMPORTANT TO use only quartz crystals. Dael Walker lists clear quartz, smoky quartz, and green quartz as the most effective for the physical body—clear as an overall energizer, smoky for grounding, and green to interact with the endocrine glands for balance and harmony.

Rose (pink) quartz and citrine work on the emotional body. Rose quartz balances the loving emotions of the upper four chakras (heart, throat, third eye, and crown).

Natural citrine (light orange to brown) balances the emotions of the lower three chakras (root, qi, and solar plexus). Tumbled golden citrine stimulates the crown chakra.

Amethyst (purple) is the spiritual stone, and it charges or transmutes lower energies into higher, more spiritual levels. It's also used in healing.

Any of these stones may be made into an amulet and suspended from your dog's collar. The stone may even be inscribed with the dog's name and/or your phone number. It may be cut to a special shape, such as a heart, cross, star, or angel. Before wearing them, be sure to wash stones in soap and water, then place them in salt water for seven days. And don't forget to program your stones with loving thoughts and emotions.

Using Crystals to Help Your Dog

TO DO AN aura scan, Dael Walker writes, gently assist your dog to lie on his right side. Hold the crystal with its point down between your thumb and first three fingers. Start at the top of the dog's head (or seventh chakra), about an inch away from the body. You are now within your dog's aura. As soon as you feel heat and some tingling emanating from the dog, move the crystal over his body from chakra to chakra, ending at the root chakra and, finally, the tip of the tail. The entire process can be done without actually touching the dog.

When you feel or sense something (coolness, resistance, more tingling, or just a hunch), stop and make a counterclockwise movement around the center of the disturbance. Keep circling in this way until the crystal feels heavy. Move your hand down to make contact with the body and touch the point of the crystal gently to the center of your circle.

Keep going over the body and making these corrections. When you reach each of the four paws, sweep from the head to the paw as if you were smoothing the coat. This aligns the energy of the aura into a smooth, even pattern.

Then turn the dog over and repeat the entire process on the left side. Once you've opened the chakras in this way, close them again by imagining a zipper at the dog's rear paws. Just pretend to pull the zipper all the way up to the top of his head. The dog should be relaxed and even sleepy, with a feeling of balance and well-being restored.

Diane Stein tells an amazing story about her fourteen-year-old poodle, Duffy, who had been diagnosed with a grade-three heart murmur on the left side. Stein had tried homeopathy and acupuncture, but, as far as treatment went, she had reached what she describes as a plateau. A recent blood profile on Duffy had showed an elevation of certain heart muscle enzymes, which indicated damage. The dog was clearly not improving.

Stein placed a quartz crystal pendant around the dog's neck at the thymus gland and applied smooth tumbled quartz crystals to the dog's halter, one crystal over each heart valve (the right and the left) and one each at the top and bottom of the chest, forming a double pyramid encircling the heart chakra. Six days later, Duffy's cough subsided, her murmur disappeared, and her blood tests showed normal heart enzyme levels. Stein continued to monitor the dog, who (at the time Stein wrote her book) continued to show no sign of the murmur.[5]

Note that Stein placed four crystals in the shape of a pyramid around the heart chakra on the inside of the halter.[6] The pyramidal design is appropriate to healing, because it focuses energy in a tight beam through the apex, or top, of the pyramid. Quartz grows in a spiral pattern, causing energy to flow out in the same pattern. When pyramid and spiral are combined, energy flows in a tight spiral beam, which may be easily focused. If you took two Kirlian photographs of an animal, with and without a halter containing crystals, you'd see that his aura had increased fivefold.

You may create a kind of gem elixir by placing a clean gem in spring water in the sun for two or three hours. The solarized water then becomes charged with its own energy—the color of the stone—and the full-spectrum electromagnetic energy of sunlight.

You may also energize your dog's food by placing a crystal underneath his food bowl. Dr. Stefanatos energizes a patient by placing a crystal at each corner of the dog's bed, under the bedding, with the base of the crystal toward outside air and the point toward the dog. She feels this procedure stimulates the immune system.

You don't need to believe that crystal therapy works for it to have an effect, but a positive attitude does provide a supportive atmosphere. Dael Walker suggests that belief consists of getting out of the way of what you want to accomplish. Regardless of what you believe, it goes without saying that you want both you and your animal companion to lead a happy, healthy life.

If one of my animals isn't feeling well, there's very little I wouldn't try to assist in his healing. I once slipped tumbled quartz crystals under the bedding of three pregnant queens during the birthing of their kittens. The three mothers produced a grand total of thirteen live births—no stillborn. I'll never know if the crystals helped, but you can bet I'd do it again!

HEALING WITH SOUND

THE VERY SAME noises—squabbling children, barking dogs, lawn mowers, traffic, television—that constantly bombard us also bombard our dogs, but it sounds much louder to them![7] Humans may learn techniques of stress control—meditation, relaxation—and tap into their own inner resources to find a moment of peace and relaxation.

Animals must deal with such noise in their own way. Their immune system, like ours, can break down amid the many unnatural influences of modern life. And soothing sounds can enhance their feeling of well-being, just as it does ours. The simple act of listening to music or other healing sounds may therapeutically augment other healing remedies.

The ancient Greeks were among the first to develop the idea of music as a healing entity. Zithers were played at mealtimes to aid digestion. Artistotle thought that flutes aroused strong emotions, leading to a cathartic release. The ancients no doubt regarded music as a type of psychotherapy that affected the body through the soul. Henry Sigerist wrote that Greek physicians restored physical balance with medicine, and mental balance with music.[8] Today it's known that some kinds of sound help integrate the functions of the left and right hemispheres of the brain.

The late John Craige, D.V.M., wrote that there's nothing in the universe of real substance. Even the most solid piece of rock consists of an arrangement of energy. All energy (whether in the smallest subatomic particle or in the largest heavenly body) is in constant rhythmic motion, such as the cycle of the moon as it revolves around Earth as it revolves around the Sun. So it follows that animals have rhythms and harmonies, too. Their health depends on their bodies being in harmony with the universe.[9]

Many years ago the engineer Royal Rife, while working with radio-wave frequencies, discovered that human cancer patients exhibited disharmonies at certain frequencies. If he subjected patients to these frequencies long enough, they came back into harmony once again, and many were reportedly cured.[10] Dr. Craige obtained a frequency generator and attempted to duplicate Rife's work, using a dowsing rod (see "The Dowsing Rod and the Pendulum") to verify that cancer patients were at the frequencies Rife reported. Dr. Craige then tested animal patients with chronic disorders and found definite reactions at specific frequencies. Moreover, the animals seemed to feel better when listening to these specific frequencies. This is not to say that he effected a cure by this means. Such work on animals is still in its infancy, although much has been published on the subject for humans.[11]

Dr. Craige and his wife, Joy Birdsall-Craige, developed several audiotapes for treating common viruses; skin allergies and severe itching; joint, tendon, and muscle disorders; circulatory and heart conditions; intestinal disorders; urinary tract disorders; and immune system weaknesses. When an animal is convalescing, I recommend placing a small tape recorder nearby and playing a therapeutic audiotape.

Using his own voice, Wayne Perry, of Signature Sound Works in Los Angeles, has made a tape that covers all the healing frequencies.[12] I had a headache when I entered the meeting room where he was demonstrating it, but as the sound enveloped me, I felt my body release the pain. Perry reports that he has successfully treated many physical and emotional problems with his tape. I play it regularly for my animals.

Perry has other materials to supplement his tapes, including a correlative healing chart for sound therapy. He has taken the twelve chromatic notes of Western music and keyed them to colors, physical conditions, emotional conditions, the twelve astrological signs, the chakras, the body's hormones, and the elements tied to the chakras and the levels of consciousness.[13] He refers to this practice as "yoga of the celestial sound within."[14] His philosophy is based on the belief that sound, light, and love are the ingredients for correcting and healing any imbalance or disease. The Sufis used sound for healing; and for millennia Tibetan bells, Gregorian chants, and mantras have been among the tools used to achieve spiritual realization.

Perry suggests that the vibration or frequency of each being is related to the notes of the scale. If the note D is missing or overemphasized in the human voice, for example, problems in digestion can arise. We (and perhaps our companion animals) are drawn to those who have our missing notes. Perhaps our animals are *toning,* and we aren't aware of it. With astrology as a guide, I use Perry's concept to see why I, a Leo, am so drawn to Romeo, my Aquarius cat, and Connie, my Leo collie; or why a Taurus, whose birth note is C-sharp and whose color is orange, could be drawn to his opposite, a Scorpio, whose birth note is G and whose color is blue-green.[15]

We can use the sounds of everyday life to heal ourselves and our animal companions. Instead of allowing the construction crew down the street to upset us, we can choose to resonate with these sounds or to deflect them, the way a martial artist redirects an opponent's force. Hear the sound. Let it come, then replicate it. Instinctively, when my animals make a sound, I imitate it. Then they usually come to me or repeat the sound, and we have a little dialogue.

I also play New Age music often in my home, to alter the mood and expand awareness. If you prefer a more conventional seventh-chakra stimulus, play some Mozart. One study found that listening to ten minutes of a Mozart piano sonata improved the scores of college students in a test of abstract reasoning. The researchers believe that the music stimulated brain cell activity.[16]

Whatever sounds or music you choose is entirely up to you. Just be sure your dog can enjoy it, too.

MAGNETIC THERAPY

THE OLDEST FORM of physical therapy known to humankind, magnetic therapy dates back to 200 B.C. Paracelsus used magnets to treat jaundice and hernias. Veterinarians Joanne Stefanatos and John Fudens use magnetic therapy to treat animals.[17] Dr. Fudens feels that biochemistry has historically overshadowed biophysics and that as this emphasis shifts, medicine will change rapidly, as illustrated by the use of magnets in healing.

A magnet is an object, such as a piece of iron or steel, that is charged with an electromagnetic field and so can attract certain substances, such as iron. Each magnet has two poles, north (yin/green) and south (yang/red).

Biophysically speaking, magnetic therapy polarizes *anions* and *cations* (negatively and positively charged ions), bringing tissue salts from a state of inactivity and stagnation to one of order and alignment. The body's polarity is normally neutral. When magnetic field lines, or lines of force, impact an organism or its various parts, they permeate and repolarize the cells, each of which acts like a microchip or miniature battery. Where injury has depolarized damaged cells, electromagnetic stimulation causes tissue fluids to flow again, as with a recharged battery (see "Radionics and Intrinsic Data Fields"). The body can then eliminate waste products; swelling (edema) and congestion are regulated, and cell metabolism reverts to normal.

Animals suffering from afflictions as diverse as arthritis and hyperactivity may benefit from magnetic therapy. The Massachusetts Institute of Technology and several European universities have found that certain magnetic devices increase the flow of blood, which may be useful in treating some orthopedic and congenital problems caused by a lack of blood flow and a disturbance of nerve tissues.

Many practitioners who use magnets believe that exposure to the north pole of a magnet slows down the processes of the body, relaxes the body, decreases blood pressure and growth of abnormal cells, treats fractures by decreasing acidity (and thus allows bones to heal faster), sedates the nervous system, decreases the growth of bacteria and viruses, decreases inflammation and assists in the healing of burns, and increases the amount of potassium ions in the body. In addition, the white blood cell count decreases and the red blood cell count increases—which when done after birth increases the life span by decreasing protein metabolism and thus increasing intelligence. (The south pole increases intelligence when used just before birth.)

The south pole increases cell growth and stimulates the production of endorphins, but it also increases the size of tumors, the growth of bacteria and viruses, the amount of sodium in the body, and the level of acidity; if used on a fracture, it lengthens the time it takes to heal. Dr. Stefanatos suggests never using the south pole to treat active infections. And don't use the south pole over the head, as it may create abnormal behavior and increase inflammatory reaction in the body by increasing the white blood cells.

In her video *Holistic Pet Care* (see "Resources"), Dr. Stefanatos demonstrates several ways to use magnetic therapy. However, I don't recommend trying it at home on your animals unless you've been instructed by a reputable veterinarian trained in this complex science. Magnets are extremely powerful and may be dangerous if used improperly. Dr. Fudens further warns that very ill or toxic animals need to be treated with extreme caution and only for short periods of time.

To treat a burn, hold the north pole of a magnet against the burn. For abnormal behavior, hold the north pole over the third-eye chakra. Treat cataracts, glaucoma, and kidneys on the verge of renal failure with little stick-on magnets. Dr. Stefanatos also employs magnetism to treat the beds of arthritic animals, who are then able to sleep peacefully and receive therapeutic treatment at the same time. She uses magnets in pairs to treat many other conditions.

Dr. Fudens has constructed a magnetic pad for animals to lie on, allowing him to treat the whole body at once. He reports that he has relieved pain and inflammation, stimulated tissues, increased circulation, increased oxygen to the tissues, and facilitated rehabilitation in his animal patients with the use of magnets. Though we can't achieve miracles with magnetic therapy, many benefits may be derived simply by improving cellular function. I purchased a similar pad for Connie; she likes to lie on it in the sun.

RADIONICS AND INTRINSIC DATA FIELDS

ORIGINATED BY AMERICAN physician Albert Abrams in the late nineteenth century, *radionics* is the study of the energy fields and centers of the body and how they are affected by health and disease.[18] Radionics is a holistic approach to healing based on the force fields that govern the function and well-being of the entire body. Its purpose is to help an organism reestablish optimum health. Physics and paraphysics, science and spirituality, meet and merge in radionics.

The basic concept is that all life-forms are submerged in the electromagnetic field of Earth and that each life-form has its own electromagnetic field. If these fields are distorted enough, disease results. Furthermore, the electromagnetic field of Earth provides the link between the practitioner and patient during analysis and treatment. It is an ancient axiom that energy follows thought, and thought is transmitted through Earth's energy field, allowing the practitioner to attune himself or herself to the patient.

Life begins and ends on the cellular level, and each organism, regardless of the size and shape of its cells, is a product of its environment. In radionics, the cell—the essential unit of organic structure—is viewed as an electromagnetic resonator capable of emitting and absorbing vibrations. Each cell has its own particular frequency.

Health is defined as equilibrium in the vibrations of the cells, and disease as the disequilibrium of these vibrations in absorbing, emitting, or transferring energy. Such disequilibrium originates from external causes, such as toxins or microbes. If a harmful external vibration is greater than the normal vibration of the cell, there is disease and pain. If the cell can adequately defend and increase its vibration, health returns; if not, the cell dies.

Many factors enter into maintaining the proper cell frequency: proper diet, clean air and water, a stress-free lifestyle, and the ability to receive divine light from a higher intelligence. All cells must be fully mineralized and balanced for optimum health and energy. The higher the rate of vibration, the higher the vitality of the cell and, by extension, the higher the being's overall state of health. Violating these factors doesn't always lead to disease, but if the violations accumulate long enough and the cells continue to be deprived of balanced energy, exhaustion sets in on the cellular level—and then disease does result.

Consider the body as if it were a car battery. If the electrical charge is drawn from the battery faster than the alternator can replace it, and if the battery is not cared for properly with water and sulfuric acid, soon it won't have enough charge to start the car. With a car, we simply replace the dead battery with a new one. Unfortunately, we can't do this with a human or animal body.

The vibration of a cell may be measured by an oscilloscope or other monitoring devices capable of registering the rate and level of an electrical impulse. Once these vibrations, or patterns of energy, have been measured, therapy can raise or lower them to the appropriate level and thus balance the energy pattern and restore health. Radionics detects potentially serious conditions at an early stage so therapy may be started before the condition manifests through physical symptoms. As the body is not physically invaded during measurement or treatment, radionics is totally harmless. New Horizons Trust prefers to use the term *intrinsic data fields* (IDFs), as *radionics* sounds similar to something it is not: radiation. The IDFs are fields or patterns of information that describe the nature and relationship of particles. Every particle has an IDF associated with it, and the connection between particles is known as an *IDF link*.

For years scientists have written about the probability of telepathic activity among particles. In 1935 Einstein, along with his colleagues Podolsky and Rosen, proposed the quantum mechanics theory known as the EPR Paradox, which states that when two particles move apart, measuring one reveals information about the other; that is, a telepathic link exists between the particles. They believed this phenomenon would occur even if the particles were separated by thousands of miles. Their theory was proved valid in tests by physicist John Bell in 1966.

By learning to read IDFs, we may access valuable information about everything in our world, including the proper intake of food and supplements by humans, animals, and plants (including livestock feeding and crop fertilization); it's also useful in problem solving and decision making. Flashes of intuition, such as knowing who is calling before you answer the phone, are apparently the result of IDFs; what we refer to as our sixth sense appears to be the ability of the human mind to read and interpret IDFs.

Government and industry have actually used the dowsing rod, an ancient but powerful instrument, to detect IDFs so as to locate wires and tunnels. Sophisticated software and electronic devices such as New Horizons's SE-5, an instrument somewhat like a biofeedback machine, are also available.[19]

My friend DeeAnne Weber, breeder of Leonbergers, uses this technology in her breeding program with excellent results. She runs programs on her pregnant dams and puppies to balance them physically and mentally. It's a fascinating study. DeeAnne has assisted me with difficult cases, and I'm certain the technique helped in every way. She needed hair samples from the animals that I felt needed assistance. Using her SE-5, she can actually prepare appropriate homeopathic remedies. I am very impressed with this technology and recommend it, along with proper supportive care.

THE DOWSING ROD AND THE PENDULUM

THE EARLIEST DOWSING rods (also known as divining rods) were forked wooden sticks used to detect underground water and metal deposits. Those interested in the history and uses of the dowsing rod and the pendulum may want to read *The Diviner's Handbook: A Guide to the Timeless Art of Dowsing,* by Tom Graves (see "Resources").

Recently I was privileged to read an unpublished manuscript entitled "Healing Hands: Energy Flow in Treating Disease," by the late John E. Craige, V.M.D. I had consulted with Dr. Craige many times and was intrigued by his diagnostic use of the dowsing rod to detect oscillating energy, the presence of which signals metabolic and traumatic disorders, throughout the meridians of the body.

Dr. Craige learned how to use this instrument from Wayne Cook, a famous water dowser. Using a handheld antenna made of spring steel with an aluminum handle and a weight on the end, Cook demonstrated his ability to detect the energy flowing through the body. He was able to discharge such oscillations (or interruptions in normal energy flow) by placing his left hand on the affected part of the body and holding the rod in his right hand. He was even able to discharge the oscillations in his own energy flow through a sort of venturi effect—like how the aerated water in kitchen faucets regulates the pressure and flow, thus cutting down on splashing. To relieve a headache, he placed his left hand on his head and discharged the oscillations accumulated there. Cook worked with Dr. Craige at his animal clinic; soon the veterinarian was practicing with a dowsing rod of his own.

The dowsing rod became invaluable to Dr. Craige in understanding and interpreting the wisdom and knowledge hidden in his unconscious mind. "The most logical explanation of [the success of] acupuncture, homeopathy, faith healing, and possibly chiropractic," he wrote, "is that these procedures manipulate the energy flow through the body, allowing normal healing processes to work effectively. The missing link in this theory is, How do they work?" He concluded that the discharge of oscillations or blocking energies might be such an explanation.

Dr. Craige began experimenting with the dowsing rod in conjunction with acupuncture. Whenever he identified an acupuncture meridian with oscillations, he placed acupuncture needles along that meridian. Ultimately, he was able to plot the course of all twenty-six meridians using the dowsing rod. Though he did observe some differences between traditional acupuncture and the results of his research, for the most part his findings confirmed what acupuncturists already believed.

Although Dr. Craige's opinions and methods were somewhat controversial, he had a long and successful track record with combining the dowsing rod technique and the use of the soft laser with acupuncture. Once when I visited his clinic, he asked to look at my throat. He used the dowsing rod to determine that I was just getting over a bout of the flu, and then he began treating my throat with the rod until the oscillations stopped. I felt better afterward, as did my cat Romeo, who was stressed from a heavy show schedule.

Tom Graves suggests that dowsing may be beneficial in conjunction with homeopathic treatment after the practitioner checks the description of symptoms. Then a pendulum may be used to find the appropriate remedy.

The pendulum should weigh about 2 ounces and hang from about 3 inches of string or links. It should swing, rather than bob around, as you hold it between thumb and forefinger. Mine has a little brass hand to hold on one end of the string, and the pendulum itself is a cylindrical gem. You can use a charm or medallion on a chain.

Rather than starting with the pendulum being at rest as your neutral position, Graves suggests beginning with an oscillation as neutral—that is, swing the pendulum lightly back and forth while you rest your mind on its oscillations, so its line (axis) of swing remains stable.

Two kinds of reaction are significant, a change from oscillation to gyration (either clockwise or counterclockwise) and the change from a side-to-side swing to one that's back and forth. The change from oscillation to gyration is the usual reaction to an object, such as a food or a remedy. Traditionally, pregnant women have used the swing of a pendulum to predict the sex of their children in utero. For this information to be useful, you must preassign values to the direction of swing or gyration. For instance, you might select a back-and-forth swing for yes and a side-to-side motion for no (a circular swing [gyration] may be read as yes or no). It's up to you to choose.

Some people place tremendous trust in energetic healing modalities. If you wish to try them yourself, it's best to keep an open mind. The dowsing rod, the pendulum, and other esoteric instruments are best left to those with integrity and a lot of experience, but novices may have success if they're willing to learn something new. As always, consult your veterinarian or holistic practitioner before embarking on any new therapy.

KINESIOLOGY

KINESIOLOGY, ACCORDING TO Wendy Volhard and Dr. Kerry Brown, is an early form of biofeedback without a machine.[20] In human medicine, *biofeedback* (a means of controlling the body through the mind by the use of a special machine) is mechanical. We've seen on ABC News (October 25, 1993) how paralyzed people in wheelchairs, with no use of their bodies, had electrodes attached to their heads to access the energy of their brains and thought processes, which was then used to drive machinery. In Russia, the authors tell us, a plane was piloted using the energy from the pilot's brain waves.

Wilhelm Reich, a disciple of Freud, introduced the idea that the body was influenced by the flow of what he called "bio-energy." It seems that without a machine, the body's energies can be tested through the muscle symptoms.

Chiropractors have used a special technique known as "applied kinesiology," which combines both Indian and Chinese medical concepts of energy to look at the body as an integrated system of muscles and nerves.

Wendy Volhard and Kerry Brown explain that Einstein's theory of mass in energy ($E = mc^2$) helps us to understand that energy fields are present in all matter. Everything has its own energy field, whose frequency can be measured with an oscilloscope or whose wavelengths can be measured with a frequency meter.

Virtually everything has an effect on the energy of all living things. We say, when we feel good, that we are full of energy, or when we don't feel well, that we are suffering from a lack of energy. We all need to be in balance. When the body is stressed from the wrong diet (see Chapter 4, "Nutrition"), the thymus gland producing the T cells in charge of our immune system shrinks. When the thymus shrinks, our immune system is impaired and we are out of balance. To see whether you are in balance, do the following with a partner ("testor"):

- Testee stands in an area that provides 16 inches of clear space all around—away from walls and furniture.

- Testee holds left hand at side, and right hand out and parallel to the ground.

- Testor faces testee and places two fingers of the left hand on testee's right wrist.

- Testor tells testee to brace himself or herself and then presses firmly down without jerking. The deltoid muscle will lock, and it will be impossible for the testor to make the arm go down. Don't use enough force to make it hurt!

A person who doesn't feel well will be projecting a smaller energy field than when he or she feels healthy. Then the arm goes down easily, telling us that the testee is out of balance. To get back into balance, the testor needs to place two fingers of the left hand over the thymus gland (found just below the V of the breastbone). Push down on the testor's right wrist, and it will go down. The testee should then thump the thymus point three times and place his or her tongue behind the upper front teeth and keep it there. Repeat. The testor should have a strong right arm. Now, repeat so that both testor and testee are in balance.

Kinesiology testing can begin with any food, drug, supplement, or even grooming products by putting each item in a plastic bag, which is then zip-locked or tied closed with a knot. Capsules can be placed directly into the hand of the testee. Liquid can be put into a small bottle. Fruit or food can be held in the hand. Put some white sugar or white flour into a bag; you will need something like this that usually tests poorly for everyone. You may test the sugar against honey, for example, or an apple. Keep in mind that jewelry can cause interference, so remove necklaces, earrings, watches, bracelets, rings—any metal that circles the body.

- Testee stands in the middle of the room, with at least sixteen inches of clear space all around.

- Left hand is at rest, at side; right arm is outstretched, like a one-winged bird. Food/product to be tested goes into the left hand and is brought down to and held at the solar plexus (middle of chest). Many believe that energy enters a body from the left side and exits through the right. Hence, the left arm holds the product, and the right deltoid is tested.

- Testor faces testee and places two fingers of the left hand on the testee's right wrist.

- Testor tells testee to brace himself or herself against the testor, who presses down on the testee's wrist.

- The arm shouldn't move much if the food/product is beneficial to the subject. There will always be a little "give" in the muscle.

Food or products that test strong (meaning the deltoid muscle didn't weaken) are in balance with the testee. When something doesn't test strong, and the arm goes down, the testee's energy is depleted, suggesting that this food or product is not in harmony with the subject at this time. Repeat these tests throughout the day when testing food or supplements. If you test an orange, for example, having just had a glass of orange juice, you may not need an orange now.

Now test your dog. The dog lies by your left side while a handler positions himself or herself on the floor next to the dog. The product is held on the dog's body (anywhere except the head). Your right arm is extended at a right angle parallel to the ground. The testor presses down on the right wrist to see if the deltoid muscle tests strong. If it is weak, the product is not resonating with the dog at this time.

I have found very few animals on fresh food who have allergy or deficiency problems. The ones who do ate commercial food for years and were excessively vaccinated or drug abused in some way. Often these sensitivities or weaknesses don't last long, once the offending substances are eliminated.

You may also use kinesiology as a diagnostic tool by asking questions of the pendulum. You can even question the remedies or therapies you are considering using. For example, while holding a pendulum over the dog, you may ask a series of questions that lead to appropriate remedies.

Just keep testing often with whichever method you choose. Personally, I prefer my little pendulum, but many veterinarians and holistic practitioners swear by this method. The pendulum method resonates for me because I often don't have a partner to involve in my testing. Although many people who have seen me demonstrate the pendulum are doubting Thomases, they usually can't believe their eyes. Don't ever include someone in this process who ridicules you. Better to choose someone with an open mind. It's exciting when you see it work. You can go all over your home testing everything your animal comes in contact with and determining sensitivities. One little tip . . . don't have a preconceived notion or attachment to the result. Just try to be a conduit for what's best for your animal.

I recommend both Diane Stein's book, *Natural Healing for Dogs and Cats,* and *The Holistic Guide for a Healthy Dog,* by Wendy Volhard and Kerry Brown, D.V.M., for in-depth discussions on kinesiology (see "Resources").

Chapter Eight

Astromedicine for Your Dog

WHY AN ASTROLOGY chapter in a book about holistic health care for dogs? I don't use astrology to chart my daily life or that of my animal companions, but I'm interested in the signs of the *zodiac* (the twelve sun signs) and their corresponding personality traits as they apply to us, our animals, and the special relationship we have with them. Astrology is much more than reading newspaper horoscopes—it can be used as a healing science.

For hundreds of years we've known that the seasons result from changes in the distance and angle of the Sun's rays relative to Earth and that the phases of the Moon affect tides, the planting of crops, even the success of fishermen. It isn't a big leap to suppose these variables affect all living things, including our dogs.

The only way we can assist them in healing and cleansing their bodies is to look for appropriate natural remedies or methods of healing. The more aware we become of canine traits and actions, the better equipped we'll be to help our animal companions. Often studying the sun signs—each of which governs a different part of the body—helps me select effective homeopathic treatments. (However, the widely respected holistic veterinarian Dr. Christina Chambreau cautions that this method diverges from the classical curative approach to homeopathy.)[1]

Dog breeders should consider carefully not only which season puppies will be born in but which sign of the zodiac will guide them. You'll be amazed to see how similar the personalities in a litter are, even taking into consideration differences in sex and pecking order.

Though the serious astrological practitioner develops a natal horoscope based on the exact time and place of the animal's birth (one of my friends actually timed the birth of her kittens with a stopwatch and has a full chart on each kitten), it isn't absolutely necessary for our purposes, although the in-depth approach can be extremely informative, and I myself have consulted periodically with experts in the field.[2] But the care, feeding, and spiritual well-being of our animal companions can benefit enormously if we simply learn about their astrological archetype; it provides a means to look past their beautiful coats and the sparkle in their eyes. On your own, you could cast a relationship chart determining your compatibility with your dog. Or you may wish to dig deeper, either learning how to set up a chart or working with those who can.

What if you don't know your dog's birthday or exact age? Well, you could figure out his sun sign by analyzing his personality and traits. If we look deeply enough, we can understand who each of our dogs is from a spiritual point of view and then explore the many healing philosophies (such as the Eastern system of yin and yang) and apply their principles to our animal friends.

AN ANCIENT HEALING SCIENCE

IT IS INTERESTING to note that the Chaldean priests of ancient Babylonia were also physicians who incorporated astrological knowledge into their medical work. They helped women organize their lives to bring their children into the world under the best possible cosmic conditions. According to astrologer and author Reinhold Ebertin, the priests took water from different-colored transparent vessels corresponding to a person's time of birth, and they sought medicinal plants that they thought resembled certain planets.[3]

In Greece during the sixth and seventh centuries B.C.—the time of the Orphic mysteries—tonal vibrations, music, and consecrated oils were important components to rituals. Even that long ago it was understood that a beautiful and harmonious environment supported self-healing. The stars were said to be the handwriting of heaven.

Empedocles (about 493–433 B.C.), the Greek philosopher, poet, and statesman, taught that all life was derived from the "root of things."[4] The four elements—earth, air, fire, and water—created various mixtures out of which arose love and hate. In turn, these active forces were continually uniting and separating the elements.

To Hippocrates (about 460–377 B.C.), "the father of medicine," has been attributed a piece of writing relating the heavens and the human body. He required that his students study astrology, stating that "the man who does not understand astrology is to be called a fool rather than a physician." When a dreamer sees the stars dimmed or obscured by atmospheric influence, Hippocrates believed, he or she can determine the severity of a disease, its cause, and the appropriate remedy.

Many other ancients were concerned with zodiacal plants, which are said to develop their full potency if gathered, prepared, and used when the sun is positioned in the appropriate sign (see "How to Make Your Own Flower Essences," in Chapter 5, "Natural Remedies").

During the reign of Alexander the Great, the theories of Eastern and Grecian astromedicine were first integrated. Two centuries later, the astronomer Hipparchus (about 190–120 B.C.) divided the zodiac into 360 degrees and expanded the concept of correlating body parts and organs to the zodiac and the planets. And about 196 B.C., through a cultural exchange between Greece and the Roman republic, astrology became known in Rome. However, it was in Rome that the practice began to deteriorate, when Augustus had all astrologers and wizards exiled. As is true today, there was a great gap between serious astrological study and superstition.

Known as the "king of astrology," the Alexandrian mathematician, astronomer, and geographer Ptolemy (Claudius Ptolemaeus, about A.D. 100–170) is considered one of the last great scientists of antiquity. His work still forms the basis of many astrological textbooks.

When the Christians entered the scene, they taught that the stars do not rule fate but act as pointers to the future. It's interesting to note that the numbers three, four, seven, and twelve are significant numerologically in both astrology and Christianity (the Trinity, the four elements, the four cardinal signs, the four evangelists, the seven days of creation, the Twelve Disciples, the twelve zodiacal signs, and so on).

Such early astrophysicians as G. W. Surya echoed what the Swiss alchemist-physician Paracelsus (Phillippus Aureolus

Theophrastus Bombast von Hohenheim, about 1493–1541) had taught: that astrology is one of the pillars of medicine. Surya quoted Cicero's dictum: "It is sufficient to experience what happens even if we do not know how it happens."

Even this brief history of astromedicine suggests that its principles are extremely deep rooted. Our ancestors had the foresight to look beyond the medical philosophy of declaring war on microbes, which is the basis of modern allopathic practice.

ASTROLOGY AND THE MODERN DOG

PEOPLE THROUGHOUT the ages have applied these principles to every aspect of their physical and spiritual lives. In much the same way, you can explore the twelve sun signs to better your relationship with your animal companions. Regardless of any suggestions given, your dog's symptoms must always be your guide. And remember, consult a holistic veterinary practitioner before embarking on any therapeutic course of action. (See Chapter 5, "Natural Remedies," for further information about the substances described below.)

Schuessler's Twelve Tissue Remedies (Cell Salts)

THE TWELVE tissue remedies,[5] or cell salts, developed by Dr. Schuessler correlate to the twelve sun signs, based on studies done by astrophysician Inez Eudora Perry, who believed that the human body was a microcosm of the cosmos.[6] With their spiritual underpinnings, Perry's choices for these remedies seem more applicable to dogs than treatments suggested by practitioners such as Dr. M. Duz and Dr. Fritz Schwab, who based their recommendations solely on *human* characteristics.

Aries	Kali phosphoricum (Kali phos.)	potassium phosphate
Taurus	Natrum sulfuricum (Nat. sulf.)	sodium sulfate
Gemini	Kali muriaticum (Kali mur.)	potassium chloride
Cancer	Calcarea fluorica (Calc. fluor.)	calcium (lime) fluoride
Leo	Magnesium phosphoricum (Mag. phos.)	magnesium phosphate
Virgo	Kali sulfuricum (Kali. sulf.)	potassium sulfate
Libra	Natrum phosphoricum (Nat. phos.)	sodium phosphate
Scorpio	Calcarea sulfurica (Calc. sulf.)	calcium (lime) sulfate
Sagittarius	Silicea (Sil.)	silica
Capricorn	Calcarea phosphoricum (Calc. phos.)	calcium (lime) phosphate
Aquarius	Natrum muriaticum (Nat. mur.)	sodium chloride
Pisces	Ferrum phosphoricum (Ferr. phos.)	iron phosphate

Bach Flower Remedies

BASED ON THE work of author Peter Damian, who states that Dr. Bach treated the personality, character, and mood of his human patients,[7] I've selected twelve of the thirty-eight flower remedies to correspond with the sun signs and Bach's twelve states of mind:

Dr. Bach's Twelve States of Mind

1. Fear
2. Terror
3. Mental torture or worry
4. Indecision
5. Indifference or boredom
6. Doubt or discouragement
7. Overconcern

8. Weakness

9. Self-distrust

10. Impatience

11. Overenthusiasm

12. Pride or aloofness

In my opinion, the twelve signs of the zodiac correlate directly to the twelve Bach states of mind because each sign involves some weakness that we can help our animals overcome as they grow and evolve. However, other remedies apply as well.

Bach's seven classifications (Seven-Step Method) may also be applicable to the sun signs. Using this method, you can prepare combinations that cover a broad spectrum of emotional states. All thirty-eight essences are employed in this system:

1. Fear: Aspen, Cherry Plum, Mimulus, Red Chestnut, and Rock Rose

2. Uncertainty: Cerato, Gentian, Gorse, Hornbeam, Scleranthus, and Wild Oat

3. Insufficient interest in present circumstances: Chestnut Bud, Clematis, Honeysuckle, Mustard, Olive, White Chestnut, and Wild Rose

4. Loneliness: Heather, Impatiens, and Water Violet

5. Oversensitivity: Agrimony, Centaury, Holly, and Walnut

6. Despondency and despair: Crab Apple, Elm, Larch, Oak, Pine, Star of Bethlehem, Sweet Chestnut, and Willow

7. Overconcern for the welfare of others: Beech, Chicory, Rock Water, Vervain, and Vine

Homeopathic Remedies

THE HOMEOPATHICS I'VE selected for each sun sign are only a sampling of remedies that might apply. I based my choices upon Ebertin's research pertaining to the sections of the body ruled by the governing sun sign, but I've made some of my own suggestions as well.

Metals

I'VE ALSO INCLUDED in the astrological listing for each sun sign the eight metallic solutions corresponding to each of the heavenly bodies (the Sun, the Moon, and the seven planets).

Gold (Aurum)	Sun
Silver (Argentum)	Moon
Quicksilver (Mercurius)	Mercury
Copper (Cuprum)	Venus
Iron (Ferrum)	Mars
Tin (Stannum)	Jupiter
Lead (Plumbum)	Saturn
Zinc (Zincum)	Uranus

Paracelsus, who was also the father of the pharmaceutical industry, became interested in metals by watching his father, a mining engineer, bring ores up from underground. He was struck by the idea of using minerals and metals as remedies.

Although we seldom hear of metallic solutions being used in modern medicine, such cures were employed in ancient times. Today we have colloidal gold available to us (see "More About

Supplements—Some Good, Some Bad" in Chapter 4, "Nutrition"). Homeopathic dilutions of metals and other colloidal mineral combinations are now appearing on the scene as well.

Aromatherapy and Sound Healing

ACCORDING TO AUTHOR Scott Cunningham,[8] there are plants and essential oils associated with each sign of the zodiac— more than one aroma for each sign because most planets and elements rule more than one sign. You can use aromas to strengthen or decrease the influence of your dog's sun sign. For example, offering a Leo dog a whiff of ginger oil would only serve to increase his inborn propensity for aggression—unless you specifically visualize otherwise.

Healing sounds are also pleasant additions to any household in which animals and humans enjoy a celestial bond.

YANG AND YIN: HEAVEN AND EARTH

IN CHARTS BASED on the astrological system already described, the horizontal plane that joins the ascendant (rising sign) and the descendant (descending sign) separates the visible from the invisible part of the heavens. The upper half is regarded as positive, and the lower half as negative. If we were to drop a line from the meridian, it would divide east and west, with the eastern half designated as positive and the western as negative.

The Chinese, relying on a five-thousand-year-old tradition, regard heaven as yang (the generation of all that exists in the world), and Earth as yin (the recipient of heaven and the bearer of heaven's progeny). Yang and yin are represented by the symbol of a circular disk divided by a wavy line. One side is dark (yin), the other light (yang), but rather than being antagonistic, they flow into each other and unite in oneness. This interrelationship is also pictured as a six-pointed star formed by overlaying of two triangles: yang with its apex pointed upward, yin with its apex pointed downward—the superimposition uniting positive and negative, male and female.

We can further classify yang as the ambient-oriented type (*ambient* referring to external surroundings) and yin as the internal- or interior-oriented type. C. G. Jung referred to them as extrovert and introvert. The ambient dog may be completely consumed with his territory, and the interior dog withdrawn and introspective, sensitive and reserved. Ambients are centrifugal (outward) in force, interiors centripetal (inward). Yang is vertical, yin horizontal. Yang corresponds to the Sun and day, yin to the Moon and night. During the day, the dog is up on all fours (vertical). At night, he is down (horizontal). At night, in the yin position, both humans and animals absorb more cosmic energy, which we emit again during the day, in the yang position.

Male and female/day and night (yang and yin) signs alternate in the zodiac. The male and female sign (positive and negative charges) form a continuous circle all around the circle of the zodiac.

Aries	Male	Libra	Male
Taurus	Female	Scorpio	Female
Gemini	Male	Sagittarius	Male
Cancer	Female	Capricorn	Female
Leo	Male	Aquarius	Male
Virgo	Female	Pisces	Female

Yang is associated with bright, warm colors; yin with dark, cool colors. The range of the spectrum falls between them, uniting the two in a kind of yang-yin rainbow:

Yang—red, orange, yellow, green, blue, indigo, violet—**Yin**

The color of your dog may be significant. For example, to create a balance, tie a brightly colored cloth or a kerchief on your yin-colored dog (red or yellow on blue, gray, or black). Buddhist monks wear saffron robes supposedly because it stimulates their minds.

Here's a summary chart of the properties of yang and yin:[9]

Yang	Yin
Male	Female
Summer	Winter
Ordered	Disordered
Day (Turns into . . .)	Night
Dry	Wet
Positive	Negative
Hard	Soft
Heavy	Light
Condensing	Dispersing
Fertilizing	Fertilized
Concentrated applied energy	Diffused misapplied energy

When the balance of yang and yin is disturbed, imbalance in the body may result. Balance may be restored through natural treatments (for instance, a yin disease may be cured with a yang remedy). However, we must not fall into the trap of thinking that yang and yin are clear-cut concepts or tendencies. Rather, they flow into each other (as day turns into night), alternate, and change from moment to moment. Both diet and healing play a big part.

We can maintain or restore balance by supplying the appropriate yang and yin foods. When planning your dog's menu, obtain guidance from his birth chart, or at least his sun sign. For example, a Jupiter type needs to be restored by yang foods.

Heating, adding salt, and seasoning with bitter herbs make foods more yang. Cooling by adding liquids, flavoring with aromatic spices, grating, and crushing makes foods more yin. When cereals are soaked in water or are sweetened, they become more yin. As for the foods themselves, some are more yang, others more yin.[10] Just think in opposites:

Yang Vegetables	Yin Vegetables
Lettuce	Asparagus
Carrots	Cauliflower
Dandelion greens	Kale
Garlic	Peas
Turnips	Cabbage (red and white)

Yang Meat	Yin Meat
Beef	Pork (I don't use pork in my animal recipes)
Chicken	
Fertilized egg	
Lamb	
Venison	
Veal	

Yang Fats/Oils	Yin Fats/Oils
Rapeseed (canola) oil	Suet (beef fat)
Sesame oil	Butter/margarine
Soy oil	Lard
Sunfloweroil	Olive oil
Wheat germ oil	Palm oil

Yang Dairy Products	Yin Dairy Products
Soft cheeses	Buttermilk

Camembert	Cream (fresh)
Goat's milk	Kefir
	Milk
	Yogurt

Yin (Miscellaneous)
Honey

ASTROMEDICINE AND THE SUN SIGNS

PLEASE STUDY THE information provided for all twelve signs, as each sign governs a different part of the body. Again, consult your holistic practitioner before beginning any treatment.

Aries (The Ram)

March 21–April 19 (also March 21–April 21)[11]

Cardinal element: fire

Ruling planet: Mars

Earth colors: cerise, magenta

Astral colors: white, rose pink

Gems: amethyst, diamond

Mineral element: iron

Bach flower: Impatiens

Cell salt: Kali phosphoricum

Aries, the first sign of the zodiac, represents birth. The ram is the newly born Lamb of God. Aries affects the cerebral nervous system and whatever is dependent on it. The spinal cord, sensory nerves, pituitary, face, and lower jaw are also influenced. The planet Mars stimulates the cells, influencing diseases related to inflammations, fevers, and organ lesions; there may be a predisposition to liver problems. An elementary quality of dry heat is associated with this cardinal fire sign.

In his mind the Aries dog, even when from a large litter, is an alpha wolf. Strong and assertive, he makes his needs known when he's hungry. When he wants something, he gets it. When he's awake, everyone's awake. If he doesn't answer when you call, it's not that he doesn't know his name—the Mars-ruled dog is simply self-absorbed and will get to you when it's convenient for him. All the world is seen from his point of view.

Aries's puppy charms and naïveté linger into old age. He's cunning and extremely hard to resist. Though he can be vulnerable, he nearly always gets his own way with people and other animals. He's also fearless and somehow always able to land on his feet. The old motto "If at first you don't succeed" fits him to a T. If he ever gets lost, he'll find his way home through the worst conditions. He perseveres to the end, even if he dies trying.

As a fire sign (he shares this element with Leo and Sagittarius), he has a sunny disposition that will cheer you in your darkest hours. Though not usually lazy, the Aries dog does seek warmth and loves to lie in your lap or by your side when you sleep.

The unneutered Aries male is the eternal stud and gets into brutal fights, as exemplified by the Greco-Roman god of war, Mars (Ares). In fact, Aries can be so aggressive that the chances of his becoming seriously injured or dying in a fight are very high. So please keep Aries dogs on a leash and spay or neuter them (unless they're part of a breeding program). Many of the aggression problems encountered in Aries dogs disappear after this simple procedure. But, no matter what, he'll never stop believing he's the alpha wolf.

The Aries dog is extremely curious and can be accident-prone. He loves you intensely and shares his possessions, but don't try to take something away from him (unless it's dangerous), because he will resent you for it. Aries is the sign of authority, after all.

As always, be gentle, as the Aries ego bruises easily. When led with love and given plenty of exercise, this dog will be a champion at everything he does. Whether pedigreed or mixed-breed, the Aries dog is very outgoing and quite the showman. He enjoys the spotlight.

To call him extremely intelligent is an understatement. If he could speak in human language, he'd have an answer for everything and would always need to be right. As it is, your life with the Aries dog will be a contest of strength and wit, with never a dull moment.

The Bach flower remedy *Impatiens* is appropriate for this willful and aggressive dog. Use either Impatiens or Rescue Remedy (which includes Impatiens) when the Aries energy and egocentric nature becomes overbearing.

The cell salt *Kali phosphoricum* (potassium phosphate) can be especially helpful when the Aries dog seems despondent, depressed and irritable, or impatient. Perhaps he is grieving the loss of some close animal or human friend, or he may be homesick after a change in residence. Cold aggravates these symptoms, and he doesn't want to be alone. He seems better after he rests, eats, and finds warmth.

The element *iron (ferrum)*, related to the planet Mars, has always been a tonic for anemia. An old folk remedy prescribed sticking a clean nail in an apple overnight and then eating the apple for breakfast. Homeopathically, iron is used for sore muscles and rheumatic disorders. It may also benefit worm infestations in puppies, symptoms of which include regurgitating food immediately after taking it in and abdominal flatulence.

Consider the following homeopathic remedies[12] for Aries:

Aconite *(Aconitum napellus)* when the head, cranial nerves, or ears ache, or if there is nasal catarrh. One of the guiding symptoms is sudden fever or inflammation with a propensity to anxiety, fear, and anguish.

Arnica for a headache or bruising condition (following surgery). Use alternately with *Hypericum.*

Belladonna for a hot head and fever (I often use it after *Aconite*), or when the skin becomes red and hot to the touch. Guiding symptoms include a full, pounding pulse and dilated pupils.

Bryonia alba when body temperature drops through exposure to cold and the dog has a great thirst. Symptoms include chills accompanied by fever.

Chamomilla for teething discomfort.

Hypericum for symptoms associated with the head and face.

Nux vomica when a symptom associated with the head, jaw, or face leads to stomach upset that produces bad breath.

Pulsatilla for conjunctivitis when yellow discharge is a guiding symptom.

Sulphur for extreme fear and aversion to light.

The plants and essential oils associated with Aries are clove, coriander, cumin, frankincense, ginger, neroli, pennyroyal, pettigrain, and pine. The ruling planet Mars is enhanced by basil, coriander, cumin, garlic,[13] ginger, hops, nasturtium, onion, and rue.

Taurus (The Bull)
April 20–May 21 (also April 21–May 21)[14]
Cardinal element: earth
Ruling planet: Venus

Earth color: cerise
Astral colors: red, scarlet, orange, lemon yellow
Gems: moss agate, emerald
Mineral element: copper
Bach flower: Gentian
Cell salt: Natrum sulfuricum

Taurus governs the cerebellum, the liver, gallbladder, thyroid, throat, and neck, with a possible relationship to the kidney. The sign of purification, Taurus is ruled by Venus, which controls intercellular fluid and influences infectious diseases. Being an earth sign means vulnerability in the back of the head and down the spine to the liver. An elementary quality of dry cold is associated with this sign.

The Taurean dog does whatever she wants whenever she wants to. Her shyness is endearing, though it may be frustrating when you'd like to show off her charming ways to friends and neighbors but she won't perform. Even to animal trainers, the stubborn Taurus proves quite a challenge. However, outside of this pigheadedness, Taurus dogs are a delight to have underfoot and love to be petted. Taurus dogs tend to bond with one person but can be magnanimous with their affection.

Taurean people are very outspoken. Without speech, the Taurus dog needs to express herself through physical means, so she needs plenty of exercise.

Vibrations and harmony are very important to Taureans' well-being. Harsh or bright lights and colors upset them, as do loud noises—so keep the stereo turned low. But they do love sound, such as those found on nature tapes and CDs. Buy one of these, or better yet, make your own audiotape, reading aloud a piece of poetry in your gentlest voice. Actually, all animals appreciate audiotapes of human companions' voices played when they're alone.

Taurus dogs have great powers of concentration. They try very hard to understand what you need, but this has to suit them or the bull emerges victorious. If you're lucky enough to adopt Taurus as a puppy, you'll delight in watching her grow into a magnificent dog. Taurean females make wonderful mothers.

The Bach flower remedy recommended for the Taurus personality is *Gentian*. Because of their typical obstinacy, they're usually slow but sure, and resistant to change—the bulls of the dog world.

The cell salt *Natrum sulfuricum* (sodium sulfate) can be used homeopathically for excess water. It occurs rather abundantly in nature (in sea water and saline springs). The mental symptoms to watch for in these dogs are wildness and irritability followed by restless, sleepless nights. The Taurus dog will seem disheartened. Since Taurus relates to the cerebellum, the nervous system, and the liver, these dogs may experience dizziness (the top of the head may be sensitive also) accompanied by the presence of bile (the tongue may be coated, and the matter produced by vomiting yellow-tinged) or diarrhea tinged with yellow. Combing or brushing the dog in this condition may be painful to her, though she'd love to be groomed when healthy. Her throat might be dry and sore, and she may develop a hacking morning cough with salty mucus. If your Taurus dog usually seeks warmth and symptoms arise during damp weather, you're at least on the right track with this remedy; Schuessler recommends the 6X potency. If these symptoms appear, though, consult a homeopathic veterinarian before administering the remedy.

Copper (cuprum) relates to the planet Venus. *Cuprum metallicum* and *Cuprum aceticum* are particularly valuable in treating kidney disease. *Cuprum arsenicum* is valuable as a therapy for diseases of the urinary tract in doses of 3X and 12X.

Consider the following homeopathic remedies[15] for Taurus:

Aesculus hippocastanum (horse chestnut) when the symptoms include dry nose and throat with scanty secretions, dry cough, catarrh of the nose and throat, throat inflammation, coughing made worse by cold air, coughing in the morning, and liver conditions affecting the general circulation. The tongue may be coated.

Alumina for nasal catarrh and sore throat due to the weakening of vocal chords from excessive calling when in estrus (heat cycle). She might strain before urinating, with a white sediment occurring occasionally. The spine may degenerate and the nails become brittle.

Arnica for sore throat when there seems to be pain (yawning seems difficult), for bruising injury when skin is unbroken. Use after surgery or during birth,[16] as it lessens the danger of difficult labor. *Arnica* can also be used externally for bruising and swelling in cream form, when the skin is not broken.

Arsenicum for laryngitis, flu, and any sore mouth condition, as well as for vomiting and diarrhea with foul smell. It is valuable in treating enteritis and skin conditions that produce dandruff-like flakes. Guiding symptom is the aggravation of conditions toward midnight.

Belladonna for dry, inflamed sore throat, thyroid conditions, or inner ear disorders. Its early use can help prevent brain damage from fever. The skin usually feels dry, with generalized redness and heat, and the dog does not want to be touched and is thirsty. The pupils dilate, and the dog shows an aversion to light, with a fixed, staring look. Use of *Belladonna* often follows *Aconite*.

Calcarea carbonica (calcium carbonate) for catarrhal involvement of mucous membranes leading to the discharge of mucus. Throat glands are enlarged and appetite is frequently irregular.

Camphora for nasal discharge and larynx-related breathing problems. Skin can be icy cold to the touch. *Camphora* is also of value for a low immune response, which creates susceptibility to salmonellosis.

Chamomilla for teething.

Hamamelis (witch hazel) for overactive thyroid and pharyngitis.

Hypericum (St. John's wort) for mucus in the throat, dry cough, scraping sound in the throat. It is also indicated for liver dysfunction with jaundice. However, its primary use, both internally and externally, is for lacerated wounds. It can be alternated with *Ledum* or alternately with *Arnica* after surgery and is ideal after spaying or neutering.

Ignatia for grief and sadness, or for when pups are taken from their protective Taurean mothers and sent to adoptive homes.

Iodum (iodine) for thyroid disorders. Symptoms may include a ravenous appetite and loss of condition.

Pulsatilla when you see bland yellow discharge from the eyes and nose, uterine discharge (tendency to pyometra and false pregnancy), influenza with eye symptoms, including yellowish discharge.

The plants and essential oils indicated for Taurus are apple, cardamom, honeysuckle, lilac, magnolia, oakmoss, patchouli, plumeria, rose, thyme, tonka, and ylang-ylang. The planet Venus corresponds to apple, cardamom, catnip, chamomile, daffodil, freesia, gardenia, geranium, hyacinth, iris, lilac, magnolia, mugwort, narcissus, palmarosa, plumeria, rose, spider lily, thyme, tuberose, tulip, vanilla, vetiver, white ginger, wood aloe, yarrow, and ylang-ylang.

Gemini (The Twins)

May 21–June 21

Cardinal element: air
Ruling planet: Mercury
Earth color: orange
Astral colors: red, white, blue
Gems: beryl, aquamarine, dark blue stones
Mineral element: quicksilver (mercury)
Bach flower: Cerato
Cell salt: Kali muriaticum

Gemini, which has a predisposition to neurosis, is governed by the planet Mercury. The nervous system, as well as the respiratory system, glands, fibers and tissues, shoulders, paws, and toes are all governed by this sign. An elementary quality of wet heat is associated with Gemini.

Gemini is male and female, extrovert and introvert, aggressive and passive—all rolled into one dog. This animal is a lesson in duality, giving you a full range of emotions and physical attributes. He gives you a nip asking you to pay attention, then she turns around and licks the same spot. He/she, she/he, back and forth. You think, "Oh well, this is a typical canine behavior." But no, it's not; it's just Gemini.

You may be hoping to have your very own animal, but the truth is, this one belongs to the world. When you leave Gemini with the house sitter, you may fret that he'll die without you.

But he's happily bonding with the sitter just in case you don't come back; and if you don't, he'll cozy up to the real estate broker, too. It's not that he's fickle, just that, as the Scorpion's nature is to sting, Gemini's is to be all things to all creatures. Maybe you should just pretend you're as special to him as he makes you feel.

The Gemini dog is a multifaceted, creative pup—poetry in motion. No doubt, he'll create something, even if it's havoc. He's ruled by Mercury, the winged-footed Greek god, so prepare to fly with him as if he were a bird. He can slip through your fingers like quicksilver. Gemini is an air sign, and air must circulate freely, so let him have the run of the garden. He loves to go for walks.

Gemini won't want to be out for long, though, since he's always in conflict. Just watch him pace back and forth. He seems to say, "I'm here, but I'd really like to be there, wouldn't I?" He rarely finishes anything, including dinner. Instead, he's off making mischief somewhere. Such curiosity!

Gemini is quick. A bird or cat doesn't have a chance. He'd like to eat it, but his twin wants to play with it. He's constantly at odds. Could we call him fidgety? No, everyone else is slow. Just let him be; he changes so fast that all his quirks are like quarks—here and gone in an instant. His mind is like a computer sifting through so much information so fast that not even the most avid nonverbal communication expert can get it all.

The Bach flower remedy to consider for Gemini is *Cerato*. In China, Gemini is known as the monkey sign because of its restless nature. However, Gemini dogs like company and are rarely loners. They're intelligent but sometimes do foolish things because of their inquisitive nature.

The cell salt *Kali muriaticum* (potassium chloride) is recommended for Gemini. Said to be in constant conflict between his yang and yin personalities, this dog might just convince one of his alter egos to starve. Since the respiratory system is governed by Gemini, it doesn't hurt to look first at such symptoms as loss of voice, white tongue, asthma, white mucus that seems difficult to bring up, a spasmodic cough, wheezing sounds, and a rattling in the chest—all signs of respiratory conditions in dogs. Usually introduced through the pup's vaccinations, this group of viruses overloads the immune system and shuts it down. As a result, respiratory symptoms may become chronic and made worse through the abuse of antibiotics. Other guiding symptoms include white mucus (could also be yellow or greenish as disease progresses) discharged from the eyes, white dandruff, white catarrh from the nose, skin eruptions after vaccination, and a sluggish constitution. Schuessler uses 6X and 12X potencies of *Kali mur.* This remedy can also be applied to the skin for burns, dry white eczema, and even warts. (*Thuja* is, however, the usual wart and/or vaccinosis remedy.)

Quicksilver (mercury) is the mineral element that corresponds to Gemini, which is ruled by the planet and god Mercury. This remedy, prepared under homeopathic guidelines, is administered for agitation with fear, restlessness, and irritability. It's also used for conjunctivitis and bronchial catarrh. The recommended doses are 3X and 12X. A guiding symptom is abundance of slimy saliva, as with spongy gums.

Consider the following homeopathic remedies[17] for Gemini:

Aconite (*Aconitum napellus,* monkshood) if there are cramping pains in the limbs, and the joints become swollen, hot, and painful when in motion. Also for pneumonic conditions with high body heat, thirst, dry cough, and nervous excitability.

Arsenicum for cough, shortness of breath, restlessness, wheezing, and even bleeding from the lungs.

Bryonia alba for gastritis, dry cough with thirst, nasal discharge, possible bleeding, extensive inflammation in the pleural surfaces. When the guiding symptom is deterioration of movement, the dog prefers to lie on the affected side during pneumonia or pleurisy.

Eupatorium perfoliatum (boneset) when the dog feels bruised or weak in the limbs. The bladder may also be affected, causing cystitis.

The plants and essential oils that Gemini responds to include benzoin, bergamot mint, caraway, dill, lavender, lemongrass, lily of the valley, peppermint, and sweet pea. Mercury corresponds to benzoin, bergamot mint, caraway, celery, clary sage, costmary, dill, eucalyptus, fennel, lavender, lemon verbena, lily of the valley, marjoram, niaouli, parsley, peppermint, spearmint, and sweet pea.

Cancer (The Crab)
June 22–July 23
Cardinal element: water
Ruling planet: Moon
Earth color: orange-yellow
Astral colors: green, russet-brown
Gems: pearl, black onyx, emerald
Mineral element: silver
Bach flower: Clematis
Cell salt: Calcarea fluorica

Cancer is ruled by the Moon, which governs cell modularity and the blood. This sign also relates to the breasts, stomach, digestive organs, spleen, and elastic tissues. It is predisposed to diseases of the head and abdomen. Wet cold is the elementary quality associated with this water sign.

The Cancer dog is a gentle creature prone to staring wistfully at you, or at what you may think is nothing, for what seems like an eternity. She's very happy to be with you, as she's most content sitting by your side. She looks like she's posing for a greeting card wherever she goes.

A strong individual, the Cancer dog often prefers to go off by herself, whether she's the only dog or one of many. However, if your spirits are low, she's more than likely to baby you. She's easy to spoil since she is an affectionate dog by nature.

The Cancer dog's tenacity is unparalleled. Usually the first to arrive at the food bowl and the last to leave, she never lets you forget that her sign rules the stomach. The Cancer dog tends to put on weight easily, so control carbohydrates and see that she exercises regularly. Cancer is also the most sentimental sign of the zodiac: she gets strongly attached to people, other animals, and things, so don't reassign a food dish or a bed without her permission.

As a puppy, the Cancer dog tends to bond with one person. She may run and hide when someone new enters or stand her ground if approached. Quite vulnerable, she can be so dedicated to protecting herself and her people that the slightest input can cause her to withdraw. But when left alone at night or separated from her companions, she's likely to cry and moan for the duration.

Lightning, thunder, earthquakes, or new people and situations can set her off, even when dogs of other signs aren't bothered at all. She's also very adept at picking up human fear, so it's important for you to remain calm through a crisis. She tends to need constant reassurance.

You may be dismayed when people come to visit and make disparaging remarks about your Cancer dog's moody or unfriendly behavior. It seems only you know that there's a loving creature behind that growl or grumpy exterior. But if you don't give this dog all the love and security she needs, she may go into her shell just like a crab.

The mythological ruler of Cancer is Diana, the Roman goddess of the hunt and the Moon. Cancer's symbol is the crab, an animal whose habits shed a lot of light on dogs born under this sign. When the crab is frightened, she runs into the sea or behind a rock, emerging only when she has resolved her feelings.

The Cancer dog can change moods quickly and dramatically. Just as the Moon, to us the fastest-moving body in the heavens, may hide behind the clouds and then emerge as a beautiful globe of light in the darkest sky, so the Cancer dog goes through her changes. When she's in touch with the emotional needs of those around her, she can be a great comfort. When she's not, or out of control, she can be miserable.

Cancer dogs make wonderful mothers. If your female Cancer dog is to be spayed, and especially if she is the only dog in the family, adopt a kitten for her to nurture. She may sulk and make a fuss at first, but the subsequent bonding will be profound. Remember, when left alone, "Moon Doggies" tend to get morose, so having their own friend is especially important. To them, being the only dog in a human family is a little like our living with a family of rhinoceroses. They may be nice to us, feed us, and play games with us, but we're not their kind. It's nice to have someone your own size to play with, someone who speaks your language. In our dog's case, fluent canine.

The Cancer dog never forgets anything and is extremely sensitive. Never laugh at her and be careful not to make her feel foolish. Your Moon Child may get clingy and overbearing sometimes, but she's so endearing that you're likely to love and need her just as much as she needs you.

The Bach flower remedy for Cancer is *Clematis*. The Cancer dog often has a faraway look in her eyes. When she withdraws, try Clematis along with something to nurture. Cancer likes solitude and, as her guardians, we must respect her space. Cancer lives more in the dream world and requires more sleep than most other signs. Cancer is the mother sign of the zodiac, and Clematis helps revive her vitality when she wears herself out caring for others.

The cell salt for Cancer dogs is *Calcarea fluorica* (calcium fluoride). One of the guiding symptoms for this remedy is deep depression. She may vomit undigested food, be prone to gastritis, and be constipated or strain during bowel movements. She may seem weak in the morning and be very fatigued all day, taking more naps than normal. When she sleeps, she dreams vividly of impending danger. She is worse in damp weather. Schuessler recommends a 12X dosage when these symptoms are present.

Silver (argentum) is governed by the Moon and is used homeopathically primarily in the form *Argentum nitricum (Arg. nit.)*. The Moon corresponds to the stomach and digestive organs, so this remedy is useful in treating gastroenteritis, usually accompanied by abdominal bloating and diarrhea after eating and drinking. Involvement of the stomach leads to vomiting. Because *Arg. nit.* acts on the central nervous system, consider administering it to dogs showing fear and nervousness toward other animals.

Consider the following homeopathic remedies[18] for Cancer:

Abrotanum (southern wood, or lad's lover) for stomachache or a constriction in the chest. It's used for eruptive skin conditions with bluish discoloration and a tendency to alopecia (hair loss). The appetite may remain good, but there may be alternating constipation, with a distended abdomen. Wasting may become progressive, developing low and traveling upward; emaciation of the lower limbs is a strong guiding symptom. The symptoms are relieved by movement. A newborn puppy in need of this remedy may show oozing from its umbilical chord. (If so, be sure to use a topical antiseptic.)

Alumina (aluminum oxide) for older dogs, especially those showing debility. Look for chronic conjunctivitis with an aversion to light, but since Cancer governs the stomach, there may be cravings for abnormal substances such as charcoal, which helps with constipation. Also good for any condition producing emaciation and vomiting; weakness of lower limbs; excessive dryness of mucous membranes; feverish states in which temperature remains elevated; cracked skin in an eczematous condition that appears rough and bleeds easily; and straining during bowel movements, with feces hard and knotty following a bout of constipation.

Arsenicum for indigestion, gas, and tremendous thirst but with minimal drinking. The abdomen could be swollen, so consider the possibility of liver and/or spleen problems. Inflammation of the lower bowel produces straining, with a dysenteric stool and a cadaverous odor. *Arsenicum* works quickly to allay vomiting and diarrhea.

Belladonna when the mouth is red, with swollen papillae, and a swollen throat makes swallowing difficult. The dog is the picture of misery, with colicky pains, noisy gas, and possibly fever.

Bryonia alba (white bryony) because Cancer also relates to fluid balance. You may wish to explore this remedy for dry cough or extensive inflammation in the lungs. The guiding symptom is the dog's worsening from movement (such as with pneumonia or pleurisy) and the dog's preferring to lie on her affected side, bringing pressure to bear and thus restricting movement. Swollen joints may also benefit from this remedy.

Chamomilla for nausea or a bloated stomach after meals (simply making the chamomile tea and setting it out in a water dish is soothing).

Ignatia (Saint Ignatius' bean) for the Cancer mother when she is grieving after her pups are taken away to their new homes.

Iodum (iodine) for pancreatitis, thyroid, or other glandular conditions, as well as for a ravenous appetite with loss of condition. The lymph glands may feel hard, the skin seems dry and withered looking, and there may be increased urination, perhaps dark and strong smelling.

Nux vomica for digestive disorders, including flatulence, indigestion, and vomiting. The area over the liver may be sensitive, and the stool is generally hard. In cases of poisoning from certain plants, *Nux vomica* has been prescribed with success when abdominal symptoms occur.

Pulsatilla for the dog with a sweet disposition, usually a feminine personality. There may be uterine discharge, bland or mucous material, or a creamy yellow discharge from the eyes, ears, and nose. Excellent remedy for pyometra and influenza, when typical eye conditions are involved.

Sulphur when there is rattling in the lungs. *Sulphur* also aids the action of other remedies.

The plants and essential oils associated with Cancer are cardamom, chamomile, jasmine, lemon, lily, myrrh, palmarosa, plumeria, rose, sandalwood, and yarrow. Those ruled by the Moon are influenced by jasmine, lemon, lily, melon, night-blooming cereus, sandalwood, stephanotis, and water lily.

Leo (The Lion)

July 22–August 21 (also July 22–August 21)[19]

Cardinal element: fire

Ruling planet: Sun

Earth colors: yellow, gold

Astral colors: red, green

Gems: ruby, peridot, sardonyx

Mineral element: gold

Bach flower: Vervain

Cell salt: Magnesium phosphoricum

Leo is the sign governing the heart, circulation, blood, eyes, and vitality. The lion is Leo's symbolic image, and this sign is ruled by the Sun. The Sun dog needs to be careful of inflammations. An elementary quality of dry heat is associated with this fire sign.

Leos love to lie in the sun—it's almost impossible to keep them out of it. But be careful, they can burn through those luxurious coats and experience excessive shedding.

It would be presumptuous of me, being a Leo myself, to refer to canine Leos as the "king of beasts," even though they (and I) think it's true! They're the only sign in the zodiac whose symbol is a beast of prey. To say canine Leos are proud and loyal is an understatement. My very own Connie, the collie, is a Leo, too!

They thrive in a positive environment and need a tremendous amount of love and admiration. They never seem to get enough scratches or pats, and their appetite for food is also insatiable. They love to be spoiled but give a great deal of love in return. However, it's usually on their terms. If you don't encourage and patronize them a bit, they'll withdraw and brood for a while. This lion must be given incredible amounts of affection.

Leo dogs are very verbal and tend to bark a lot. One woof is seldom enough. They're rarely shy.

Always the instigator, Leo marches around your home and yard like the Pied Piper, with everyone following behind. If another dog usurps his position, the lion will most likely stalk off and sulk, awaiting the fond caresses of his "subjects"—you and other members of your household. Leo plays many roles, including your mother or your baby, depending on whether he's in a giving or a receiving mood. He's sunny by nature and will play and bark at all who enter his kingdom.

Leo usually takes center stage. If you're giving affection to another person or animal, he's sure to get in the middle. I suggest you make a special effort not to let him become overbearing or possessive, correcting him gently and telling him he'll have his turn. He hates to be demeaned publicly. Leo doesn't understand the meaning of "wrong" or "bad"—he thinks he's always right. However, he does have a great sense of fair play.

Leo dogs have a great sense of dignity. Just like Leo people, they're as theatrical as they are regal, so they often show off with acrobatics and high jumps. Leo dogs need a lot of stimulation and love new toys and games, tiring of old ones quickly. Guard against accidents with Leos, as they often don't think before they act—they just like to be watched and admired.

His independent nature will sometimes make you feel you can never get him to do what you want. Be patient and remember to lavish praise and affection on him. You've got a star on your hands, so be prepared to be his fan.

The Bach flower remedy suited to Leos is *Vervain*. Dogs born under this sign may suffer from exhausting overenthusiasm. Strong-willed Leos possessed of great courage (the heart of the lion) exemplify Vervain. They tend to be overly concerned for others (such as their puppies and close pals). When this trait becomes overbearing, Vervain is an excellent choice.

Magnesium phosphoricum (magnesium phosphate) is the cell salt for Leo when symptoms call for its use. This is a remedy for cramps, convulsions, and other such contractive disturbances. When involuntary twitching of the legs, general tendency to nervous chorea, or spasmodic movements occur, this cell salt is one to look into. The eyelids may be twitchy, becoming heavy or droopy with tearing, and stomach cramps may cause the animal to paw at his abdomen. The heart may become easily excited, palpitating when spasmodic. Schuessler recommends the 6X trituration; for dogs, dissolve 1 or 2 tablets or pellets in an ounce of distilled water at room temperature and just pop them into the fold of skin at the side of the mouth. The guides for the use of this cell salt are symptoms relieved by pressure and rubbing, or those aggravated by cold air, cold food, and so on. The mental state of the Leo dog may seem constrictive, fearful, sorrowful, grieving, or worried. If a *simillimum* occurs (that is, the remedy corresponds to the totality of symptoms), try *Mag. phos.*

The Sun is represented by the element *gold (aurum),* which is a normal constituent of the body primarily found in the brain, through which it enters the central nervous system and enhances vitality. As the ruler of Leo, the Sun has to do with the heart. *Aurum* is beneficial in treating palpitations and constriction around the heart indicated by the dog's drawing deep breaths. *Aurum iodatum* and *Aurum sulfuratum* are also prescribed in 3X to 12X dosages.

Consider the following homeopathic remedies[20] for Leo:

Aconite when there is cardiac anxiety, a full pulse, and increased heartbeat, and in the early stages of all feverish states, when symptoms come on suddenly. Animals that exhibit fear of crowds or strange places will also benefit from *Aconite.*

Aesculus hippocastanum (horse chestnut) when the heart action is full and heavy, or for liver conditions associated with venous congestion affecting the general circulation.

Arnica when the heart becomes enlarged while a generalized cardial dropsy appears. As a heart remedy, it restores tone to the weakened muscle. *Arnica* reduces shock and should be a routine prescription after surgical procedures and birthing because it lessens the danger of difficult labor. It can be used externally as well in cream form, when the skin is *not* broken.

Arsenicum for diarrhea and vomiting, with symptoms worse after midnight, and for skin conditions with dry, scaly, itchy patches, loss of hair, and dandruff-like flakes. Also for restlessness, with the dog frequently changing positions and being thirsty for small sips of water.

Camphora (camphor) in the event of shock when the pulse becomes weak and heart failure is threatened. Also for salmonella.

Hamamelis (witch hazel) for any condition showing venous congestion and passive hemorrhage from veins.

Plants and essential oils associated with Leo are basil, bay, cinnamon, frankincense, ginger, juniper, lime, nasturtium, neroli, orange, pettigrain, and rosemary. Bay, bergamot, calendula, carnation, cedar, cinnamon, copal, frankincense, juniper, lime, neroli, orange, pettigrain, rosemary, and saffron are attributed to the Sun.

Virgo (The Virgin)

August 22–September 22 (also August 23–September 22)[21]

Cardinal element: earth

Ruling planet: Mercury

Earth color: chartreuse

Astral colors: gold, black

Gems: pink jasper, sapphire

Mineral element: mercury

Bach flower: Centaury

Cell salt: Kali sulfuricum

The Virgo dog is ruled by Mercury, which maintains the nerves. Virgo dogs are prone to infections. Virgo governs the bowels, intestines (and everything dependent on them), and solar plexus. This earth sign has an elementary quality of dry cold.

Though quick and alert, Virgos tend to be the most tranquil of all dogs, their personality making them the most able to handle unfavorable conditions. If you live in constant stress and chaos, the Virgo dog is probably well suited to your lifestyle. But don't forget that even she has her limits, so try not to overload her. She can distress you and then exhibit her own contradictory moods, such as wanting to be with you but not wishing to be held against her will. Win her trust by avoiding the use of force. She is naturally friendly and has a warm disposition but can be irritable if you make fun of her. Perceptive and steadfast, she responds best to a gentle approach.

It's been said that contact with animals actively reduces stress in humans. When humans stroke an animal, their bodies almost instantaneously release stress, providing a kind of animal psychotherapy. But it's more than just touching the animal. When you earn a dog's love, the bond is so deep that even people with deep emotional scars, who find it hard to trust, often find their way back through their relationship with an animal. Such companionship may actually reduce blood pressure and calm the overworked heart.

Like the Leo dog, Virgo usually follows you all over the house and yard as you do chores, content just to see you and be near you.

She may be shy with visitors or at crowded dog shows, but with family and regular visitors this dog certainly won't be at a loss for something to say. She tries to communicate with you with sound just as you do with words, but she'll also send you pictures with her beautiful eyes—so listen with your heart as well as your ears. She may have a wonderful story to tell. She chatters away nonverbally but then buttons up the minute a stranger appears. Mercurial is the word, as she is ruled by Mercury.

She is so well mannered and easy to be with, you may tend to favor her. She announces herself when she's ready to play. However, if rebuffed, she'll be hurt, so always be gentle and sensitive with this beautiful creature. She understands "no" very well and usually doesn't need to be scolded, but if she does, send a positive mental picture (see "Nonverbal Communication" in Chapter 2, "Interacting with Your Dog").

The Virgo dog loves routine and dislikes having the furniture moved, let alone her food or water bowl, so leave things where they are. However, being a Virgo, she adapts to change when necessary. She loves to be well groomed, so take pride in her appearance.

She'd probably love a little puppy or kitten as a friend, but don't consider a breed of dog that will grow larger than she is unless you introduce the new arrival as a young puppy. Virgo likes to mother things smaller than herself and doesn't want her position to be usurped.

Inquisitive at all times, the Virgo dog loves balls, Frisbees, and lots of exercise. She delights in something new.

The Virgo dog loves to learn and often surprises us by mastering new tricks—such as bringing in the newspaper—on the first try. However, if you don't help develop Virgo's potential fully, she can become a sad little introvert.

This dog needs physical affection and encouragement and loves human companionship. Often she can't wait until you sit down so she can lie at your feet. If another animal or person in the house infringes on her one-on-one time with human companions, Virgo is likely to sulk. She gets lonely easily, so remember to give her quality time in great quantities. Virgos also have a fear of falling and will usually shy away from edges.

Since she's a good traveler, take her with you when you go on vacation. She'll really appreciate that.

The Virgo dog may be prone to actually acquiring the same physical maladies her human companions have or fear the most, so stay as positive as you can.

Centaury is the Bach flower choice for Virgos who are shy, timid, or anxious to please. You may not even know when Virgos are out of sorts since they rather calmly accept their plight. When your Virgo dog has difficulty standing up for herself and gets browbeaten by her pals, try Centaury.

The cell salt for the Virgo constitution is *Kali sulfuricum* (potassium sulfate). As with *Sulphur,* a guiding symptom is irritability. Virgos are not irritable by nature, only when they don't feel well. When they are out of sorts, they really don't want to be fussed with. And that's the beauty of homeopathy: sometimes one dose is all it takes; the remedies are easy to administer and don't taste bad. You might notice that Virgo dogs in need of *Kali sulf.* feel better in the open air. *Kali sulf.* has been used in the treatment of bronchial pneumonia. Certain types of fungi may benefit from this treatment when the skin shows a shedding or peeling action, is scaly looking, or shreds—a kind of casting off known in homeopathy as *desquamation.* Because Virgo rules the intestines, you may find symptoms such as slimy yellowish diarrhea, excessive thirst, vomiting, mucus, and serous discharges that are profuse and yellow (slimy or watery). Loss of smell is typical when these symptoms are present. You may notice a hacking cough, indicating dryness and constriction. Kennel cough could be the culprit. The latter stages of inflammation are served by this remedy. Schuessler recommends 6X and 12X dosages. Compare with *Pulsatilla* in your materia medica and choose whichever remedy is more appropriate. Symptoms for both are aggravated in a warm room, discharges are yellow to yellowish-green, and there may be pressure and a feeling of fullness (bloating) in the stomach.

The more books you can collect on homeopathy (for both animals and people), the better equipped you'll be to self-diagnose and diagnose for your dogs. I always confer with my homeopathic practitioner prior to taking or giving a remedy, but what I read and observe can help the practitioner and me find the best remedy. Virgo can be an especially sensitive dog, so choosing the wrong remedy, or even the right remedy in the wrong potency, can produce an aggravation.

Quicksilver (Mercurius hydrargyrum) is the mineral to consider when Virgo's nerves are fraying. Just as the planet Mercury corresponds to the element, the element responds to the central nervous system.

This said, *consider the following homeopathic remedies[22] for Virgo:*

Abrotanum because Virgo rules the intestines. You may notice anxiety and depression from digestive disorders, with alternating constipation and diarrhea. Symptoms worsen at night.

Agaricus for treatment of postdistemper chorea (irregular spasmodic movements of the limbs or facial muscles) as well as eczema with nervous involvement.

Aloe to combat allopathic drug use in congestive states of liver disease. It will help the portal circulation and restore a normal bowel action.

Alumina when constipation occurs, or for any condition producing emaciation and vomiting, together with weakness of the lower limbs.

Arsenicum, with its all-embracing quality, is useful in the treatment of many well-defined sets of symptoms or conditions. In gastroenteric conditions *Arsenicum* generally will allay vomiting and diarrhea quickly.

Belladonna when the guiding symptom is a full, bounding pulse during any feverish condition, or when thirst is prominent along with abdominal pain and gas.

Bryonia alba when a yellowish discharge covers the tongue or there is tenderness over the liver area; in chronic conditions the stool becomes hard and dry. *Bryonia alba* is useful when the dog seems worse for movement, as with pneumonia or pleurisy. The animal prefers to lie on her affected side, bringing pressure to bear and thus restricting movement.

Calcarea carbonica (calcium carbonate) if your young Virgo is fat and lazy, with slow dentition. This remedy, made from the middle layer of the oyster shell, is an excellent way for establishing calcium in the system.

Eupatorium purpureum for inflammation of the ovaries, together with a tendency to miscarry; pain and tenderness over the kidneys; and cystitis with blood-stained urine. This remedy seems to have an affinity with the urogenital system of both male and female.

Nux vomica for many digestive disturbances and congestions, or when there is gas and indigestion, when vomiting takes place, there is tenderness over the stomach, and the liver region is sensitive to the touch. Stool is generally hard, but diarrhea and constipation may alternate. *Nux vomica* has proved of value in the treatment of umbilical hernia in young dogs.

Pulsatilla when the mucous membranes are involved. This is predominantly a female remedy, especially for mild, gentle, yielding dispositions. *Pulsatilla* types, like Virgo, are changeable. They usually feel better in open air, worse in warm or damp closed areas. A thick, bland, creamy yellow discharge; lacrimation of the eyes; and stoppage of the right nostril often occur.

Sulphur is an excellent clearing remedy that also aids the actions of other remedies. The *Sulphur* type can display irritability. The action of this remedy is centrifugal (outward from within). If Virgo's abdominal (or other) conditions don't respond to other remedies, *Sulphur* may give your dog the push she needs to complete the healing process.

The plants and essential oils associated with Virgo are caraway, clary sage, costmary, cypress, dill, fennel, honeysuckle, lemon balm, oakmoss, and patchouli. Mercury's influential aromas are benzoin, bergamot mint, caraway, celery, clary sage, costmary, dill, eucalyptus, fennel, lavender, lemon verbena, lily of the valley, marjoram, niaouli, parsley, peppermint, spearmint, and sweet pea.

Libra (The Scales)
September 23–October 22
Cardinal element: air
Ruling planet: Venus
Earth color: green
Astral colors: black, crimson, light blue
Gem: opal
Mineral element: copper
Bach flower: Scleranthus
Cell salt: Natrum phosphoricum

Libra, ruled by Venus, governs the bladder and kidneys. A cardinal air sign, it has an elementary quality of wet heat.

The eternal judge, the Libra dog is part angel, part devil. Usually the peacemaker, he has to be right in the thick of it or you'll find him surveying his territory from every conceivable angle. That way, he can represent all sides of the equation. Only then can he make a decision—but Libra defines "decisions" as things you change your mind about constantly. He loves harmony but remains a paradox himself.

The lesson of this sign, if you will, is never to give Libra a choice. He hates to make decisions. It's so difficult to choose, and it's so difficult to get him into the groove of a routine, but this is exactly what he needs. Just feed him the same well-balanced fresh foods at the same time in the same place every day because change will upset his sense of well-being.

Libra tends to be a bit slow. You call him and call him for breakfast, but he's more interested in watching something out the window—a butterfly or the mailman. It's not that he's stubborn; it's just that he'll come when he wants to. If he doesn't come for meals, let him miss a few. This won't hurt as long as he has fresh purified water. Perhaps at this moment some serious meditation is more beneficial to his psyche than eating, and this self-imposed fast will be cleansing.

All dogs need basic obedience training, but Libras thrive on it! Always use a firm, gentle tone when obedience training and, after a session, sing to him. Libras tend to be auditory and like music. If you whistle a little tune, he'll come running. Try "Pop Goes the Weasel" or "You Are My Sunshine" or whatever you like. If you have to leave him alone in your house or apartment, call him often and let him listen to your soothing voice on your answering machine.

Loving and sweet, Libra tends to be a verbal dog who talks to you. He drives you crazy, but you end up living to please him and loving every minute. It's hard to say no to a Libra. And he's difficult to train, as he loses interest quickly, but stick with it. He needs the discipline.

He loves to please you, but he'd rather please himself. If you have more than one dog, your Libra eats out of everyone else's bowl and snoozes in everyone else's bed. He curls up on your favorite chair even though you've said, "No chair!" a thousand times. All he hears and sees in his mind's eye is "chair." Don't even try to yell at him; it hurts his ears. If you do, he'll forget what he's been doing anyway.

In the Bach flower repertory, *Scleranthus* is perfectly suited for Libras because they are hesitant, uncertain, and seesaw between moods. The Venus-ruled dog may benefit from Scleranthus when indecision is part of the picture. Scleranthus combined with Rescue Remedy or Centaury can restore balance to his life during stressful times.

Natrum phosphoricum (sodium phosphate) is the cell salt for Libra, treating the blood, muscles, nerve and brain cells, and intestinal tissues. *Nat. Phos.* is the remedy for conditions arising from an excess of lactic acid. The liver is the prime and master laboratory of the animal body, and since this remedy emulsifies fatty acids, it's indicated for liver upsets, such as when the dog has eaten fatty cooked meat or poultry (see Chapter 4, "Nutrition," for more about the harmful effects of such a diet). Often simply changing his diet to fresh raw foods restores the dog's health, but if the symptomatic picture fits this cell salt, it's worth considering. Only the fresh food diet ensures resistance to parasites in the heart and intestinal tract, so if your dog has been on some other diet, you may want to take a stool sample to the veterinarian to check for worms. Anxiety and fear, or a kind of dullness with irritability, may be present; the Libra dog may become upset easily. Other guiding symptoms may be a creamy, golden yellow discharge on the eyelids in the morning; yellow nasal discharge; and yellow coating on the tongue, palate, back of the throat, and tonsils, along with inflammation. The dog may strain when eliminating. Libra governs the bladder and kidneys, so diabetes is something to watch for in its hepatic form.

Copper (cuprum) is the metallic element suited to those ruled by Venus. It occurs naturally in blood serum as a catalyst for a series of enzymes, is a component of cellular protoplasm, and controls the activity of the blood-building cells. It is valuable in the treatment of kidney disease accompanied by spasms. The 3X and 12X potencies are usually recommended.

Consider the following homeopathic remedies[23] for Libra:

Aconite if the urine is hot and assumes a reddish color.

Agaricus muscarius when conditions affect the central nervous system. The renal system may be involved when polyurine (large amounts of urine) accompanies a mucous urethral discharge in the male's urinary tract.

Aloe to combat use of allopathic drugs as well as the effects of free feeding dry food, both of which often lead to urological problems. When the urine is scanty and high colored and urging is frequent, particularly at night, think of *Aloe.* It is also indicated for congestive states of the liver, helps portal circulation, and restores normal bowel action.

Arsenicum album, along with all of its other beneficial uses, for Bright's disease, a kind of chronic nephritis (inflammation of the kidneys). Urinary dribbling may also be noted.

Camphora for the dog that's unable to void a full bladder; for shock, when the pulse becomes weak and heart failure is threatened; or for salmonellosis.

Nux vomica if the urine is scanty and frequently contains blood.

Pulsatilla, besides all of its applications, for creamy yellow discharge from eyes, nose, and so on if increased urination is an additional symptom. Young (often female) animals of gentle but changeable dispositions are well suited to *Pulsatilla*.

Plants and essential oils pertaining to Libra are chamomile, daffodil, dill, eucalyptus, fennel, geranium, palmarosa, peppermint, pine, spearmint, and vanilla. Aromas attributable to Venus are apple, cardamom, catnip, chamomile, daffodil, freesia, gardenia, geranium, hyacinth, iris, lilac, magnolia, mugwort, narcissus, palmarosa, plumeria, rose, spider lily, thyme, tuberose, tulip, vanilla, vetiver, white ginger, wood aloe, yarrow, and ylang-ylang.

Scorpio (The Scorpion)
October 23–November 21
Cardinal element: water
Ruling planets: Pluto, Mars
Earth color: blue
Astral colors: golden brown, black
Gems: topaz, malachite
Mineral element: iron
Bach flower: Chicory
Cell salt: Calcarea sulfurica

Ruled by Pluto, Scorpio governs the reproductive organs. Symbolized by the scorpion (and sometimes by the white eagle or the gray lizard), this fixed water sign has an elementary quality of wet cold.

Scorpio is ruled by Pluto, lord of the underworld. The myth that describes Scorpion is that of the phoenix rising from the ashes. She seems to know that she can achieve whatever she wants, visualizing the goal before she begins.

The most invincible of signs, she loves a good contest. Such an incredible animal, with a strong body and a strong will, she scraps with her mates and usually wins. Scorpio loves a good fight, but mostly, she likes to win and possesses the necessary strategy. If she loses the battle, just wait; she'll be hiding around the corner ready to fight and won't quit until she succeeds.

The Scorpio dog is very athletic. To maintain her sinewy muscles, feed her fresh foods and keep her active. She needs to release tension with lots of play and jogs around the block, but it's not unusual for her to sit by the sidelines watching others make fools of themselves, whether they're dogs or humans.

Scorpio needs firm but loving discipline. So say it with conviction, right now, out loud, "I am the boss"; otherwise, your Scorpio dog will get what she wants when she wants it! But remember, the Scorpion can sting, so handle her with care and give her lots of love and affection along with your discipline. Be the alpha wolf, or you'll be in big trouble.

Don't let this aloof being fool you. She needs your love in lavish amounts. And how can you resist when she stares deep into your soul as only a Scorpio can? Her penetrating eyes express an almost unfathomable depth, and she never reveals everything to you. That's part of her mystery and her charm. Her eyes follow you wherever you go, just like the Mona Lisa; she'll even hypnotize you if she can. If you think she's enchanted, you just may be right!

Though you'll never completely understand her, she seems wise to things humans can only guess at—forces operating on different levels of consciousness. If you're blue, she's likely to be there for you, licking away your tears before anyone else has an inkling that something's wrong. She loves to share this little secret with you, and you'll be laughing out loud sooner than you think. But don't take it seriously if sometimes she ignores you. She'll be ready to be social again before long.

She's loyal but can be tough, too. When crossed, she warns you, but only enough to let you know she isn't pleased. Don't push then. She may be fun and outgoing, but she never forgets and can hold a grudge against anyone who inflicts pain, accidentally or otherwise. She'll get back at you by jumping on you when you least expect it. Afterward, she'll lick your hand, so there's no way you can stay angry with her.

The Scorpio dog loves company but is okay as an only dog also. She bonds with one person easily. If you work at home, she's content to be with you. If not, she'd like a friend to torment—just a little. Get her a challenging companion, maybe an Aries or a Sagittarius. However, Scorpio dogs are fond of the opposite sex, so be sure to spay or neuter them unless you're a conscientious, natural breeder.

Scorpio is a sensuous sign, and these dogs love to be groomed. If she's short-haired, polish her gleaming coat; she'll love it. She needs lots of stroking, and she'll thank you for it.

She's likely to be a pack rat. Your favorite powder puff, hair ribbon, sport socks, or slippers may disappear and later be found behind the dresser. If you retrieve them, give her a toy or raw, juicy, turkey neck in its place. On the other hand, the Scorpio dog may rediscover a treasured item you thought was gone forever; she may bury it out in the yard along with that bone.

The Bach flower remedy *Chicory* is ideally suited for dogs whose energy is drawn inward. Chicory types can be jealous, controlling, and possessive, keeping those in love with them in a state of constant attachment. Even though we all cherish the unconditional love animals offer, Scorpios seem to have a few strings attached. Humans who are Chicory types harbor a strong need to be thought as significant, so they enjoy company that supports this need. If you find yourself worshiping your Scorpio or start to feel as if you're in bondage, consider Chicory and a little Walnut (the remedy for advancing stages and breaking the tie that binds) for yourself. A loving relationship with your Scorpio is based on mutuality: "I am in your debt; you are in my heart. I am in your heart; you are in my debt."

Calcarea sulfurica (calcium sulfate) is the cell salt selected for Scorpio. Consider it for septic conditions (the presence of toxins) in general, the chief guiding symptom being pus that has found an outlet (as in an anal gland abscess). Other symptoms include mucous diarrhea with occasional pus, yellow discharge, and purulent crusts; a slimy discharge with the stool; changeable mood; and fear. Schuessler recommends 6X and 12X, low potencies for purulent eye troubles with a yellow discharge. The dog is better in open air.

Iron (ferrum) is the metallic element related to Pluto. Prepared homeopathically, this remedy is used to raise hemoglobin and red blood cell counts. It stimulates the bone marrow and accelerates the circulation of blood.

Consider the following homeopathic remedies[24] for Scorpio:

Alumina is for conditions producing both emaciation and weakness of the limbs. A craving for an abnormal substance (such as charcoal) may be seen, as well as straining at stool, with hard, knotty feces.

Arnica is often used both before and after surgery. It can be used prophylactically prior to spaying or neutering and in any condition where bruising and injury occur, when the skin remains unbroken.[25] It reduces shock. Consider using *Arnica* after teeth cleaning or extraction. (I've found that the teeth and gums of raw-meat-eating dogs stay much cleaner and healthier, especially if they get plenty of raw turkey necks, wings, and backs to gnaw on. However, routine dental care is always advised; try to find a practitioner who doesn't use anesthesia.) This remedy is also appropriate if hunger is constant but food is rejected; for gastric bleeding; and for dysenteric stools accompanied by colicky pain and much straining. The dog may have difficulty expelling urine because of a weakness in the bladder wall.

Arsenicum album for foul-smelling diarrhea. When *Arsenicum* is indicated, the dog exhibits thirst for small quantities of water, and other symptoms exacerbate toward midnight.

Belladonna for retention of urine, with straining to pass. Urine could be dark and turbid owing to presence of blood. Use *Belladonna* for feverish conditions, when the dog's pupils are markedly dilated and she assumes a staring look. Glands may show swelling and tenderness. The skin is usually red and hot, and the dog resents being touched.

Chamomilla for a teething pup. Also of value to the dam when there is tenderness and swelling of the mammary glands.

Hamamelis for venous congestion and passive hemorrhage from veins, and possibly blood in the urine. The eyes may appear bloodshot due to congestion of blood vessels.

Hypericum for lacerated wounds. When Scorpio gets into a brawl with another dog, it can be serious. Wounds that may lead to tetanus indicate the use of this remedy, along with *Ledum* for punctures (*Hypericum* for lacerations or incisions). These remedies can also be used externally. I often make a topical lotion of *Hypericum* and *Calendula*,[26] and I keep *Ledum* ointment on hand as well as standardized grapefruit extract ointment.[27]

Ignatia for postpartum Scorpio mothers if they become

depressed when separated from their pups. This remedy also has an affinity with rectal conditions such as prolapse.

Iodum for gland conditions in general. The keys are a loss of condition and a ravenous appetite, though loss of appetite may also be an indication.

Iris versicolor to control sluggish action of the liver. Can be used to control some types of vomiting.

Pulsatilla for the dam with a tendency to yellow vaginal discharge; ovarian underactivity leading to infertility; influenza, with typical bland yellow discharges from one or both eyes or nostrils, usually the right.

Plants and essential oils influential to Scorpio are cardamom, galangal, hyacinth, hops, pennyroyal, pine, thyme, tuberose, and woodruff. Pluto is affected by basil, broom, coriander, cumin, deerstongue, galangal, garlic, ginger, hops, nasturtium, onion, pennyroyal, pine, rue, and woodruff.

Sagittarius (The Archer)
November 23–December 21
Cardinal element: fire
Ruling planet: Jupiter
Earth color: blue
Astral colors: gold, red, green
Gems: turquoise, diamond
Mineral element: tin
Bach flower: Agrimony
Cell salt: Silicea

Sagittarius is ruled by Jupiter, the planet of expansion, which also affects cell regeneration. This sign relates to the musculature, the cardiac system, and the blood vessels. A mutable fire sign and the friendliest sign in the zodiac, Sagittarius has an elementary quality of dry heat.

Happy, playful, and clownlike from birth, the Sagittarian dog lives to be loved, petted, and appreciated. The eyes of this archer are trusting, and he'll be your loving, faithful friend always, especially if you keep him busy learning new things and meeting new people. He's independent but never denies your divine right to give him pleasure. This optimistic dog steals your heart and keeps you smiling.

He doesn't possess a mean bone in his body and never rejects you, your friends, or other animals. He cries and whines if you leave him alone, so don't. He needs a companion from birth and it's best to adopt a sibling from the same litter, as two Sagittarians are better than one.

He'll go for a ride in the car (he loves to travel) and may enjoy dog shows. He's happy if you leave an article of your clothing on the floor or in his bed for him to sleep with when you're at work. Better yet, take him with you if possible. If not, he'll probably drag that clothing of yours all around the house. Basically, he loves to be wherever you are. But his need for attention is balanced by his desire for freedom, so never let him roam from home.

Obedience-train him to heel by your side and take him for long walks. The Sagittarian dog may just think he's a person. He's happy to be friends with your other animal companions if you start him young. Dogs and cats can make wonderful companions, despite what many people think. But if you have a doggie door, be careful your cat doesn't sneak out and call every feline in the neighborhood to come over and play.

He's forever curious. If this dog could talk, he'd never stop asking questions. If he knew what hypocrisy meant, he wouldn't stand for it. If he sees you do something, he wants to do it, too. He may be clumsy, knocking over vases and pulling down tablecloths in his path.

A Sagittarian can also be obstinate and likes to challenge your authority, especially if he's a big dog. As he grows, he may become a bit overbearing. He simply doesn't realize how heavy he is and wants to cuddle like a puppy. Don't throw him off when he jumps on you, just give him the bear hug he seems to crave.

At dog shows, people and commotion don't frighten a Sagittarian one bit. If you're interested in showing him, get him used to being handled from an early age. The judges will love him as he shows off himself beautifully.

The Bach flower remedy for Sagittarius is *Agrimony*. The Agrimony type is good spirited and carefree, but these attributes may disguise inner worries, nervousness, and anxiety. Peace loving and good companions, they love freedom and adventure but may worry that you'll forget about them and lock them up somewhere or that you won't ever come home and feed them. They are dichotomous like the archer, which illustrates triumph over his animal nature. He knows he's an animal, but you treat him as if he were a person. Agrimony can work wonders for oversensitivity, too.

The cell salt attributed to Sagittarius is *Silicea* (silica). It is recommended when the dog seems irritated, definitely a symptom that something is wrong, either mentally or physically. Could this clumsy dog have fallen and injured himself? *Silicea* may be used for everything from acne to bronchitis. The dog may experience a loss of power in the legs and/or a contraction of the tendons. Caries (decay, ulceration, or inflammation of the bone) of spinal processes may indicate the use of this remedy. Symptoms are always worse at night and during a full moon. Schuessler recommends the 6X and 12X potencies.

Tin (stannum) is Jupiter's element. Like Jupiter, tin has a close connection with the respiratory system as well as the digestive organs, including the liver. Tin is used for a hoarse throat, with accompanying rawness, obstruction of the air passages, and yellow-green phlegm. The recommended dosage is 3X.

Consider the following homeopathic remedies[28] for Sagittarius:

Arnica because of the potential for the dog to injure himself. *Arnica* is a good remedy to keep on hand for both internal and external use before and after surgery, including tooth extraction.[29]

Bryonia alba for a feeling of weakness in the limbs. This remedy is extremely useful in the treatment of many conditions when the main guiding symptom grows worse from movement (such as with pneumonia or pleurisy), and the animal prefers to lie on his affected side, bringing pressure to bear and thus restricting movement.

Chamomilla for mild pain in the extremities and for teething in the young pup.

The plants and essential oils associated with Sagittarius are bergamot, calendula, clove, hyssop, lemon balm, mace, nutmeg, oakmoss, rosemary, and saffron. Jupiter is enhanced by clove, honeysuckle, hyssop, lemon balm, meadowsweet, nutmeg, oakmoss, sage, star anise, and tonka.

Capricorn (The Goat)
December 22–January 20
Cardinal element: earth

Ruling planet: Saturn

Earth color: blue-violet

Astral colors: garnet, silver, gray, brown, black

Gems: garnet, white onyx, moonstone

Mineral element: lead

Bach flower: Mimulus

Cell salt: Calcarea phosphoricum

Ruled by Saturn and represented by the goat (and sometimes the fish or the unicorn), Capricorn rules the digestive tract and the bones. This sign has an elementary quality of dry cold.

Capricorn is an elegant dog, with one of the most intriguing personalities. Because of her depth and complexity, she may appear aloof or remote, but this only masks an inherent shyness and introspection.

Saturn indicates security, caution, and reliability. Capricorn, represented by the mountain goat, takes one step at a time, checking for sure ground or a firm foundation before making a move.

Capricorn is a feminine sign and forever youthful, but there's something stoic about her even when she's playing. Such intense eyes when she looks at you, they tell the whole story. Just be receptive to it.

She's strong willed and tenacious, with a mind of her own. She doesn't like to be embarrassed and hates to lose. Though she's the most conservative sign in the zodiac, energy is one thing she doesn't conserve. Like the mountain goat, she likes to climb to the highest vantage point and assume dominion over everything and everyone. When it comes to play, she's nonstop and downright silly.

The Capricorn dog tries hard to be a person for you, but

remember, she's still a dog. A tidy animal, she rarely gets dirty or breaks anything. If she does, she's very sorry, as she wants to be liked and admired.

Watch her weight—she loves to eat. She loves to let you groom her, bathe her, and brush her teeth, but if she thinks your guard is down, she'll bolt in a flash and head for the hills. Take her for frequent walks on a leash. She dreams about birds, chasing rabbits, and anything that keeps her agile body and quick mind moving. She seems to sleep less than most dogs, but boredom will knock her right out.

The Capricorn dog matures quickly but still wants to be the baby and may be jealous of a new puppy, so think twice before bringing home a pal. She'd rather have you all to herself. But when her supremacy isn't threatened, Capricorn loves other animals, perhaps more than she does people. And when she challenges another animal companion, she ends up on top through sheer persistence, and the former ruler won't even realize his position has been usurped. If you do bring home a new friend, be patient. The Capricorn will come around eventually, but she'll growl at the intruder every chance she gets and may even ignore you for a while. She's quite serious about her aggression and can do damage to the new pet, so be careful. Try changing the subject by giving her a toy or a raw turkey neck.

The Capricorn in need of *Mimulus,* the Bach flower remedy selected for this sign, suffers from fears of unknown origin and from insecurities caused by past experience. Her home, human guardians, and animal friends are all-important to her sense of security. She may be withdrawn yet dislike being alone. Unless you look closely, you may think she's not the warmest dog you've ever known, but her sense of play will usually warm your heart. When fear gets the better of her, incorporate Mimulus into her regimen, along with Rescue Remedy for extreme situations.

The cell salt for Capricorn is *Calcarea phosphoricum* (calcium phosphate). When Dr. George W. Carey allocated *Calc. phos.* to Capricorn, he may have done so because the Latin word *calcium* means (in addition to "lime") "end" or "goal." This corresponds beautifully to the sign of Capricorn, as its season closes out the Roman calendar year. Capricorn rules the limbs and the digestive tract. Discuss this remedy with your practitioner if your dog seems especially anxious, has been grieving a loss, or is vexed. A change in weather may exacerbate rheumatism in the joints, accompanied by pain and swelling; there may be pain in the extremities during movement. Symptoms are worse from cold, wet, or motion; the dog feels better lying down. There may even be brittleness of bones. Corneal opacities and ulceration of the eyes, with a tendency to cataracts, may be present. A young dog may display colicky diarrhea after feeding. In the adult, diabetes insipidus may benefit from this remedy. Think of *Calc. phos.* for an animal whose development was delayed because of improper diet. This remedy has an affinity with tissues concerned with the growth and repair of cells. The lower potencies of 3X and 6X are usually prescribed.

The metal for Saturn is *lead (plumbum)*. This remedy has proved useful for intermittent limping and for arteriosclerosis (a painful disorder in which fibrous tissue thickens the arteries, so smaller ones may become blocked). This condition can lead to others, such as epilepsy and kidney disorders. Since lead is not broken down metabolically (yet another reason not to feed food from cans, which contain lead), this element is eliminated from the body with great difficulty. Only dilutions from 6X and up should ever be considered.

Consider the following homeopathic remedies[30] for Capricorn:

Bryonia alba when there's a weakness in the limbs or pain with any movement. Joints are painful and swollen.

Calcarea carbonica (calcium carb.) for joint pain and poorly developed bones due to calcium deficiency. This is a good constitutional remedy for the treatment of skeletal disorders, perhaps exacerbated by too-close breeding of pedigreed dogs. It's essential to include adequate bonemeal for calcium in the diets of pregnant and nursing dams. They, as well as nursing pups, can require twice what other dogs need on a daily basis. (Some giant breeds, however, may require less.)

Pulsatilla for influenza with typical eye symptoms. Again, pain in the limbs accompanies other symptoms.

Plants and essential oils influencing Capricorn are cypress, honeysuckle, lilac, mimosa, myrrh, patchouli, tonka, tulip, and vetiver. Cypress, mimosa, myrrh, and patchouli are attributed to the ruling planet, Saturn.

Aquarius (The Water Carrier)

January 21–February 19

Cardinal element: air

Ruling planets: Uranus, Saturn

Earth color: violet

Astral colors: blue, pink, nile green

Gems: amethyst, sapphire, opal, turquoise

Mineral element: zinc

Bach flower: Water Violet

Cell salt: Natrum muriaticum

Ruled by Uranus (a planet added to the astrological literature after its discovery in the eighteenth century), Aquarius is a fixed air sign, with an elementary quality of wet heat. This sign governs the legs, ankles, circulatory system, and blood.

Aquarius is strong, trusting, fearless, and courageous but also sensuous and sensitive. The Aquarian dog is incredibly psychic—he seems to know, without knowing how he knows. There is nothing average about Aquarius. He's the most precocious dog in the house and becomes top dog before you know it. He knows when he's being good and when he's being bad—and has extremes in both directions. He loves freedom and is very independent.

Male or female, Aquarian animals talk to you incessantly—verbally and nonverbally. They love people and tolerate other animals nicely, but they know you love them best and share that secret with you. They ignore you sometimes when you call but come running when they're ready (just a few moments later than you'd like). They're unpredictable and contradictory—one moment calm and docile, then suddenly wound up like a tornado.

Great eaters as well as very good athletes, they love to roll over on their backs (sometimes falling asleep in that position, a hilarious sight).

With this perpetual clown, you never know what to expect. Your Aquarian can become best friends with a cat, a potbellied pig, even a horse or a goat! He's so outgoing and fearless that these other creatures just accept him as one of their own. Aquarius has a capacity to love beyond that of any other sign in the zodiac.

Matilda was an Aquarian half-basset who shared her life with Dr. Scanlan.[31] The only surviving puppy from a dying mother who had been in labor far too long, her first precocious act was to start yelling when only her head had emerged from Momma. Everyone was her friend. She regularly left home to visit the neighbors nearby but always came back home. Her best buddies were a cat and a Doberman, and she regularly made friends with dogs that wanted to eat all other dogs.

The Bach flower remedy selected for Aquarius is *Water Violet* because, despite his wonderful charms, this dog can be proud and aloof. He also can feel lonely if there's no one around to give him constant admiration. If he suddenly withdraws a bit, consider Water Violet, which will, when used with Rescue Remedy, help him handle whatever he's going through. He may also be quite headstrong and a bit indifferent. Water Violet may assist with any of these negative states of mind.

The cell salt selected for Aquarius is *Natrum muriaticum* (sodium chloride). Symptoms may include acrid lacrimation of the eyelids, which may be swollen. Cataracts or generalized opacities of the cornea may occur. There may be a thin watery discharge from the nasal passages, with difficulty breathing and an attendant cough. The dog may vomit a whitish gray material. An indifferent appetite and constipation may be present, as well as a generalized weakness of limbs. The skin may be itchy, and bald spots may occur on various body parts. *Nat. Mur.* is useful in the treatment of eczema in debilitated dogs. Salt retention leads to thirst, which may indicate kidney problems.

Associated with Uranus, *zinc (zincum)* is a relatively new metal. The amount of zinc in organs seems to be higher when cell growth is vigorous. Uranus relates to the cerebellum, and many have regarded zinc as a brain remedy. Its main action is on the central nervous system, when tiredness and weakness alternate with restlessness and excitement. There is a tendency for the animal to lean to the left side. Lameness and weakness in the legs, with trembling and twitching, may be noticeable. Vomiting can occur, as well as enlargement of the liver, with signs of gas and colic. Eyes may twitch, and the conjunctiva become red and inflamed. This is a useful homeopathic remedy in veterinary practice for suppressed feverish conditions with long-standing septic (toxic) states.

Consider the following homeopathic remedies[32] for Aquarius:

Abrotanum for circulatory disorders and for emaciation of the legs.

Aconite, as it relates to the veins.

Arnica for injuries, especially to the legs.

Ceanothus for conditions involving the spleen.

Kali iodatum or *Kali hydriodicum* for various symptoms indicating eye and respiratory conditions, such as pneumonia or kennel cough. Stiffness of the joints, with pain that makes the dog cry out suddenly, is also a symptom. The skin may produce nodules, with swelling. I have used Kali for incessant itching when nothing else seems to help.

Ledum when the extremities become swollen and the feet feel hot. There can be tenderness and stiffness in the shoulder area.

Rhus toxicondedron for stiffness in joints alleviated by moving.

Plants and essential oils associated with Aquarius are cost-mary, hops, lavender, lemon verbena, parsley, patchouli, pine, star anise, and sweet pea. Uranus is influenced by cypress, mimosa, myrrh, and patchouli.

Pisces (The Fish)
February 20–March 20

Cardinal element: water
Ruling planets: Neptune, Jupiter
Earth colors: cerise, magenta
Astral colors: white, pink, emerald green, black
Gems: chrysolite, pink shell, moonstone
Mineral element: tin
Bach flower: Rock Rose
Cell salt: Ferrum phosphoricum

Pisces, the twelfth and last sign of the zodiac, is ruled by Neptune and Jupiter and represents change and the consciousness of the soul. This sign governs the arterial blood, the red corpuscles, and the feet. Dogs born under this sign may be susceptible to diseases of the chest. Pisces is a mutable water sign, with an elementary quality of wet cold.

Sweet, gentle, endearing, and magical—part elf, part leprechaun—she grabs at your heartstrings, and before you know it, you're the proud adoptive parent of a Pisces puppy.

The Piscean is a truly fanciful creature. You expect to see her leaping from lily pad to lily pad in pursuit of the elusive butterfly. And, oh, those dreamy eyes—made of stardust, to be sure. She sees, hears, and smells many things, such as spirits, that we don't know are there.

The Piscean is the keeper of thousands of years of secrets. Tune into her, and you'll be amazed at what she tells you. When you see her sleeping body twitch, she's dreaming of chasing brightly colored birds, rainbows, and rabbits, for color is extremely important to them. She needs it to express the higher attributes of her spirit. Try it yourself sometime, and maybe you'll meet your Pisces on the astral plane playing in the cool blue-green grass among the buttercups.

The Pisces dog needs to remain still for periods of time and, through this occasional stillness, can bring the correct response directly to the surface of the psychic sea. Otherwise, she's pulled in opposing directions, constantly in conflict. Her sign is symbolized by two fish—one swimming toward the source of the water, the other toward the sea.

Her tendency to be dreamy makes it easy for her to leave her body. Your Pisces dog may learn this technique early in life in order to avoid reprimands. She simply tunes out, traveling to realms of safety on the wings of fantasy. Give her lots of attention and encourage her to be outgoing. If you don't, she'll be shy forever. But respect her privacy when she's in a mysterious mood, and let her be.

Pisces loves to love, but she gets stressed easily. Fortunately, you rarely need to reprimand her. She seems perfect—though you might be letting her get away with a lot. She can charm you into getting her own way, so you may as well surrender. But she never abuses you for this or lets you spoil her too much—she's too loving for that. Because she makes up her own rules, you must gently let her know what yours are. Use positive reinforcement and avoid the negative. Tell her she's good, and that's what she'll be.

Pisces dogs have their own schedules. They sleep when they want to, eat when they want to, play when they want to—so you may just have to adjust your schedule to theirs.

It's important to protect your Piscean from bullies, animal or human, as she doesn't understand and can't tolerate aggression or violence. The music of Chopin or Mozart (both Pisceans) soothes her.

Rock Rose is the Bach flower remedy of choice for Pisces.

One of the five ingredients in Rescue Remedy, Rock Rose is usually prescribed for acute or accumulated fear. The Pisces dog can be a target for abuse and is easily panicked. A hotbed of neuroses renders them prone to diseases of the psyche. For these reasons, also consider Rescue Remedy for the Pisces dog.

Ferrum phosphoricum (iron phosphate) is the cell salt attributed to Pisces. This remedy is especially useful in the early stages of inflammatory conditions that develop less quickly than those calling for *Aconite,* and a soft, full pulse is symptomatic, as opposed to the *Aconite* type. Throat involvement may be a consideration. *Ferrum phosphoricum* may prove useful in the treatment of heat stroke, ailments of the feet, and muscular stiffness, when joints become swollen.

Neptune also responds to the element *tin (stannum).* This metal has a close connection with the respiratory system, and so is employed for hoarseness and raw conditions of the throat, a weak chest, obstruction of air passages, and when yellow/green phlegm is expectorated with each cough. Tin is also associated with digestive organs such as the liver. The mental state of the Pisces dog may seem sad or anxious, and she may hide from people. Her symptoms worsen with anger, a loss of fluids, and even the slightest touch on affected parts. She feels better after her breakfast. She seeks warmth and is improved by rest at night.

Consider the following homeopathic remedies[33] for Pisces:

Aconite because of Pisceans' propensity to fear.

Bryonia alba when chills and fever accompany a thirst for large quantities of water. Nasal discharge may show bleeding, a yellowish deposit may cover the tongue, and vomiting may occur. The liver may be affected, leading to hepatitis, with jaundice and swelling or tenderness over the liver.

Calcarea carbonicum (*Calc. carb.*) can be used for muscular spasms, since Pisces controls the feet. Its application to the extremities in general is beneficial. *Calcium,* in homeopathic potency, is the only sure way to establish this element in the system.

The plants and essential oils influencing Pisces are apple, cardamom, gardenia, hyacinth, jasmine, lily, mugwort, myrrh, palmarosa, sandalwood, vanilla, and ylang-ylang. Neptune's essential aromas are clove, honeysuckle, hyssop, lemon balm, meadowsweet, nutmeg, oakmoss, sage, star anise, and tonka.

IN SUMMARY

THIS SECTION TOUCHES on only a few homeopathic remedies, Bach flowers, cell salts, and plant essences,[34] each of which may or may not have specific relationships to various aspects of the twelve sun signs. I encourage you always to look to your dog's specific symptoms, referring to your homeopathic repertory book (I use J. T. Kent's) and then working with your materia medica to find which remedy is the best to try (I use Boericke).

This is the homeopathic approach, so rather than trying to conquer disease, you may match as many symptoms as you can to the descriptions given for the homeopathic types in order to discover the constitutional and acute remedies that fit the overall picture of your dog's condition. Again, be sure to consult your homeopathic veterinarian or practitioner prior to administering any remedy.

Chapter Nine

Saying Good-bye to the Ones We Love

COPING WITH THE LOSS OF AN ANIMAL COMPANION

FOR ME, THE loss of an animal companion is as agonizing an experience as anything I can imagine. My animal companions are every bit as important to me as my human family. I meet so many people at cat shows or through referrals who have lost an animal companion or who have an old or infirm animal for whom they would like a young friend, but I know in my heart that they want that young animal to be there to help them grieve when the inevitable happens.

I've grieved the loss of many animal friends. My mother tells me the first death I ever witnessed was that of a sparrow in my backyard. She says I stood right over that little bit of fluff and feathers. When asked what I was doing, I responded that I was waiting to be sure its soul would fly up to heaven.

As a cat breeder now, I still cry on the rare occasion when I lose a kitten, at birth or days later. There never seems to be enough time for these precious little spirits. It can be hard to find people who understand such a deep attachment, but I've been blessed with friends and clients who love their animal companions and so can truly empathize with me.

The mourning process, the time needed to grieve, is a personal thing, but we must go through it—as denial is even more painful. I feel flower remedies are helpful at such times. The Grief Recovery Hotline (800-445-4808) may be of help to some. For others, adopting a kitten, puppy, or adult cat or dog from the pound or Humane Society may be the answer, for surely our love doesn't die with our loved ones. With so many animals dying needlessly at shelters every day, these adoptions are beneficial to both the adopter and the adoptee. You may find the image of your deceased companion, or you may adopt a very different little being. Either way, trust yourself and follow your heart.

Allow yourself to progress through the stages outlined by Elisabeth Kübler-Ross in her excellent book *Death: The Final Stage of Growth* (see "Resources"). They are, not necessarily in this order (1) denial and isolation, (2) bargaining, (3) anger and depression, and (4) acceptance. Barbara Meyers, a certified grief therapist at the Holistic Animal Consulting Center in New York City, adds reinvestment to this list. After all, what good is love if you don't give it away? Other stages commonly experienced are guilt and the feeling of not being able to go on.

The decisions that plague us at the end are heavy burdens to bear—for instance, is it too late to seek alternative healing therapies when the animal has been through so much? Should we choose euthanasia or permit our animals to endure until the end? Most holistically treated animals can die at home and do not need to be euthanized unless their disease causes great discomfort.

COMMUNICATE WITH YOUR SICK OR AGING DOG

ULTIMATELY, YOU AND your animal friend need to make these choices together. Now is the time for spiritual work: meditation, prayer, and nonverbal communication. You'll receive guidance when your heart and mind are open. Do what you think is best, then let it go. Animals have their own paths and their own spiritual journeys, according to Dr. Christina Chambreau. So when the end is near, the best thing you can do is release them. Tell them, out loud, that it's okay for them to pass on. This helps them follow their own path.

The psychic Laurel Steinhice says that animals reincarnate in tandem with their human companions and with one another. The closer the interspecies bonding, the more likely and more frequent such reincarnation is to occur. Steinhice believes that the species are interchangeable. The Egyptians must have known this, too: their cats were often mummified and entombed with their human guardians. Steinhice also recommends telling your animal companions that you understand they wish to leave this body and that you will welcome them in their new one, so their spirit may continue its bond with you.[1]

Someone once told me I might view death as a departure on a great ship. Just as the ship sails away from us, and we wave good-bye from the shore, so it is that someone waits on the other side and is waving hello. Our animals make this journey with such grace only when we allow them this dignity, which is their birthright. So, before you allow your beloved animals to be drugged, poked and prodded, or surgically explored, communicate with them and try to ascertain what they want. There may be a brand-new healthy body waiting just around the corner for their spirit to slip into in order for them to be with you again.

When my collie Lonnie was so desparately ill with bone cancer, we communicated constantly. Having her put to sleep was one of the most difficult decisions I have ever made in my life. However, she told me when it was time. It was the right time because more time in her broken little body would have injured the dignity of this magnificent soul. Heaven must be a better place because she's there.

However, as with living, we can learn so much from our animal friends about death and dying. They have no fear of it but seem to view it as a natural progression. I'm sure they're sad to leave us (just as we're sad to lose them), but finally we must, after our grief, say farewell to the dead and concentrate on giving our love to the living and watching for a clue to help us recognize their return. It may not always be convenient for us. However, when they come back, you will open your heart and allow them to come home.

Dr. Chambreau says we've been changed permanently by living with our animals, and in that way they live forever in how we interact with the world. Machaelle Small Wright suggests that animals, like humans, are not of this earth, but rather souls that have chosen to use this planet as their setting for an evolutionary experience. Animals have chosen not to operate in the same complicated way as humans, but rather to participate through nature. This, of course, does not make them lesser beings than us—it simply makes them different.[2]

As long as we remain in our steward relationship with them, they must trust us to do what's best for them. And that, of course, is all we can do.

Animals have feelings very close to our own (as we learn by reading books like *When Elephants Weep* [see "Resources"]). The only difference seems to be that we are the only species that has feelings about our feelings. This does not make their pain, their sorrow, their losses any less than ours. We need to take an active interest in how animals are treated. If they could speak to us in our own language, what would they say about our stewardship? Would they implore us in laboratories to cease drilling holes in them, dissecting them with agonizing experiments? Would they beg to be returned to their homes and families and state their unalienable rights? How can we destroy them in the name of anything? No, we do not have the right, only the power. Let's work together to free them from exploitation and profit and join with them in a deeper emotional connection across the species barrier.

I cherish every moment I spend with these precious spirits, and every one of them has taught me that we are all one family on this planet. This planet and our lives are made better because they are here.

Conclusion

I HOPE THE information in this book benefits your dog. Perhaps it will even motivate you to explore, both for you and for your companion animal, the fascinating world of nutrition and holistic health care. I trust you can feel the passion and excitement I have for this ever expanding field, which I believe is every bit as important as mainstream medicine.

Though along the way I've probably offended some well-meaning institutions and their schools of thought, my intent has merely been to present the many alternative treatments and therapies. I am in no way attempting to prescribe, give medical care, or replace anyone's veterinary practitioner. I just wish to arm you with all the information you need to make well-informed choices.

Indeed, many conventional veterinarians and pet-food manufacturers mean well. They've spent years studying their specialties, and they deserve to profit from our use of their goods and services as long as we and our companion animals benefit from their care or products.

Isn't it time we took back the responsibility for our health and that of our animals? I would never be so narrow-minded as to deny completely the usefulness of allopathic medicine, but I make sure that I exhaust every natural method available before I risk the use of drugs or surgery. And when I must resort to these methods of treatment, I'm glad I know how to help the body and spirit repair whatever toll or side effects they induce. The wonderful thing about holistic health care is that it can be used in conjunction with allopathic medicine.

Many of the things discussed may seem a little "far out" to you, and nothing works for everyone. Explore the "Resources" section that follows, and call or write for more information about whatever seems appropriate or interesting. In conjunction with your veterinarian, make your own determination when working with alternative consultants and practitioners. Always ask for references.

Finally, share this book, as well as your insights and concerns, with your health care providers; such a partnership benefits you, them, and your animal. You may be surprised at how open to new ideas your providers will be. Even if they're not, the decision about whether to use holistic care is still yours.

I welcome you to the world of *Natural Dog Care* and want you to know that I'm committed to continuing my journey and sharing my findings with those who have an open mind and heart and are willing to listen. Just remember, the truth is not of much use if it comes too late.

Notes

Chapter One: Getting to Know Your Dog

1. Bruce Fogle, D.V.M., *Encyclopedia of the Dog,* pp. 10–11.
2. Ibid., p. 19.
3. My discussion of the seven groups of dogs was obtained from Tetsu Yamazaki's *Legacy of the Dog,* pp. 8–9.
4. Roger De Haan, D.V.M., "What Is Holistic Veterinary Care?" *Natural Care of Pets: Alternative Therapies in Companion Animal Health,* 1982, p. 23.

Chapter Two: Interacting with Your Dog

1. Machaelle Small Wright, *Behaving As If the God in All Life Mattered,* p. 65.
2. According to Yolanda LaCombe in "On the Floor with Cats: Cindy Wood's Feline Communication Advice," *Tiger Tribe,* Mar.–Apr. 1993, p. 19.

Chapter Three: The Dangers of Conventional Care

1. Deepak Chopra, *Perfect Health* (New York: Crown Publishing,1991), p.14.
2. Unless otherwise noted, all further quotations of Dr. Chambreau come from her conversations/correspondence with the author.
3. John Fudens, D.V.M., "Vaccinations," *Natural Pet,* pp. 9–11.
4. W. Jean Dodds, D.V.M., DVM, Dec. 1990.
5. Richard Pitcairn, D.V.M., address to the American Holistic Veterinary Medical Association (AHVMA), September 1993; text available from the AHVMA on audiotape or in written proceedings of conference. This condition has also been identified in people and was written about extensively by J. Compton Burnett, M.D., in *Vaccinosis and Its Cure by Thuja, with Remarks on Homeoprophylaxis,* and in his other books.
6. Richard Pitcairn, D.V.M., "A Foolish Practice," *Tiger Tribe,* Jan.–Feb. 1994, pp. 24–26.
7. C. Edgar Sheaffer, D.V.M., "Hooked on Homeopathy," *Tiger Tribe,* Nov.–Dec. 1993. pp. 8, 15–17.
8. Wendy Volhard and Kerry Brown, D.V.M., *Holistic Guide for a Healthy Dog,* pp. 99–100.
9. Sue Marston, *The Vaccination Connection,* p. 4.
10. Ibid., p. 5.
11. Ibid., p. 30.
12. Ibid.
13. Ibid., p. 9.
14. Ibid.
15. Ibid., p. 6.
16. Viera Scheibner, Ph.D., *Vaccination: A Medical Assault on the Immune System,* back cover.

17. Marston, *The Vaccination Connection*, p. 6.

18. Ibid., p. 28.

19. Ibid.

20. Ibid.

21. Fudens, "Vaccinations," pp. 6–9.

22. Elizabeth Terrell, "Post-Vaccinational Tumor Development in Cats," *Cat Fanciers Almanac*, CFA Health Committee News, Dec. 1993, p. 90.

23. Tom R. Phillips D.V.M., Ph.D., and Ronald D. Schultz, D.V.M., Ph.D., "Canine and Feline Vaccines," *Kirk's Current Veterinary Therapy*, 1992, pp. 202–6.

24. Personal communication with Dr. Christina Chambreau.

25. Ibid.

26. Proving is the homeopathic procedure for ascertaining the effects of substances by administering them to healthy subjects in order to observe and record symptoms.

27. In a speech at the 1993 AHVMA convention, Dr. Pitcairn addressed research on and clinical experience using nosodes, mentioning the writing of Hahnemann (cholera), Boenninghausen (thuja in smallpox), Shepherd (homeopathy in epidemic diseases), Jervis (treatment of canine distemper), and Day (stillbirths in pigs and bovine mastitis). Other studies on nosodes (or microdoses) conducted with human and animal subjects include those by Bastide, Daurat, Carriere, Karouby, Doucet-Jaboeuf, and Saxton. Don't confuse the prophylactic use of nosodes with their use in treating different diseases, as they are often used as remedies.

28. Christopher Day, M.R.C.V.S., "Isopathic Prevention of Kennel Cough—Is Vaccination Justified?" *International Journal for Homeopathy*, Apr. 1987, pp. 45–50.

29. Personal communication with Dr. Chambreau.

30. Dr. Pitcairn's address at the 1993 AHVMA meeting.

31. Dr. Chambreau suggests that you determine which disease your puppy is most likely to contract and start with that nosode and then alternate with the other most likely nosode. Distemper and parvovirus are the two diseases most common in young puppies, unless you have a particular epidemic of something else in your kennel. It is best, again according to Dr. Chambreau (personal communication from Dr. Chambreau, July 23, 1996), to start at age eight weeks or older. If there is a lot of risk, you may start as young as four weeks. Explore with your holistic veterinarian the rationale for giving nosodes on an ongoing basis. Dr. Chambreau feels they are more effective when given after exposure (as both the virus and the nosode are rushing to the receptor sites). Dr. Chambreau feels that it is better to build up the overall health and well-being of our pets than to erect walls of protection the same way conventional veterinarians do with vaccines. You must, as your animal's guardian, ask yourself if you are willing to deal with and treat symptoms as they arise, even those from infectious disease. Or is this too scary a proposition? Personally, the side effects of vaccines are more frightening to me than the risk of acute disease episodes.

32. Marina Zacharias, *Natural Rearing Newsletter*, Vol. 1, Issue 4, May 1995, p. 6.

33. The source of the information in this section is "Danger: Toxic Chemicals in the Home," *Natural Pet*, July–Aug. 1993, pp. 18–19.

34. Volhard and Brown, *Holistic Guide for a Healthy Dog*, p. 98.

35. Baby meats make excellent bribe foods for finicky or convalescing pets, so many of us have switched to Beachnut since Gerber has recently added onion and garlic powder.

36. Diane Stein, *Natural Healing for Dogs and Cats,* p. 180.

37. Joanne Stefanatos, "Holistic Pet Care."

38. Ann Martin, "Does Your Dog Food Bark? A Study of the Pet Food Fallacy," *Natural Pet,* Mar.–Apr., 1995, pp. 58–59.

39. Ibid., p. 59.

40. Ibid.

41. Deborah Belgum and David Ferrell, "Elephant Deaths Draw Spotlights' Glare," *Los Angeles Times,* Aug. 10, 1996.

42. Richard Pitcairn, D.V.M., and Susan Hubble Pitcairn, *The Complete Guide to Natural Health for Dogs and Cats,* p. 13.

43. Pat McKay, *Reigning Cats and Dogs,* p. 3.

44. Stein, *Natural Healing for Dogs and Cats,* p. 13.

45. Douglas Kappstatter, D.V.M., "Enzymes, Raw Food, and Kitty's Hat Size," *Tiger Tribe,* Mar.–Apr. 1995, p. 17.

46. Ibid.

47. Francis M. Pottenger, Jr., M.D., *Pottenger's Cats,* pp. 39–42. This book is available through the Price-Pottenger Nutrition Foundation (see "Resources"), as are edited versions of Dr. Pottenger's many research reports, books, pamphlets, and tapes. The foundation is a nonprofit educational organization that conducts worldwide research and disseminates information about natural nutrition.

48. "Effects of Food Processing on Amino Acids," *The Cornell Book of Cats: A Comprehensive Medical Reference for Every Cat or Kitten,* p. 73.

49. Alfred Plechner, D.V.M., and Martin Zucker, "Pet Allergies: Remedies for an Epidemic," *D.V.M.,* Mar. 1985, p. 11.

50. Ibid., p. 13.

51. "Effects of Food Processing on Amino Acids," p. 73.

52. Volhard and Brown, *Holistic Guide for a Healthy Dog,* pp. 255–81.

53. R. L. Wysong, D.V.M., *Fresh and Raw* (available from the Wysong Company, see "Resources").

54. Ibid.

55. *Animal Protective Institute of America's Investigative Report,* p. 8.

56. Tribal News, "Don't Zap the Cat," *Tiger Tribe,* Nov.–Dec. 1993, p. 9.

57. Ibid.

58. Ibid.

59. Ibid.

Chapter Four: Nutrition

1. Barry Sears, Ph.D., *Enter the Zone,* p. 77.

2. Personal communication with Dr. Barry Sears.

3. Sears, *Enter the Zone,* p. 77.

4. Ibid., Preface pp. xiii–xiv.

5. Personal communication with Dr. Christina Chambreau.

6. Sears, *Enter the Zone,* p. 14.

7. Ibid., p. 15.

8. Ibid., p. 16.

9. Ibid., p. 103.

10. Wendy Volhard and Kerry Brown, D.V.M., *Holistic Guide for a Healthy Dog,* p. 17.

11. Ibid., p. 20.

12. Ibid., p. 19.

13. Cats require higher protein. See my other book, *Natural Cat Care,* p. 69.

14. Volhard and Brown, *Holistic Guide for a Healthy Dog,* p. 255.

15. Ibid., p. 11.

16. Sears, *Enter the Zone,* p. 85.

17. Personal communication with Dr. Russell Swift.

18. Personal communication with Dr. Sears.

19. Personal communication with Dr. Nancy Scanlan.

20. Volhard and Brown, *Holistic Guide for a Healthy Dog,* p. 90.

21. Conversation with Dr. Chambreau.

22. Personal communication with Dr. Sears.

23. This diet is based on Dr. Swift's recipe for homemade pet food. His recipe was printed in *Healthy Pets, Naturally,* Feb.–Mar. 1996, p. 8. I have modified it slightly to conform to "The Zone" principles. Your individual dog may need a touch more or less of the different ingredients, so check with your holistic veterinarian before deviating from these guidelines.

24. Conversation with Dr. Sears.

25. Personal correspondence with Dr. Scanlan.

26. Personal correspondence with Dr. Chambreau.

27. Ibid.

28. Personal communication with Dr. Scanlan.

29. Personal communication with Dr. Chambreau.

30. Pat McKay, *Reigning Cats and Dogs,* pp. 17–18.

31. See section on supplements for a partial list of organisms that this invaluable addition controls, as well as a discussion of other uses to which it may be put.

32. McKay, *Reigning Cats and Dogs,* p. 19.

33. Marina Zacharias, *Natural Rearing Newsletter,* May 1996, p. 6.

34. Beth M. Levy, *Dr. John Willard's Catalyst-Altered Water: A Health Learning Handbook.*

35. Volhard and Brown, *Holistic Guide for a Healthy Dog,* pp. 66–67.

36. "Neutraceuticals vs. Pharmaceuticals," *Natural Pet Magazine,* July–Aug. 1995, pp. 46–48.

37. Personal communication with Dr. Scanlan.

38. Ibid.

39. Montmorillonite clay is also known as Redmond clay. It contains the following trace minerals: antimony, arsenic, barium, beryllium, bismuth, boron, bromine, cadmium, calcium, cerium, cesium, chlorine, chromium, cobalt, copper, dysprosium, erbium, europium, fluroine, gadolinium, gallium, germanium, gold, hafnium, holmium, indium, iodine, iridium, iron, lanthanum, lithium, lutecium, magnesium, manganese, molybdenum, neodymium, nickel, niobium, osmium, palladium, phosphorus, platinum, potas-

sium, praseodymium, pihenium, rhodium, rubidium, ruthenium, samarium, scandium, selenium, silicon, silver, sodium, strontium, sulfur, tantalum, tellurium, terbium, thallium, thorium, thulium, tin, titanium, tungsten, uranium, vanadium, ytterbium, yttrium, zinc, zirconium.

40. Personal communication with Dr. Charles Loops.

41. Personal communication with Dr. Scanlan.

42. The oil should be decreased to 1 tablespoon if the fat content of the meat is greater than 15 percent. Two tablespoons for extra lean meat and poultry.

43. Sears, *Enter the Zone,* p. 123.

44. Sunrider's excellent line of herbal foods was created for people, and I've taken them for years. (See "Resources.")

45. I recommend holistic therapy, such as homeopathy or herbs, over the use of antibiotics and steroids, which are suppressive and push disease back into the system only to resurface as something else more serious later on. However, both are necessary in emergency treatment. Obviously, you should follow the advice of your dog's veterinarian, or the consequences could be extremely life threatening. We can rebalance the dog holistically when the animal is through the crisis.

46. Alfred J. Plechner, D.V.M., and Martin Zukor, *Pet Allergies: Remedies for an Epidemic,* p. 20.

47. Zacharias, *Natural Rearing Newsletter,* Oct. 1994.

48. Michael Lemmon, D.V.M., "Your Pet's Health," *Animal Guardian,* 1994, pp. 11–12.

49. Zacharias, *Natural Rearing Newsletter,* July 1995.

50. Robert S. Goldstein, *Pet Talk,* winter 1996, p. 16.

51. Zacharias, *Natural Rearing Newsletter,* May 1995, p. 4.

52. Zacharias, *Natural Rearing Newsletter,* July 1995, p. 5.

53. Zacharias, *Natural Rearing Newsletter,* Nov. 1995, p. 8, with a follow-up on p. 4, May 1995.

54. Personal communication with Dr. Chambreau.

55. Conversation with Dr. Swift.

56. Zacharias, *Natural Rearing Newsletter,* Mar. 1996, pp. 3–4.

57. Luke Granfield, "Super Blue Green Algae—Not Just for Fish," *Tiger Tribe,* Nov.–Dec. 1994, pp. 14–16.

58. Richard A. Passwater, Ph.D., *The New Super Antioxidant Plus: The Amazing Story of Pycnogenol, Free Radical Antagonist and Vitamin C Potentator.*

60. Dr. Scanlan suggests that gold could be toxic to the kidneys if improperly used.

61. Pat McKay, "Have You and Your Cat Had Your Oxygen Today?" *Tiger Tribe,* Sept.–Oct. 1993, pp. 21–22.

62. With various other brands of O_2, such as Homozon, the package directions give suggested dosages for humans. Make sure to adjust the dosage appropriately for your dog.

63. Research on DMG and the immune response was conducted at the Medical University of South Carolina under the directorship of Charles D. Graber, Ph.D. Dr. Graber's group demonstrated that DMG may enhance both humeral (antibody production) and cellular (cellular lymphocyte production) immunity, making an individual less prone to infections and able to respond more quickly to invasion by various viral and bacterial organisms. The research also showed a normalized or substantially raised immune response in the blood of patients with diabetes and sickle-cell anemia. Many health

practitioners are reporting that DMG is an effective anti-infectious agent for their patients. See Charles D. Graber, Ph.D., *Journal of Infectious Diseases* 143, pp. 101–5.

64. J. W. Meduski, M.D., Ph.D., at the University of Southern California School of Medicine.

65. Including bacteria *(salmonella, E. coli, streptococcus, bacillus, vibrio cholera, staphylococcus, clostridium, corynebacteria, diplococcus, lactobacillus, mycobacterium, shigella dysenteria, chlamydia, brucella, cloaca, hemophilus, klebsiella, legionella, moraxella, neisseria, pseudomonas, sarcina, proteus, alcalingenes, campylobacter, pasteurella, serratia, aerobacter, helicobacter)*; fungi *(candida albicans,* trichophyton, epidermophyton, aspergillus, niger, chaetomium, deratinomyces, *Monilia albicans,* trichoderma, saccharomyces, fusarium, pencillium, neurospora); and virus/amebiasis *(Giardia lamblia,* influenza a, African swine fever, *Entamoeba histolytica,* swine vesicular, herpes simplex, foot-and-mouth disease).

Chapter Five: Natural Remedies

1. John Fudens, D.V.M., *The Affinity Holistic Veterinary Clinic's Layman's Handbook to Holistic Care,* p. 21.

2. The "resources" section contains names of organizations that can help you find holistic veterinarians.

3. John Fudens, D.V.M., *Layman's Handbook,* "Herbal Medicine and Pet Health."

4. Note that powdered herbs are also sold in capsule form. You may remove the contents of the capsules to use in herbal recipes.

5. Concentrated herbs are also available. They are processed in the same way as extracts but are subjected to dehydration to remove the moisture, resulting in a solvent-free product. Concentrated herbs are four to six times more potent than extracts.

6. There are three companies whose products I use often, both for myself and for my pets, and distribute to my clients: Sunrider Whole Food Herbs, Nature's Sunshine, and Systemic Formulas, Inc. See "Resources" for further information.

7. See "More About Supplements—Some Good, Some Bad" in Chapter 4, "Nutrition," for information about the dangers of preservatives used with aloe vera.

8. Check with your own health practitioner before fasting.

9. Deepak Chopra, M.D., *Quantum Healing,* p. 17.

10. Other examples of functional disturbances include a lot of scratching, but no evidence of bumps, redness, or scabs; a slight red line along the tooth-gum margin; appetite changes or finickiness at mealtime; behavioral changes (too sweet, too aggressive); vomiting (or gagging); and any other symptoms out of the normal range for healthy dogs.

11. Marina Zacharias also uses combination remedies, which I have found to be very helpful (see "Resources").

12. Homeopathic Education Services (which reports that homeopathy is sometimes called the "royal medicine" because the British royal family has used these remedies since the 1830s) produces a catalog and has a store in Berkeley, California. Standard Homeopathics and Washington Homeopathic Products are also quite reliable, according to Dr. Christina Chambreau.

13. Conversation with Dr. Chambreau.

14. There are now many excellent holistic and homeopathic veterinarians across the country. A number of them may be of help by phone even though they're not local (see

"Resources" or contact me for help).

15. See "Books, Publications, Tapes" in "Resources" for further sources of information on the preparation of homeopathic remedies.

16. Remedies made from diseased tissue are known as nosodes and are discussed in more detail in the section on vaccination (in Chapter 3, "The Dangers of Conventional Care").

17. Recommended readings and sources for purchasing cell salts are included in "Resources." See also Chapter 8 for the relationship of cell salts to the sun signs.

18. H. G. Wolff, D.V.M., *Your Healthy Cat: Homeopathic Medicines for Common Feline Ailments,* p. 7.

19. Marina Zacharias, *Natural Rearing Newsletter,* May 1995.

20. Dr. Chambreau demonstrates this technique on her video (see "Resources").

21. Wendy Volhard and Kerry Brown, D.V.M., *Holistic Guide for a Healthy Dog,* p. 225.

22. Ibid p. 224

23. Kirlian photography allows us to see this energy field, which surrounds all living things. A Kirlian photograph of a leaf, part of which has been cut off, shows light still glowing around the portion that's no longer there (see the "The Aura and Chakras of a Dog" in Chapter 7).

24. Many flower remedies contain alcohol as a preservative. Always dilute them in purified or spring water, as recommended on the label.

25. Numerous human case studies are detailed in Phillip M. Chancellor's book *Bach Flower Remedies.* If you're interested in studying Dr. Bach's approach in depth or in prescribing his remedies for yourself or your dogs, I recommend his book *The Bach Flower Remedies* as well as *Practical Uses and Applications of the Bach Flower Remedies,* by Jessica Beal, Ph.D., N.D. (see "Resources").

26. The founders of FES, Richard Katz and Patricia Kaminsky, have written *Flower Essence Repertory,* a comprehensive selection guide for the natural health practitioner. This book describes the FES remedies and English flower essences produced by Bach's company as well as those by Healing Herbs (see "Resources").

27. Sheehan publishes a booklet entitled *A Guide to Green Hope Farm* (see "Resources").

28. I consult with Yolanda LaCombe (see "Resources"), who prefers to work with healing herbs and North American flower essences, but I use the Bach remedies as well.

29. The remedies are preserved in alcohol, so you must dilute them in spring water before administering, especially orally, as most dogs will have a strong negative reaction to the taste.

30. You can get this type of dosage bottle wherever you purchase your flower remedies, or you may order them directly from Ellon USA or FES (see "Resources").

31. Researched from *Practical Uses and Applications of the Bach Flower Remedies,* by Jessica Beal, Ph.D., N.D.; *The Flower Remedies Handbook,* by Donna Cunningham; and *Flower Essence Repertory,* by Flower Essence Services.

32. I feel that 5 Flowers is even more effective than Rescue Remedy; however, I use them both.

33. I also make up special formulas for my clients by appointment and through telephone

consultation.

34. Diane Stein, *Natural Healing for Dogs and Cats*, pp. 146–47.

35. Diane Stein suggests placing the bottles under a copper pyramid for two hours. Again, do this one flower essence at a time. In my opinion, this step is optional.

36. Contact Perelandra Flower Essences for a catalog and information about its books and remedies (see "Resources").

37. The Burton Goldberg Group, *Alternative Medicine: The Definitive Guide*, pp. 52–61. The authors of this work also cite information from John Steele, Ph.D., and Robert Tisserand, both leaders in the field of aromatherapy. I use John Steele's oils myself, available through Capital Drugs (see "Resources").

38. Scott Cunningham, *Magical Aromatherapy*, pp. 25–39.

39. One source for live aromatic plants, herbs, seeds, and other products is Capriland's Herb Farm in Connecticut (see "Resources").

40. Eye of the Cat in California is a good source of quality dried herbs.

41. You may also purchase essential oils from Aroma Vera, Inc., in California (see "Resources").

42. Hydrosol is a type of homeopathic aromatherapy.

43. Nelly Grosjean, *Veterinary Aromatherapy*, p. 30. This is an excellent work to keep on hand for reference and recipes.

44. A poultice made of some powder, such as clay, mixed with water to form a thick paste. It's applied with gauze and secured with a bandage. See also "Herbs" in this chapter.

45. Personal communication with Joan Clark, June 5, 1996.

46. Grosjean supplies diffusers and natural mixtures for them through La Chevêche (see "Resources").

47. Cunningham, *Magical Aromatherapy*, p. 45.

Chapter Six: Hands-On Healing

1. Nancy Scanlan, D.V.M., "Needles for Cats, or How I Saw the Light and Became Holistic with the Help of Acupuncture," *Tiger Tribe*, Mar.–Apr. 1993, pp. 15–17; Jeanne Demyan, D.V.M., "The Case of Murasaki," in ibid., p. 18.

2. The validity of the meridian system was verified by the French researcher Pierre de Vernejoul, who injected radioactive isotopes into the acupoints of humans and tracked them with a gamma-imaging camera. These injections traveled 30 cm along the known acupuncture meridians within four to six minutes. Vernejoul then injected the isotopes into blood vessels at random places in the body; these injections did not travel in the same manner. Thus, Vernejoul saw that the meridians constitute a system of distinct pathways within the body (researched from the Burton Goldberg Group, *Alternative Medicine: The Definitive Guide*, p. 37). Moreover, Kirlian photographs of the energy field emanating from the body show changes after acupuncture treatment.

3. Richard H. Pitcairn, D.V.M., and Susan Hubble Pitcairn, *Complete Guide to Natural Health for Dogs and Cats*, pp. 148–50. See "Yang and Yin: Heaven and Earth," in Chapter 8.

4. Ibid.

5. Diane Stein, *Natural Healing for Dogs and Cats*, p. 125. Stein's source for this information

was Edith A. Uridel, "Alternative Therapies," *Dog Fancy,* Mar. 1992, p. 46.

6. In an article entitled "Animal Acupuncture" previously published in *Natural Pet Magazine* and reprinted with permission of the author.

7. Personal communication with Dr. Nancy Scanlan, November 28, 1995.

8. Alan M. Schoen, D.V.M., and Pam Proctor, "Acupressure," *New Age Journal,* July–Aug. 1995, pp. 39–43.

9. Developed by Moshe Feldenkrais, this method is based on the concept that each cell, through its life force or vital intelligence, is connected with the whole body and with other life-forms.

Chapter Seven: Other Healing Approaches

1. From *Alternative Medicine: The Definitive Guide,* p. 465. It's amazing how few practitioners are aware of the miracles that occur on a daily basis when alternative holistic care is practiced on both people and animals. You may wish to share this book with your veterinarian as a gift.

2. Joanne Stefanatos, D.V.M., *Holistic Pet Care* (videotape); see "Resources."

3. From Stanley Burroughs, *Healing for the Age of Enlightenment,* pp. 116–19.

4. Dael Walker, *The Crystal Book,* p. 13.

5. Diane Stein, *Natural Healing for Dogs and Cats,* p. 174.

6. Dr. Stefanatos shows an example of an energy halter, originally designed by Dr. Gloria Dodd, in her videotape *Holistic Pet Care* (see "Resources").

7. Human beings hear at approximately 20 kilohertz (kHz). Dogs' hearing is much more sensitive.

8. Henry Sigerist, *Civilization and Disease,* p. 149.

9. John Craige, D.V.M., "Therapeutic Sound for Animals," *Pet and Horse Exchange,* July 1993.

10. Conversation with Dr. Craige.

11. Such as Richard Gerber, M.D., *Vibrational Medicine* (see "Resources").

12. Wayne Perry, "Cosmic Choir" (audiotape). See "Resources."

13. You may obtain the chart and tape by contacting Musikarma Productions (see "Resources"); the materials are meant to be used together.

14. Conversation with Wayne Perry.

15. This is detailed in Perry's chart.

16. Study conducted by Frances Rauscher, University of California, Irvine; reported in "Tribal News," *Tiger Tribe,* Nov.–Dec. 1993, pp. 10–11.

17. See John Fudens, D.V.M., "Magnetism," *The Affinity Holistic Veterinary Clinic's Layman's Handbook;* and Joanne Stefanatos, D.V.M., "Holistic Pet Care" (videotape; see "Resources").

18. Fudens, "Radionics," *The Affinity Holistic Veterinary Clinic's Layman's Handbook.*

19. New Horizons also offers intensive seminars on identifying the vitamins, minerals, herbs, and homeopathic substances that fit your specific body chemistry and on combating the "electronic pollution" in our environment. Both the equipment and the training are expensive. The SE-5 sells for approximately $2,500, and a six-day training course costs $700. You may obtain more information by contacting New Horizons Trust ("see

Resources").

20. Volhard and Brown, *The Holistic Guide for a Healthy Dog,* p. 145.

Chapter Eight: Astromedicine for Your Dog

1. Throughout this chapter there are Dr. Chambreau's cautionary notes regarding the astrological use of homeopathy. Always consult a doctor of veterinary medicine before administering any remedy to your dog.

2. Though sun sign astrology can be entertaining and fun, it by no means provides the scientific depth or insight available through consultation with a trained astrologer. With the advent of computer technology, interdimensional astrological readings (which incorporate information from the several different systems of the zodiac) can now be offered at a reasonable cost. An astrological profile varies depending upon the system used, so combining perspectives allows us to understand more completely the personality, soul, and social aspects of an individual (human or animal). Interdimensional astrologer Eleanor Haspel-Portner, Ph.D., offers all levels of astrological consultations, some of which include the interdimensional use of color (see "Resources").

3. Reinhold Ebertin, *Astrological Healing: The History and Practice of Astromedicine,* pp. 3–4. Ebertin's books contain a wealth of data documenting how, historically, astrology has been incorporated into most healing sciences.

4. Ibid., pp. 37–38.

5. See William Boericke, M.D., and Willis A. Dewey, M.D., *The Twelve Tissue Remedies of Schuessler,* pp. 29–30.

6. Ibid., pp. 39–45. Perry observed that the work of Dr. George W. Carey, who wrote *The Relations of the Mineral Salts of the Body to the Signs of the Zodiac* (see *The Zodiac and the Salts of Salvation* in "Resources"), upon which Perry's work is based, unlocked the door to mental and physical well-being.

7. Peter Damian, *The Twelve Healers of the Zodiac,* pp. 2–3.

8. Scott Cunningham, *Magical Aromatherapy,* pp. 167–68.

9. Ebertin, *Astrological Healing: The History and Practice of Astromedicine,* p. 138.

10. Jeffrey Levy, D.V.M., of Williamstown, Massachusetts, has incorporated the yang/yin philosophy into his natural diet for cats. He refers to the protein portion of raw meat and organ meat as yang, the carbohydrate portion as neutral, and the vegetable portion as yin. He uses both yang and yin supplements.

11. The dates in parentheses are those given by Inez Eudora Perry in *The Zodiac and the Salts of Salvation.* Perry's astrological dating of this and certain other sun signs varies from the traditional system used by most prominent astrologers.

12. Dr. Chambreau reminds us that the best way to use homeopathy is to treat the animal with professional help, at the deepest (constitutional) level. This means giving one dose of a remedy and then often waiting weeks or months. Do not use these remedies without consulting your homeopathic veterinarian.

13. I give my animals only Kyolic garlic, because fresh garlic seems too bitter.

14. See note 11, above.

15. Dr. Chambreau points out that the goal is not to need these remedies. Ideally, your dog

should be healthy enough to get a cough or cold and get well on his own within two to seven days.

16. *Caution:* Do not use *Arnica* if anesthesia is to be used (such as with cesarean section).

17. As Dr. Chambreau reminds us, our homemade diet and the care of a homeopathic practitioner (both begun when the puppy is only a few weeks old) should keep your dog so healthy that he probably won't need to be given any remedies.

18. You can help your homeopathic prescriber by noticing the characteristics of your dog's condition, even if the practitioner ends up choosing a different remedy. Always ask him or her about your selection before administering it.

19. See note 11.

20. See note 12.

21. See note 11.

22. As long as the dog is not already receiving deep constitutional treatment with another homeopathic remedy. Always consult your homeopathic veterinarian before giving a remedy to your dogs.

23. See note 15.

24. See note 17.

25. I don't recommend using *Arnica* on the day of surgery itself. Consider using *Aconite* the night before and the morning of surgery, and resume with *Arnica,* alternating with *Hypericum,* after surgery. However, Dr. Chambreau has stopped routinely recommending *Arnica* or *Aconite,* using them only if dogs are sore. Often, they recover well without this treatment.

26. One part tincture to 10 parts distilled water.

27. One drop of the liquid to one ounce of distilled water.

28. See note 18.

29. See note 25.

30. See note 22.

31. Personal communication with Dr. Scanlan.

32. See note 12.

33. See note 15.

34. See Chapter 5, "Natural Remedies," for more complete information about all these substances.

Chapter Nine: Saying Goodbye to the Ones We Love

1. Cited in Diane Stein, *Natural Healing for Dogs and Cats,* p. 166.

2. Machaelle Small Wright, *Behaving As If the God in All Life Mattered.*

Resources

PLEASE NOTE: At the time of this writing, the companies and practitioners listed supply one or more products and/or services that are acceptable within the guidelines of this book. This does not mean that I necessarily recommend all products and/or services made, sold, or provided by these companies and/or practitioners. Product and service quality can change. Management, policies, and standards can change. I urge you to keep this in mind and to be alert. Read labels and product brochures carefully, even for products you have been using for a long time. Conduct your own interviews. There may be other fine suppliers and practitioners not listed here. My not listing certain suppliers and practitioners does not necessarily mean that I wouldn't recommend them if I knew about them.

Associations

American Holistic Veterinary Medical
  Association
2214 Old Emmorton Road
Bel Air, MD 21014
(410) 569-0795
Referrals and information.

American Veterinarian Chiropractic
  Association
623 Main Street
Hillsdale, IL 61275
(309) 658-2920
A 150-hour course is taught on animal chiropractic to veterinarians and chiropractors. Leave a message with your area code and phone number for a referral of a chiropractic veterinarian in your area.

Animal Protection Institute of America
P.O. Box 22505
Sacramento, CA 95822
2831 Fruitridge Road
Sacramento, CA 95820
(916) 731-5521
FAX (916) 731-4467
National nonprofit animal-welfare organization working through legislation and

education. Call or write for their pet-food investigative report.

American Society for the Prevention of Cruelty to Animals (ASPCA)—National Animal Poison Control Center
1717 Philo Road
Urbanal, IL 61801
(900) 680-0000
$20 for the first five minutes; $2.95 each minute thereafter.
(800) 548-2423—you may still incur a consultation charge in calling this number.

Bio-Integral Resource Center
P.O. Box 7414
Berkeley, CA 94707
(510) 524-2567
Nonprofit organization researching and promoting information on the least toxic methods of pest management.

Delta Society
289 Perimeter Road East
Renton, WA 98055-1329
(206) 226-7357
National directory of grief counselors, books

on grief, Pet Partners, and the National Service Dog Center.

Flower Essence Services
P.O. Box 459
Nevada City, CA 95959
(800) 548-0075
Classes in flower essences and a newsletter.

Food and Water, Inc.
R.R. 1, Box 68D
Walden, VT, 05658
(800) EAT-SAFE/(802) 563-3300
FAX (802) 563-3310
Food and Water is a natural nonprofit consumer-education and advocacy group waging grassroots campaigns to stop the use of food irradiation, pesticides, and bovine growth hormone.

The Foundation for Homeopathic
   Education and Research
5916 Chabot Crest
Oakland, CA 94618
(510) 420-8791
Sponsors homeopathic research and educates health professionals and the general public about research on homeopathic medicine.

Grief Recovery Help Line
Grief Recovery Institute
(800) 445-4808
Monday–Friday, 9–5 P.M. EST

Homeopathic Educational Services
2124 Kittridge Street
Berkeley, CA 94704
(800) 359-9051 for orders/(510) 649-0294 for info and catalogs
Extensive list of books (including third edition [1997] *Everybody's Guide to Homeopathic Medicine,* by Stephen Cummings, M.D., and Dana Ullman, M.P.H.), tapes, information, homeopathic kits, and helpful service.

Institute for Traditional Medicine
2017 S.E. Hawthorne

Portland, OR 97214
(800) 544-7504
Chinese herbs and books.

International Bio-Oxidative Med.
   Foundation (Ed Baker)
P.O. Box 610767
Dallas/Fort Worth, TX 75261
(817) 481-9772
Promotes use of intravenous hydrogen peroxide infusion.

International Foundation for Homeopathy
2366 Eastlake Avenue E., Suite 329
Seattle, WA 98102
(206) 324-8230
Directory of homeopaths who are graduates of IFH courses. Their journal, *Resonance,* contains occasional articles by veterinary homeopaths, including Dr. Pitcairn and Dr. Levy. Also publishes a yearly collection of "cured cases," which are very useful in studying homeopathy.

International Veterinary Acupuncture
   Society
2140 Conestoga Road
Chester Springs, PA 19425
(610) 827-7245
FAX (610) 827-1366
Referrals and information. Send SASE for listing of veterinarians in your area.

National Center for Homeopathy
801 N. Fairfax Street, #306
Alexandria, VA 22314
(703) 548-7790
Directory of homeopathic practitioners, pharmacies, resources, and study groups.

National College of Naturopathic Medicine
11231 S.E. Market Street
Portland, OR 97216
(503) 255-7355
A national center for homeopathic education.

Network Chiropractic Veterinarians
P.O. Box 119
Oldenbury, IN 47036
(812) 934-2410
Contact Dr. Mark P. Haverkos for referrals
and information.

New England School of Homeopathy
356 Middle Street
Amherst, MA 01002
(800) 637-4440 / (203) 763-1225 / (413)
529-2245 for journal
Courses, seminars, and journals.

Ohio Parents for Vaccine Safety
251 W. Ridgeway Drive
Dayton, OH 45459
(513) 435-4750 (phone and FAX)
Kristine M. Severyn, R.Ph., Ph.D., Director
Call or write for free general information
packet.

The Pacific Institute of Aromatherapy
P.O. Box 6723
San Rafael, CA 94903
(415) 479-9121
Courses available to individuals and companies interested in becoming certified in
aromatherapy practice.

Price-Pottenger Nutrition Foundation
P.O. Box 2614
La Mesa, CA 91943-2614
(619) 574-7763
"A nonprofit tax-exempt education organization dedicated to the promotion of
enhanced health through an awareness of
ecology, lifestyle, and healthy food production for good nutrition." Catalog of books,
pamphlets, and tapes.

Practitioners

Marc Bittan, D.V.M.
11673 National Blvd.
Los Angeles, CA 90064

(310) 231-4415
Holistic veterinarian specializing in homeopathics, acupuncture and Chinese herbal
medicine.

Christina Chambreau, D.V.M.
908 Coldbottom Road
Sparks, MD 21152
(410) 771-4968
Member Academy of Veterinary Homeopathy. Gives courses on veterinary
homeopathy.

W. Jean Dodds, D.V.M.
938 Stanford Street
Santa Monica, CA 90403
(310) 828-4804

John Fudens, D.V.M.
29296 U.S. 19N, #104
Clearwater, FL 34621
(813) 787-6010
Affinity holistic clinic.

Marty Goldstein, D.V.M.
Smithridge Veterinary Center
400 Smithridge Road
S. Salem, NY 10590
(914) 533-6066 / FAX (914) 533-6405

Linda Goodman
2023 Chicago Avenue, #B-25
Riverside, CA 92507
(909) 784-9070
Animal communicator and behavior consultant.

Carol Gurney
3715 N. Cornell Road
Agoura, CA 91301
(818) 597-1154
Animal communicator and bodywork.

Donald K. Hamilton, D.V.M.
P.O. Box 67
Ocate, NM 87734
(505) 666-2091

Eleanor Haspel–Portner, Ph.D.
(310) 459-1886
Astrologer, psychologist, and Reiki master.

Lydia Hibby
18810 Bert Road
Riverside, CA 92508
(909) 789-0330
Animal analyst available for consultations,
lectures, and seminars. Newsletter:
Pet Network News.

Linda Johnson, D.V.M.
Commonwealth Animal Hospital
1941 W. Commonwealth
Fullerton, CA 92633
(714) 525-2355

Douglas Kappstatter, D.V.M.
15 Sewall Street
Marblehead, MA 01945
(617) 639-8013
Acupuncture, homeopathy, Bach flower
remedies, and nutritional consulation.
Available for phone consultations.

Samantha Khury
1251 10th Street
Manhattan Beach, CA 90266
(310) 374-6812
Therapist and educator available for lectures,
seminars, workshops, and private therapy.

Yolanda LaCombe/John Lowry
Glendale, CA
(818) 845-6570
Yolanda is a consultant working with healing
herbs and North American flower essences.
John does energy balancing.

Dan Lavach, D.V.M., M.S.
Eye Clinic for Animals
13132 Garden Grove Boulevard
Garden Grove, CA 92643
(714) 971-8271
FAX (714) 971-1963
Practice limited to diseases of the animal eye.

Laurel Leach, D.V.M.
Beverly Oaks Animal Hospital
14302 Ventura Boulevard
Sherman Oaks, CA 91423
(818) 788-5246
FAX (818) 788-2022
Emergency veterinary medicine.

Douglas Lemire, V.M.D.
Mobile Alternative Veterinary Care
P.O. Box 40521
Santa Barbara, CA 93140
(805) 565-3985
Traditional medicine and holistic therapy.
Acupuncture (pets, horses), herbs, homeo-
pathy, and natural remedies, including
chiropractic.

Michael W. Lemmon, D.V.M.
1409 Union Ave. N.E.
Renton, WA 98059
(425) 226-8418

Charles E. Loops, D.V.M.
Route 2, Box 568
38 Waddell Hollow Road
Pittsboro, NC 27312
(919) 542-0442
FAX (919) 542-0535

Loving Touch Animal Center
1975 Glenn Club Drive
Stone Mountain, GA 30087
(770) 498-5956
Michelle Tilghman, D.V.M., manufacturer of
Homeopathic Animal First Aid Kit.

Bea Lydecker
Bea Lydecker's Naturals
15443 S. Latourette Road
Oregon City, OR 97045-9432
(503) 631-7389 Consults and information.
(800) 258-8589 FAX and orders only for
natural herbs and supplements.
Product catalog and natural healing information. Nonverbal communication. Author of

Seasons, What the Animals Tell Me and *Stories the Animals Tell Me* (self-published).

Pat McKay
396 W. Washington Boulevard
Pasadena, CA 91103
(626) 296-1120
Holistic practitioner and author of *Reigning Cats and Dogs*.

Barbara Meyers
Holistic Animal Consulting Center
29 Lyman Avenue
Staten Island, NY 10305
(718) 720-5548
Grief therapist, certified Bach flower remedies counselor.

Laura Mignosa
912 Corbin Avenue
New Britain, CT 66052
(860) 666-5064
FAX (860) 667-2075
Certified Chinese herbalist/consultant and formulator.

Lisa Newman
7334 E. Broadway
Tucson, AZ 85710
(800) 497-5665
Holistic animal practitioner and owner of holistic animal care stores.

David B. Nielsen, D.V.M.
Advanced Veterinary Dentistry
1401 N. Sepulveda Boulevard
Manhattan Beach, CA 90266
(310) 546-5731
FAX (310) 546-5636

Richard Pitcairn, D.V.M., Ph.D.
1283 Lincoln Street
Eugene, OR 97401
(541) 342-7665

Jeanne Rose
219 Carl Street
San Francisco, CA 94117
(415) 564-6785
Author, teacher, aromatherapist, herbalist. Has created a network of organic farmers to distill hydrosols.

Nancy Scanlan, D.V.M.
750 S. Beach Boulevard
La Habra, CA 90631
(714) 691-7751
Acupuncture, trigger point therapy, nutritional therapy, Chinese herbs. Author of *Stop That Itch!, Safe Detox for Dogs and Cats, Holistic Options for Companion Animals with Cancer,* and *Arthritis—Natural Treatments for Companion Animals.* Other holistic health books available. Send for free catalog.

Viera Scheibner, Ph.D.
178 Govetts Leap Road
Blackheath, NSW, Australia 2785
(047) 87-8203
FAX (047) 87-8988

Barry Sears, Ph.D.
Surfactant Technologies, Inc.
21 Tioga Way
Marblehead, MA 01945
(800) 346-2706
Author of *The Zone.*

Sis Sewell
c/o *Healthy Pets Naturally*
1895 New Franklin Church Road
Canon, GA 30520
(706) 356-7031
Holistic practitioner and publisher of *Healthy Pets, Naturally.*

Robert Silver, D.V.M.
Holistic Wellness Center
4660 Table Mesa Drive
Boulder, CO 80303
(303) 494-7877
FAX (303) 494-4496

John Steele
3949 Longridge Avenue
Sherman Oaks, CA 91423
(818) 986-0594
Aromatic consultant, archaeologist. John specializes in environmental fragrancing. He distributes a line of high-quality essential oils and has some hydrosols, too. He also has some very rare flower essential oils that are widely used by the perfume industry.

Joanne Stefanatos, D.V.M.
1325 Vegas Valley Drive
Las Vegas, NV 89109
(702) 735-7184

Laurel Steinhice
6712 Currywood Drive
Nashville, TN 37205
(615) 356-4280
Channeling and psychic work. Reiki master for animals and people, and past-life therapy.

Russell Swift, D.V.M.
5871 N. University, Suite 720
Tamarac, FL 33321
(800) 868-1009 / (954) 720-0794 / (954) 720-0978
Also see Pet's Friends.

Linda Tellington-Jones
P.O. Box 3793
Santa Fe, NM 87501-0793
(800) 854-TEAM
T-Touch therapy.

Marion Webb-Former
340 The Circle
Queen Elizabeth Street
London, England SE1 2ND
Channeling and psychic work.

DeeAnne Weber
(909) 360-1685
FAX (909) 360-9485
Naturally raised Leonbergers and IDF practitioner.

Marla Wilson
2313 Pullman Lane
Redondo Beach, CA 90278
(310) 372-3737
Certified aromatherapy teacher and consultant. Custom blending, Bach flowers, tarot.

Celeste Yarnall, Ph.D.
9875 Gloucester Drive
Beverly Hills, CA 90210
(310) 278-1385; (888) CEL-PETS
http://www.celestialpets.com
e-mail: celeste@celestialpets.com
Available for consultation on the fresh food diet and supplementation, as well as alternative healing therapies for cats and dogs. We distribute most of the products discussed throughout the book. Feel free to call for shipping and delivery information and price sheet.

Marina Zacharias
Ambrican Enterprises, Ltd.
P.O. Box 1436
Jacksonville, OR 97530
(541) 899-2080
FAX (541) 899-3414
e-mail: ambrican@cdsnet.net
Supplier of Juliette de Bairacli Levy's original herbal formulas imported from England. Many other items are also available, including nutritional supplements, homeopathics, flower remedies, and a complete herbal wormer. Publishes *Natural Rearing Newsletter* and *Natural Rearing Breeders' Directory*.

Suppliers

Acuspark
P.O. Box 366
Swanee, GA 30174
(770) 822-0752
EMS unit (for practitioners), which provides electro-muscle stimulation for pain relief.

Agape Video Systems, Inc.
1325 Vegas Valley Drive
Las Vegas, NV 89109
(702) 735-7184
Holistic Pet Care video by Dr. Joanne
Stefanatos.

Ainsworth Homeopathic Pharmacy
36 New Cavendish Street
London, England WIM 7LH
44-171 935-5330
Large choices of remedies, many that are not
available in the United States, and animal
nosodes.

Ambrican Enterprises, Ltd.
P.O. Box 1436
Jacksonville, OR 97530
(541) 899-2080
FAX (541) 899-3414
e-mail: ambrican@cdsnet.net
Marina Zacharias, President
Supplier of Juliette de Bairacli Levy's origi-
nal herbal formulas imported from England.
Many other items are also available, includ-
ing nutritional supplements, homeopathics,
flower remedies, and a complete herbal
wormer. Publishes: Natural Rearing
Newsletter and Natural Rearing Breeders'
Directory.

Anaflora
P.O. Box 1056
Mt. Shasta, CA 96067
(916) 926-6424
Sharon Callahan. Flower essence therapy for
animals.

Analytical Research Labs
8650 N. 22nd Avenue
Phoenix, AZ 85021
(800) 528-4067 / (602) 995-1580
Heavy-metal analysis and mineral analysis.

Animal Health Options, Inc.
1724 Langhorne-Yardley Road
Yardley, PA 19067

(215) 493-0621
Manufacturers of Chinese herbal food supplements.

Animal Magnetism
c/o the Human Touch
10061 Riverside Drive
Suite #325
Toluca Lake, CA 91602
(818) 344-7393
Magnetized Pet Pads.

Animals' Apawthecary
P.O. Box 212
Conner, MT 59827
(406) 821-4090 (phone and FAX)
Complete line of herbal tinctures.

Annandale Apothecary
3299 Woodburn Road
Annandale, VA 22003
(703) 698-7411
Homeopathic remedies, books.

AromaPet
117 N. Robertson Boulevard
Los Angeles, CA 90048
(800) 677-2368 / (310) 276-1191
Joan Clark. Aromatherapy.

Aromatherapy Seminars
1830 S. Robertson Boulevard
Los Angeles, CA 90035
(800) 677-2368 / (310) 838-6122
Certificate programs provided through
correspondence courses, and specialty classes
offered to those individuals already certified.
Videotapes and blending materials also
available.

Aroma Vera, Inc.
5901 Rodeo Road
Los Angeles, CA 90016
(310) 280-0407
Essential oils.

Australian Bush Flower Essences
Box 531

Spit Junction NSW
Australia 2088

Beckett's Apothecary
1004 Chester Pike
Sharon Hill, PA 19079
(800) 727-8188
Homeopathic remedies. Mail order.

Belle Haven Pharmacy, Inc.
1451 Belle Haven Road
Alexandria, VA 22307
(703) 765-5656
Homeopathic remedies, kits, books, UPS
delivery.

Best Friends Supplements
C/o Celeste Yarnall
(310) 278-1385 (888) CELPETS
FAX (310) 278-1385

Bierer's Pharmacy
146 S. Main Street
Lexington, VA 24450
(800) 552-6779 / (703) 463-3119
Homeopathic remedies, mail-order service.

Biogenetics Food Corporation
Naples, FL 33942
(800) 926-5100 / (941) 643-7188
Manufacturers of nutritional and antioxidant
supplements.

Biovet International/Pacific Botanicals
1440 Kapiolani Boulevard, #108-186
Honolulu, HI 96814
(800) 468-7578 or (800) 304-4240
Antioxidants from organically grown wheat
sprouts.

Boericke and Tafel
2381 Circadian Way
Santa Rosa, CA 95407
(800) 876-9505
Homeopathic remedies, kits, books.

Boiron-Borneman
6 Campus Boulevard

Newtown Square, PA 19073
(800) 258-8823
Suppliers of homeopathic remedies.

Boiron, The Natural Pharmacy (East Coast)
1208 Amosland Road
Norwood, PA 19074
(800) BLU-TUBE
Homeopathic remedies, kits, books, educational materials.

Boiron, The Natural Pharmacy (West Coast)
98C W. Cochran Street
Simi Valley, CA 93065
(800) BLU-TUBE
(805) 582-9094
Homeopathic remedies, kits, books, educational materials.

Books from India, Ltd.
45 Museum Street
London, England WC1A1LR
011-44-171405-3784

Capitol Drugs
8578 Santa Monica Boulevard
West Hollywood, CA 90069
(310) 289-1125

4454 Van Nuys Boulevard
Sherman Oaks, CA 91403
(818) 905-8338
Homeopathic remedies, herbs, and books.

Capriland's Herb Farm
534 Silver Street
Coventry, CT 06238
(203) 742-7244
Live aromatic plants, herbs, seeds, and products. Send SASE for catalog ordering
information.

CC Pollen Company
5455 N. 51st Avenue, #17
Glendale, AZ 85301
(800) 875-0096

Celletech Ltd./National Homeopathic
Products

518 Tasman St.
Madison, WI 53714
(608) 221-9413 or (800) 888-4066
Ships single-dose homeopathics, and more.

Deva Flower Remedies
C/o Natural Labs Corp.
P.O. Box 230229
Encinitas, CA 86341
(800) 233-0810

Gloria Dodd, D.V.M.
Everglo Ranch
P.O. Box 1242
Gualala, CA 95445
Audiocassettes. Dr. Dodd no longer offers
consultations.

Dolisos America, Inc.
3014 Rigel Avenue
Las Vegas, NV 89102
(800) 365-4767 / (702) 871-7153
Homeopathic remedies. Free catalog.

Dr. Goodpet Laboratories
P.O. Box 4489
Inglewood, CA 90309
(800) 222-9932 / (213) 672-3269
Homeopathics and vitamins.

Ellon USA, Inc.
644 Merrick Road
Lynbrook, NY 11563
(800) 433-7523
Bach flower remedies.

Energy Refractors
53166 State Route 681
Reedsville, OH 45772
(614) 378-6155
Hydrogen peroxide.

En Garde Health Products
7702 Balboa Boulevard, Building #10
Van Nuys, CA 91406
(818) 901-8505 / (800) 955-4633
Producers of oxygen supplements.

Enhanced Water Products, Inc.
8337 Penn Avenue South
Bloomington, MN 55431
(612) 881-7314
Crystal-enhanced water.

Environmental Lighting Concepts, Inc.
3923 Coconut Palm Drive
Tampa, FL 33619
(813) 621-0058
OTT-Lite full-spectrum, radiation shielded,
natural light supplement.

Fairfax Medical Center Pharmacy
10721 Main Street
Fairfax, VA 22030
(800) 723-7455 / (703) 273-7311
Homeopathic remedies, mail-order service.

Five Elements Center
115 Route 46, Building D, Suite 29
Mt. Lakes, NJ 07046
(201) 402-8510
Homeopathic remedies, educational
materials.

Fleabusters, Inc.
(800) 779-3532 / (310) 470-3532
Nonpesticide flea product.

Flower Essence Services
P.O. Box 1769
Nevada City, CA 95959
(800) 548-0075
Flower essences, aromatherapy, and books
available through mail order.

Frontier Cooperative Herbs
P.O. Box 69
Norway, CA 52318
Bach flower remedies. Source of gelatin cap-
sules, herbs, combination homeopathics, and
more.

Green Foods Corporation
320 N. Graves
Oxnard, CA 93030
(800) 777-4430 / (805) 983-7470

FAX: (805) 983-8843
Manufacturers of Green Magma and Barley
Dog and Cat.

Green Hope Farm
P.O. Box 125, True Road
Meriden, NH 03770
(603) 469-3662
Flower essences by Molly Sheehan, including Bermuda essences, Adirondack essences,
and vegetable/flower essences from her
divinely directed garden.

Green Terrestrial Herb Farm
P.O. Box 266
Milton, NY 12547
Pam Montgomery
Wild crafted, common, and hard-to-find
tinctures. Catalog.

Gurudas
P.O. Box 868
San Rafael, CA 94915
Flower essences, gem elixirs, and books.

Hahnemann Pharmacy
828 San Pablo Avenue
Albany, CA 94706
(510) 527-3003
Supplies the nosodes for animal disease
prevention (sold only to veterinarians).
Herbal formulas and remedies up to 30C.

Halo Products, Purely for Pets
3438 East Lake Road, #14
Palm Harbor, FL 34685
(800) 426-4256 / (813) 854-2214
Manufacturers of Dream Coat, Derma
Dream, Natural Herbal Ear Wash, and other
natural pet-care products.

Harmony Farms
2824 Foothill Boulevard
La Crescenta, CA 91214
(818) 248-3068
Bruce Oxford, owner.
Naturally grown meat and poultry.

Health Concerns
8001 Capwell Drive
Oakland, CA 94621
(510) 639-0280
FAX (510) 639-9140
Herbal products.

Helios Pharmacy
97 Camden Road
Turnbridge Wells
Kent, England TN1 2QR
011-44-1-892-536393/ 537254
FAX 011-44-1-892-546850
Homeopathic remedies, including LM
potencies.

Holistic Pet Care Catalog for Dogs, Cats,
    and Horses
Patty Swygert
1811 Franklin Avenue
McLean, VA 22101
(703) 536-2515
FAX (703) 536-4070
The catalog includes natural foods, supplements, first aid, treats, homeopathic
remedies, herbs, aromatherapy products,
flower essences, books, and suggested magazines, classes, and events.

HomeoVetiX
P.O. Box 8243
Naples, FL 33941
(800) 677-4439 / (813) 643-4439
FAX (813) 643-7370
Homeopathy for animals.

Interproduct, Inc.
858 Third Avenue, #126
Chula Vista, CA 91911
(619) 427-7231
FAX (619) 425-2989

International Office: Elecsystem
IBS Inductive-Bio-Stimulation
GMF Corporation AG
Alpenstr. 4

CH-6304 Zug (Switzerland)
041-7107554
FAX 041-7107618
Magnetic field therapy.

Jade / East Earth Herb, Inc.
P.O. Box 2802
Eugene, OR 97402
Chinese herbal products and information.

K & K Pet Products
2901 W. Bartlett
Tucson, AZ 85741
(520) 887-4926

Kyolic Garlic
Wakunaga of America Co., Ltd.
23501 Madero
Mission Viejo, CA 92691
(800) 421-2998 / (800) 544-5800 (in CA)
Manufacturers of high-potency garlic in
capsule, tablet, and liquid form.

McZand Herbal
4143 Glencoe Avenue
Marina Del Rey, CA 90292
(310) 822-0500
Herbal products.

Magnet Sales and Manufacturing, Inc.
11248 Playa Court
Culver City, CA 90230
(800) 421-6692
Magnetic specialties and more.

Mannatech, Inc.
C/o Celeste Yarnall
(310) 278-1385
ManAloe (Acemannon).

May Way Trading Company
San Francisco, CA 94607
(510) 208-3123
Chinese herbs and patent medicine.

The Medicine Shop
6307 York Road
Baltimore, MD 21212-2699

(410) 323-1515
Homeopathic remedies.

Merz Apothecary
4716 N. Lincoln Avenue
Chicago, IL 60625
(800) 252-0275 / (312) 989-0900
Homeopathic and herbal remedies, books.

Metagenics
971 Calle Negocio
San Clemente, CA 92673
(800) 638-4362
Herbal and vitamin products, including
mycelized vitamin A oil. Or you may contact Celeste Yarnall, distributor (310)
278-1385.

Michael Scholes School for Aromatic
    Studies
117 N. Robertson Boulevard
Los Angeles, CA 90048
(310) 276-1191
Carries books, newsletters, bottles, and supplies for the aromatherapist. Essential oils by
Laboratory of Flowers, John Steele, and
Aroma Vera. Also has an aromatherapy pet-
care line. White Rose of Provence spa for
aromatherapy treatments.

Mid-America Homeopathic Medicine Shop
(800) 552-4956
Homeopathic pharmacy.

Mid-America Marketing
P.O. Box 124
Eaton, OH 45320
(800) 922-1744
Complete source for magnet therapy prod-
ucts.

Minimum Price Homeopathic Books
250 H Street
P.O. Box 2187
Blaine, WA 98231
(604) 597-4757 for info / (800) 663-8272
for orders

Morrill's New Directions
P.O. Box 30
Orient, ME 04471
21 Market Square

Houlton, ME 04730
(800) 368-5057 / (207) 532-9501
FAX (207) 532-0895
Natural pet-care products. Free catalog available. Publishes Your Newsletter . . . Naturally.

Multi-Pure Drinking Water Systems
Solid carbon block technology certified by
NSF International and the state of California
to remove 99 percent of potential health
hazards, including asbestos, chlorine, trihalomethanes, lead, pesticides such as
Lindane, as well as volitile organic chemicals
(VOCs) such as TCE and PCE, in addition
to turbidity and microscopic organisms such
as cysts and giardia lamblia.
C/o Celeste Yarnall
(310) 278-1385

Musikarma Productions/Wayne Perry
8391 Beverly Boulevard, Suite 333
Los Angeles, CA 90048
(213) 655-7781
Healing charts and tapes for sound therapy.

Natural Care Catalog for Animals
See Holistic Pet Care Catalog for Dogs,
Cats, and Horses.

Nature's Own Environmental Services
899 Brentwood
Venice, FL 34292
(941) 483-9032
Melinda Leeson consults on homeopathy,
nutrition, and herbs for animals.

Nature's Sunshine
P.O. Box 1000
Spanish Fork, UT 84660
(800) 278-7214 / (801) 798-9861
Chinese herbs, supplements, and homeopathics. To become a distributor, give my

name (Celeste Yarnall) as a referral, and you
will be part of my down-line, or contact me
for product sales and information.

Nature's Way Products, Inc.
10 Mountain Spring Parkway
Springville, UT 84663
(801) 489-1500

Nelly Grosjean's Natural Products
La Chevêche
13690 Graveson-en-Provence, France
(33) 90 95 81 72 /
FAX (33) 90 95 85 20

In the United States:
Vie Arôme distributed by Aromatherapy
    International
3 Seal Harbor Road, Suite 437
Winthrop, MA 02152
(617) 846-0285
FAX (617) 846-5474
Natural and organic quality aromatic essential oils, hydrosols, aromatic diffusers, books,
and Nelly Grosjean's aromatic specialties.
Mail-order facility. Delivery within fortyeight hours in France; five days elsewhere.

New Horizons Trust
53166 Street, Route 681
Reedsville, OH 45772
(800) 755-6360
Alternative health and all natural products.
Free catalog available.

Newton Laboratories
P.O. Box 936
Lithonia, GA 30058

612 Upland Trail
Conyers, GA 30207
(800) 448-7256 / (404) 922-2644
Homeopathic remedies and educational
materials.

Norfields
632-3/4 N. Doheny Drive
Los Angeles, CA 90069

(800) 344-8400
Manufacturers of magnetic health care
products.

Northeast Homeopathic Products
563 Massachusetts Avenue, Route 111
Acton, MA 01720-2903
(800) 551-3611
Standard homeopathic distributor pharmacy.

Nu Age Laboratories
4200 Laclede Avenue
St. Louis, MO 63108
(314) 533-9600
Suppliers of homeopathic remedies.

Nutri-Dyn Products, Inc.
   (New Biologics)
2470 Wisconsin Street
Downers Grove, IL 60515
(708) 969-6700
Glandular supplements, herbals, homeopathics, amino acid supplements, and
nutritionals.

Nutritional Enzyme Support Systems
   (NESS)
2903 N.W. Platte Road
Riverside, MO 64150
(800) 637-7893 for catalog
Manufacturers of Vet-Zimes (digestive
enzymes for pets). Sells to veterinarians.
Newsletter and product catalog, including
water-filtration systems through reverse
osmosis. They also carry Acuspark for pain
relief.

Ocean Health Products
5 Canal Street
Bellows Falls, VT 05101
(800) 477-5108
Cartilade (shark cartilage).

Orcon Organic Control, Inc.
Los Angeles, CA
(213) 937-7444
Beneficial nematodes as well as other
beneficial insects to help rid your garden of
fleas, naturally.

Oshadi
32422 Alipaz, Suite C
San Juan Capistrano, CA 92675
(714) 240-1104
Carries the finest quality essential oils,
hydrosols, diffusers, and other aromatherapy
products. Organic and wild essential oils and
the Atr pro diffuser (best nebulizer on the
market).

Palmetto
1034 Montana Avenue
Santa Monica, CA 90403
(310) 395-6687
One of the first natural skin-care stores in
California. They carry Oshadi, John Steele,
Aroma Vera, and Tisserand essential oils, and
the best Bulgarian rose hydrosol, Bach
flower remedies, herbs, natural soaps, skin-
care products, and an array of holistic books.
Will ship UPS.

Peeskill Pet Products—PVT
2306 N.E. 7th Avenue
Ft. Lauderdale, FL 33305-2128
(800) 551-1495
PVT, a complete health care line for dogs
and cats. Organic vitamin supplements,
protein shampoo, and skin cream.

Pegasus Products, Inc.
P.O. Box 228
Boulder, CO 80306
(800) 527-6104
Flower and gemstone essences.

Perelandra Flower Essences
P.O. Box 3603
Warrenton, VA 22186
(540) 937-2153
FAX (803) 937-3360
Flower essences, books by Machaelle Small
Wright.

PetGuard, Inc.
P.O. Box 728
Orange Park, FL 32067-0728
165 Industrial Loop S.
Orange Park, FL 32073
(800) 874-3221/ (904) 264-8500
Provides one of the natural commercial pet foods.

Pet Sage
(800) PET-HLTH
Natural medicines, alternative therapies, and specialty products designed for pet health and safety.

Pet's Friends, Inc.
5871 N. University, Suite 720
Tamarac, FL 33321
(800) 868-1009 / (954) 720-0794
FAX (954) 720-0978
Dr. Russell Swift's enzyme products (FloraZyme EFA and FloraZyme EFA, Ani-Minerals, Pet Glandulars, and other natural healing products).

Pets Naturally
13459 Ventura Boulevard
Sherman Oaks, CA 91423
(818) 784-1233
Health-food store that carries natural products, homeopathics, and natural supplements.

Prima Fleur Botanicals
1201-R Anderson Drive
San Rafael, CA 94903
(415) 455-0956
Carries the Jeannie Rose organic hydrosols and some organic essential oils.

Professional Health Products
Nutritional Specialties, Inc.
P.O. Box 80085
Portland, OR 97280
Homeopathic and nutritional supplements.

Puppy Go Potty™
14431 Ventura Boulevard, #137

Sherman Oaks, CA 91423-2606
(818) GO POTTY / (818) 467-6889
Complete housebreaking system for puppies.

Rainbow Vacuum Cleaners
(800) 870-5770
For the Greater Los Angeles area, contact Catherine Shaffer at D.H.D. Marketing
7242 Sepulveda Boulevard, Suite. #1-A
Van Nuys, CA 91405
(818) 243-4463 / (213) 427-5888

RX for Fleas
6555 N.W. Ninth Avenue, #411
Ft. Lauderdale, FL 33309
(800) 666-3532
Nonpesticide flea product.

Santa Monica Homeopathic Pharmacy
629 Broadway
Santa Monica, CA 90401
(310) 395-1131
Homeopathic remedies, Chinese herbal food supplements.

Seven Forests
U.S. Distribution
I.T.M. 2017 S.E. Hawthorne
Portland, OR 97214
Chinese herbal products.

Sherpa's Pet Trading Company
357 E. 57th Street, Suite 15A
New York, NY 10022
(800) 743-7723 / (212) 838-9837
FAX (212) 308-1187
Travel carrier bags for pets accepted on most major airlines.

Standard Books
210 W. 131st Street
P.O. Box 60167
Los Angeles, CA 90061
(800) 624-9659
(213) 321-4284
Complete selection of titles; Jain Indian homeopathic books.

Standard Homeopathic Company
P.O. Box 61067
Los Angeles, CA 90061
(800) 624-9659 / (310) 321-4284
FAX (212) 308-1187
Standard and Hylands Homeopathic Remedies. Remedies sold in amber bottles from 2-dram to 2-ounce size. You can request any size pellet, from #10 to #35, or tablets. Wide selection of lotions and creams, too.

Standard Process Laboratories
1200 W. Royal Lee Drive
Palmyra, WI 53156
(800) 558-8740
Immuplex, thyrotropin, glandulars.

Systemic Formulas
P.O. Box 1516
Ogden, UT 84402
(800) 445-4647
Food supplements, glandulars with herbs, and homeopathics (for veterinarians only). Free catalog available, or contact Celeste Yarnall for product information.

Taylor's Pharmacy
230 North Park Avenue
Winter Park, FL 32789
(407) 644-1025
Homeopathic pharmacy.

Tea Garden
9001 Beverly Boulevard
West Hollywood, CA 90069
(800) 288-HERB
Promoters of radiant health through Chinese herbs.

Top Dog Training School
30 Besaw Road
Phoenix, NY 13135
Write for information on training camps, instructor schools, and holistic dog-care camps.

Turtle Mountain and Jade Pharmacy
   Products
K'An Herbs
339 Rio Del Mar Boulevard
Aptos, CA 95003

2425 Porter Street, #18
Soquel, CA 95073
Chinese herbal products.

Vetri Science Labs
20 New England Drive
Essex Junction, VT 05453
(800) 882-9993
Manufacturers of pet supplements with digestive enzymes, and vetri-liquid DMG.

VideoRemedies
P.O. Box 290866
Davie, FL 33329-0866
(800) 733-4874
Homeopathic instructional videos. Dr. Chambreau's video: homeopathic first aid for pets and two for treating humans (see "Books, Publications, and Tapes").

Vita-Lite Duro-Lite Lamps, Inc.,
Duro-Test Corp.
9 Law Drive
Fairfield, NJ 07004
(800) 526-7193 / (201) 808-0902
Full-spectrum natural lighting.

Washington Homeopathic Products
4914 Del Rey Avenue
Bethesda, MD 20814
(800) 336-1695 / (301) 656-1695
Makes veterinary nosodes and carries remedies, ointments, and some books, including Natural Cat Care, by Celeste Yarnall.

Weleda Pharmacy, Inc.
175 N. Route 9W
Congers, NY 10920
(914) 268-8572
Homeopathic remedies, mail order.

Whole Foods Markets
General Office:
15315 Magnolia Boulevard, Suite 320
Sherman Oaks, CA 91403
(818) 501-8484
FAX (818) 990-7089

Wysong Corporation
1880 N. Eastman
Midland, MI 48640
(517) 631-0009
Educational materials and tapes. Natural pet foods and supplements.

Books, Publications, Tapes

Alternative Health Care Resources
by Brett Jason Sinclair.
Englewood Cliffs, N.J.: Parker Publishing Co., 1992. Although this directory contains only two listings for veterinary care (the AHVMA and the IVAS, both listed in this section), its five hundred-page list of resources contains organizations, journals, and practitioners that could prove useful.

Alternative Medicine: The Definitive Guide
The Alternative Medicine Yellow Pages:
  A Comprehensive Guide to the New World of Health
The Alternative Medicine Digest, the Voice of Alternative Medicine
Puyallup, Wash.: Burton Goldberg Group/Future Medicine Publishing, Inc., 1994.

Alternatives in Healing
by Simon Mill and Steven J. Finando.
New York: Plume/NAL Books, 1988.

Alternatives for the Health Conscious Individual (newsletter)
Mountain Home Publishing, P.O. Box 829, Ingram, TX 78025. (512) 367-4492.

The Animal Guardian
Distributed by the Doris Day Animal League

227 Massachusetts Avenue N.E.
Suite 100, P.O. Box 96829
Washington, D.C. 20090-6829.

Animal Press
1815 Hancock Street
San Diego, CA 92122
(619) 297-7092
FAX (619) 297-5233
Jay Runzi, General Manager

Are You Poisoning Your Pets?
by Nina Anderson and Howard Peiper.
New Canaan, Conn: Safe Goods East, 1995.

Aromatherapy: To Heal and Tend the Body
by Robert Tisserand.
Santa Fe, N. Mex.: Lotus Light Press, 1988.

Astrological Healing: The History and Practice of Astromedicine
by Reinhold Ebertin.
York Beach, Maine: Samuel Weiser, Inc., 1989.

The Bach Flower Remedies
by Edward Bach, M.D., and F. J. Wheeler, M.D.
New Canaan, Conn.: Keats Publishing, Inc., 1979. Available through Ellon USA, Inc.

Bach Flower Therapy: Theory and Practice
by Mechthild Scheffer.
Rochester, Vt.: Inner Traditions Int'l, Ltd., 1984.

Behaving As If the God in All Life Mattered
by Machaelle Small Wright.
Warrenton, Va.: Perelandra, Ltd., 1987. A beautifully written book dealing with the story of the author's ability to see and hear the invisible forces of nature.

The Betrayal of Health: The Impact of Nutrition, Environment, and Lifestyle on Illness in America
by Joseph D. Beasley, M.D.
New York: Times Books, 1991. A highly readable condensation of a report made to the Kellogg Foundation.

The Biochemic Handbook
by J. B. Chapman and Edward L. Perry, M.D.
St. Louis: Formur International, 1976.

A Cancer Battle Plan
by Anne E. Frahm with David J. Frahm.
Colorado Springs, Colo.: Pinon Press, 1992.

*Chinese Herbal Patent Formulas, A Practical
    Guide*
by Jake Fratkin.
Boulder, Colo.: Shya Publications, 1986.

Chinese Tonic Herbs
by Ron Teeguarden
Tokyo: Japan Publications, Inc., 1985.

Civilization and Disease
by Henry Sigerist.
Chicago: University of Chicago Press, 1962.

*Common-Sense Pest Control: Least Toxic
    Solutions for Your Home, Garden, Pets, and
    Community*
by William Olkowski, Sheila Daar, and Helga
    Olkowski.
Newtown, Conn.: Taunton Press, Inc., 1991.

*The Complete Herbal Handbook for the Dog
    and Cat* (6th ed.)
by Juliette de Bairacli Levy.
Winchester, Mass.: Faber and Faber, 1991.

*The Complete Medicinal Herbal: A Practical
    Guide to the Healing Properties of Herbs with
    More Than 250 Remedies for Common
    Ailments*
by Penelope Ody.
New York: Dorling Kindersley, 1993.

The Consumer's Guide to Homeopathy
by Dana Ullman, M.P.H., and Jeremy P.
    Tarcher.
New York: Putnam, 1996.

The Crystal Book
by Dael Walker.
Sunol, Calif.: The Crystal Co., 1983.

Cunningham's Encyclopedia of Magical Herbs
by Scott Cunningham.
Saint Paul, Minn.: Llewellyn Publications,
1985.

Death: The Final Stage of Growth
by Elisabeth Kübler-Ross.
Englewood Cliffs, N.J.: Prentice-Hall, 1976.

*Discovering Homeopathy: Medicine for the
    21st Century*
by Dana Ullman.
Berkeley, Calif.: North Atlantic Books, 1991.

*Divided Legacy: The Conflict Between
    Homeopathy and the AMA*
by Harris L. Coulter.
Berkeley, Calif.: North Atlantic Books, 1981.
This is volume 3 in a series of four books.

*The Diviner's Handbook: A Guide to the
    Timeless Art of Dowsing*
by Tom Graves.
Rochester, Vt.: Destiny Books, 1990.

Dogs: Homeopathic Remedies
by George Macleod, M.R.C.V.S., D.C.S.M.
Saffron Walden, England: C.W. Daniel,
Reprinted 1994.

Don't Dine without Enzymes
by Victor P. Kulvinskas, M.S.
Hot Springs, Ariz.: L.O.V.E. Foods, Inc.

*Dr. Pitcairn's "Complete Guide to Natural
    Health For Dogs and Cats"*
by Richard Pitcairn, M.D., Ph.D., and Susan
    Hubble Pitcairn.
Emmaus, Pa.: Rodale Press, 1995.

Echo, Inc. (Educational Concern for
    Hydrogen Peroxide). A newsletter.
P.O. Box 126, Delano, MN 55328.

Encyclopedia of the Dog
by Bruce Fogle, D.V.M.
New York: Dorling Kindersley, 1995.

Resources: Books, Publications, Tapes

Encyclopedia of Magical Herbs
by Scott Cunningham.
St. Paul, Minn.: Llewellyn Publications,
1992.

Enzyme Nutrition: The Food Enzyme Concept
by Dr. Edward Howell.
New York: Avery Publishing Group, Inc.,
1985.

*Essential Reiki: A Complete Guide to an Ancient
Healing Art*
by Diane Stein
Freedom, Calif.: The Crossing Press, 1996.

The Essentials of Chinese Acupuncture
by Foreign Language Press.
Beijing: Foreign Language Press, 1980.

Everybody's Guide to Homeopathic Medicines
by Stephen Cummings, M.D., and Dana
Ullman, M.P.H.
Los Angeles: Jeremy P. Tarcher, 1991.

The Family Guide to Homeopathy
by Alain Horvilleur, M.D.
Norwood, Pa.: Health and Homeopathy
Publishing, Inc., 1986.

The Family Guide to Homeopathy
by Andrew Lockie.
New York: Fireside, 1993.

The Family News (quarterly newsletter on
Oxygen Therapies), 9845 N.E. Second
Avenue, Miami Shores, FL 33138, (800)
284-6263.

Flower Essence Repertory
by Richard Katz and Patricia Kaminsky.
Nevada City, Calif.: Flower Essence Society,
Division of Earth-Spirit, 1992.

*Flower Essences: Reordering Our Understanding
and Approach to Illness and Health*
by Machaelle Small Wright.
Warrenton, Va.: Perelandra Ltd., 1988.

*The Flower Remedies Handbook: Emotional
Healing and Growth with Bach and Other
Flower Essences*
by Donna Cunningham.
New York: Sterling Publishing Co., Inc.,
1992.

*Food Enzymes: The Missing Link to Radiant
Health*
by Humbart Santillo.
Prescott, Ariz.: Hohm Press, 1987.

Food Is Your Best Medicine
by Dr. Henry G. Bieler and Maxine Block.
New York: Ballantine Books, Inc., 1987.

*Four Paws, Five Directions: A Guide to Chinese
Medicine for Cats and Dogs*
by Cheryl Schwartz, D.V.M.
Berkeley, Calif.: Celestial Arts, 1996.

*Free Radicals, Stress and Antioxidant Enzymes:
A Guide to Cellular Health* (booklet)
by Peter R. Rothschild and William J. Fahey.
Honolulu: University Labs Press,1991.

Fresh and Raw
by Dr. Wysong.
Midland, Mich.: The Wysong Company,
1990.

*Healing for the Age of Enlightenment: Balanced
Nutrition, Vita Flex, Color Therapy*
by Stanley Burroughs.
Newcastle, Calif.: Self-published, 1976.

*The Healing Herbs: The Ultimate Guide to the
Curative Power of Nature's Medicines*
by Michael Castleman.
Emmaus, Pa.: Rodale Press, 1991.
A "user-friendly herbal guide."

*Healing Music: The Harmonic Path to Inner
Wholeness*
by Andrew Watson and Nevill Drury.
Dorset, England: Prism Press, 1989.
A Nature and Health Book.

*The Healing Touch: The Proven Massage
    Program for Cats and Dogs*
by Michael W. Fox.
New York: Newmarket Press, 1981.

Healing Wise
by Susan Weed.
Woodstock, N.Y.: Ash Tree, 1989.
P.O. Box 64, Woodstock, New York 12498
(914) 246-8081.
Susan consults on Tuesday evenings between
7:30 and 9:30, Apr.–Oct., or you can send
her $1.00 for a catalog or newsletter.

Health and Healing
by Andrew Weil, M.D.
Boston: Houghton Mifflin, 1988.

*Healthy Homes, Healthy Kids: Protecting Your
    Children from Everyday Environmental
    Hazards*
by Joyce M. Schoemaker, Ph.D., and Charity
Y. Vitale, Ph.D.
Washington, D.C.: Island Press, 1991.
What's good for your kids is even better for
your animal companions.

*Healthy Pets, Naturally: The Holistic Newsletter
    with Natural Remedies for Treatable Ailments*
1895 New Franklin Church Road, Canon,
GA 30520
Sis Sewell, N.D.
(706) 356-7031
FAX (706) 356-7031 ★51

The Herb Book
by John Lust.
New York: Bantam Books, 1974.

Herbal Handbook for Farm and Stable
by Juliette De Bairacli Levy.
Emmaus, Pa.: Rodale Press, 1976.

Herbally Yours
by Penny C. Royal.
Hurricane, Utah: Sound Nutrition, 1982.

The Holistic Guide for a Healthy Dog
by Wendy Volhard and Kerry Brown, D.V.M.
New York: Macmillan, 1995.

*Holistic Pet Care: A Video with Dr. Joanne
    Stefanatos.*
Produced by Agape Video Systems, Inc., Las
Vegas, Nev.
An amazing survey of the holistic therapies
available for animals.

The Holographic Universe
by Michael Talbot.
New York: Harper-Perennial, 1991.
About physics, with lots of miracle stories.

Homeopathic First Aid for Pets (video)
Features Christina Chambreau, D.V.M.,
explaining the use of six homeopathic remedies for animals. The videotape and the
remedies she describes can be ordered
through Video Remedies, Inc., P.O. Box
290866, Davie, FL 33329-0866,
(800) 733-4874.

Homeopathic Medicine in the Home
by Jonathan Brewlow.
Ojai, Calif.: Ashwin Publications.
This book was intended to be used as part of
a correspondence course, but it can stand
alone. It uses as a companion volume, *Homeopathic Medicine at Home,* by Maesimund B.
Panos, M.D., and Jane Heimlich (Los Angeles: Jeremy Tarcher, Inc., 1980), which
includes a section on homeopathy and animals. Topics covered in the Brewlow book
include materia medica, use of the repertory,
and use of remedies in acute conditions.
Short section on prescribing for animals.
Useful resource listings.

The Homeopathic Treatment of Children
by Paul Herscu.
Berkeley, Calif.: North Atlantic Books, 1991.
Modern, in-depth work on eight remedies.
Gives insights that are applicable to animals.

*The Homeopathic Treatment of Small Animals—
    Principles and Practice*
by Christopher E. Day.
Saffron Walden, England: C.W. Daniel, 1992.

How to Heal the Earth in Your Spare Time
by Andy Lopez.
Malibu, Calif.: The Invisible Gardener.

How to Live the Millenium: The Bee Pollen Bible
by Royden Brown.
Prescott, Ariz.: Hohm Press, 1993.
Encyclopedic examination of research done
on bee products by the founder of CC
Pollen. Available through CC Pollen (800–
875-0096).

How Natural Remedies Work
by Jo Serrentino.
Point Roberts, Wash.: Hartley & Marks,
1991.
Interesting discussions of the "active" ingredients in natural remedies, including
vitamins, minerals, nutrients, and homeopathic and naturopathic remedies.

How to Talk to Your Dog
by Jean Craighead George.
New York: Warner Books, 1985.

Immunizations: The Reality behind the Myth
by Walene James.
New York: Greenwood, 1988.
Available through the American Natural
Hygiene Society, P.O. Box 30630, Tampa, FL
33630, (813) 855-6607.

Inventing the AIDS Virus
by Peter H. Duesberg.
Washington, D.C.: Regency Publishing, Inc.,
1996

Keep Your Pet Healthy the Natural Way
by Pat Lazarus.
New Canaan, Conn.: Keats Publishing, 1986.
Contains references to many holistic
veterinarians.

Kinship with All Life
by J. Allen Boone.
San Francisco: Harper San Francisco, 1976.

Kirk's Current Veterinary Therapy
by Robert W. Kirk.
Philadelphia: W. B. Saunders Co., 1994.

Lectures on Homeopathic Philosophy
by James Tyler Kent, M.D.
Berkeley, Calif.: North Atlantic Books, 1979.
If you are going to care for your animal
companions holistically, you have to change
your thinking. This book, written in 1900,
explains how homeopathy works and how
best to use it.

Legacy of the Dog
by Bruce Fogle, D.V.M.
San Francisco: Chronicle Books, 1995.

Love of Animals Newsletter
by Robert S. Goldstein, V.M.D., and Susan
    Goldstein.
7811 Montrose Road, Potomac, MD 20854,
(800) 861-5969.
Natural care and healing for dogs and cats.

Love, Miracles, and Animal Healing
by Alan M. Schoen, D.V.M., and Pam Proctor.
N ew York: Simon and Schuster, 1996.

*The Magic of Massage: A New and Holistic
    Approach* (3d rev. ed.)
by Ouida West.
Mamaroneck, N.Y.: Hastings House Publishers, 1990.

Magical Aromatherapy: The Power of Scent
by Scott Cunningham.
Saint Paul, Minn.: Llewellyn Publications,
1989.

*The Magical Staff: The Vitalist Tradition in
    Western Medicine*
by Matthew Wood.
Berkeley, Calif.: North Atlantic Books, 1992.
An understanding of how the use of energy

medicines came about historically. Offers an interesting perspective on homeopathy from someone trained in both homeopathy and herbalism.

Mother Knows Best—The Natural Way to Train Your Dog
by Carol Lea Benjamin.
New York: Howell Book House.

The Natural Dog
by Mary L. Brennan, D.V.M., with Norma Eckroate.
New York: Plume, 1994

Natural Healing for Dogs and Cats
by Diane Stein.
Freedom, Calif.: The Crossing Press, 1993. Everything from physical anatomy to non-physical anatomy and reincarnation. Very useful book Includes surveys of nutritional, herbal, and homeopathic approaches to healing animals.

Natural Health, Natural Medicine
by Andrew Weil, M.D.
Boston: Houghton Mifflin, 1990.

Natural Pet Magazine
P.O. Box 57900, Los Angeles, CA 90057-0900
(213) 385-2222

Natural Rearing Breeders Directory / Natural Rearing Newsletter
c/o Marina Zacharias at Ambrican Enterprises, Ltd., P.O. Box 1436, Jacksonville, OR 97530, (541) 899-2080 / FAX (541) 899-3414

The Natural Remedy Book for Dogs and Cats
by Diane Stein.
Freedom, Calif.: The Crossing Press, 1994

Nature Healing Conings for Animals
by Machaelle Small Wright.
Warrenton, Va.: Perelandra, Ltd., 1993.

The New Holistic Herbal
by David Hoffman.
Rockport, Mass.: Element Books, Inc., 1990. Contains a precise and detailed herbal as well as good sections on the preparation of herbs, the actions of herbs, the chemistry of herbs, and an overview of each body system and its relationship to herbs.

A New Model for Health and Disease
Berkeley, Calif.: North Atlantic Books, 1991. Gives greater understanding of the dangers of overusing antibiotics.

The New Super Antioxidant Plus: The Amazing Story of Pycnogenol, Free-Radical Antagonist and Vitamin C Potentiator
by Richard A. Passwater, Ph.D.
New Canaan, Conn.: Keats Publishing, Inc., 1992.

Nontoxic, Natural and Earthwise
by Debra Lynn Dadd.
Los Angeles: Jeremy P. Tarcher, 1990. More than six hundred mail-order sources for nontoxic, recycled, cruelty-free, natural, and other products. See also her book, The Nontoxic Home and Office. Los Angeles: Jeremy P. Tarcher, 1992.

On Death and Dying
by Elisabeth Kübler-Ross.
New York: Macmillan, 1969.

The Organon of Medicine
by Samuel Hahnemann, M.D. Translated with preface by William Boericke, M.D.
New Delhi, India: B. Jain Publishers, 1976. From the master's mouth. A must for the serious student.

Perfect Health: The Complete Mind-Body Guide
by Deepak Chopra, M.D.
New York: Crown Publishing Group, 1991.

Resources: Books, Publications, Tapes

Pet Allergies: Remedies for an Epidemic
by Alfred J. Plechner, D.V.M., and Martin
 Zucker.
Inglewood, Calif.: Very Healthy Enterprises,
Inc., 1986.

Pottenger's Cats: A Study in Nutrition
by Francis M. Pottenger Jr., M.D.
San Diego: Price-Pottenger Foundation,
1983.

*Practical Uses and Applications of the Bach
 Flower Remedies*
by Jessica Beal.
Las Vegas: Balancing Essentials Press, 1989.

Prescription for Nutritional Healing
by James F. Balch, M.D., and Phyllis A. Balch.
New York: Avery Publishing Group, 1990.

The Principles of Light and Color
by Dr. Edward D. Babbitt.
Santa Fe: Sun Publishing Co., 1992.

A Quick Guide to Food Additives
by Robert Goodman.
San Diego: Silvercat Publications, 1990.

*Quantum Healing: Exploring the Frontiers of
 Body, Mind, Medicine*
by Deepak Chopra.
New York: Bantam Books, 1990.

Raw Energy
by Leslie Kenton and Susan Kenton.
London: Ebury Press (Random House).

Reigning Cats and Dogs
by Pat McKay.
Pasadena, Calif.: Oscar Publications, 1997.

*The Reiki Handbook: A Manual for Students
and Therapists of the Usui Shiko Ryoho System
of Healing*
by Larry Arnold and Sandy Nevius.
Harrisburg, Pa.: PSI Press, 1982.

Rodale's Illustrated Encyclopedia of Herbs
Claire Kowalchik and William H. Hylton, eds.
Emmaus, Pa.: Rodale Press, 1987.

I Talk To Animals (video).
by Samantha Khury
1251 10th Street, Manhattan Beach, CA
90266, (310) 374-6812.

The Science of Homeopathy
by George Vithoulkas.
New York: Grove Atlantic, 1980.

Stories the Animals Tell Me
by Beatrice Lydecker
San Francisco: Harper San Francisco, 1979.

*The Tellington T-Touch: A Breakthrough
 Technique to Train and Care for Your Favorite
 Animal*
by Linda Tellington-Jones with Sybil Taylor.
New York: Viking Penguin, 1992.
A system of bodywork based on Feldenkrais
for people.

Today's Herbal Health
by Louise Tenney.
Woodland Books, P.O. Box 160,
Pleasant Grove, UT, (800) 777-BOOK.

The Twelve Tissue Remedies of Schuessler
by William Boericke and Willis A. Dewey.
New Delhi: B. Jain Publishers, 1982

*Vaccination: A Medical Assault on the Immune
 System*
by Viera Scheibner, Ph.D.
Maryborough, Victoria, Australia: Australian
Print Group, 1993; U.S. distributor: New
Atlantean Press, P.O. Box 9638, Santa Fe,
NM 87504, (505) 983-1856.

The Vaccination Connection
by Sue Marston.
Woodland Hills, Calif.: People for Reason in
Science and Medicine (PRISM), 1993.

Veterinary Aromatherapy
by Nelly Grosjean.
Saffron Walden, England: C. W. Daniel, 1994.

Vibrational Medicine: New Choices for Healing Ourselves
by Richard Gerber, M.D.
Santa Fe: Bear and Co., 1988.

The Web That Has No Weaver
by Ted Kaptchuk.
Congdon & Weed, 1983.

What Is Holistic Veterinary Care? Natural Care of Pets
by Roger De Haan, D.V.M.
This is a booklet available from Dr. De Haan at (508) 521-1899.

What Your Doctor Won't Tell You
by Jane Heimlich.
New York: HarperCollins, 1990.
A tremendous overview of alternative medical therapies. Contains a good listing of resources for further exploration.

When Elephants Weep
by Jeffrey Moussaieff Masson and Susan McCarthy.
New York: Delacourt Press, 1995

Wolf Clan Magazine
Wolf Clan Publications, Inc.
3952 N. Southport Avenue, Suite 122
Chicago, IL 60613
(847) 546-1400

Your Body Doesn't Lie
by John Diamond, M.D.
New York: Warner Books, 1980.
Also published under the title BK: Behavioral Kinesiology.

The Zodiac and the Salts of Salvation
by G. W. Carey and Inez E. Perry.
York Beach, Maine: Samuel Weiser, Inc., 1989.

The Zone
by Barry Sears, Ph.D., with Bill Lawren.
New York: HarperCollins, 1995.

Repertories and Materia Medica

Allen, H.C. M.D. *Allen's Keynotes.: Keynotes and Characteristics with Comparisions of Some of the Leading Remedies of the Materia Medica.* New Delhi, India: B. Jain Publishers, 1977. Nosode materia medica.

Barthel, H. *Synthetic Repertory,* vol. 2. Heidelberg, Germany: K.F. Haug Verlag, 1973. A modern repertory, many additions. Volume 2 is general and very useful with animals.

Boericke, William. *Materia Medica with Repertory.* St. Louis: Formur International, 1982.

Clarke, J.H. *Clinical Repertory.* New York: Beekman Publications, Inc., 1979. Three-volume set with detailed symptoms from provings.

Coulter, Catherine. *Portraits of Homeopathic Medicine,* 2 vols. Berkeley, Calif.: North Atlantic Books, 1986, 1988. On human personality of remedies.

Hahnemann, S. Trans. by R. E. Dudgeon. *Materia Medica Pura,* 2 vols. New Delhi, India: B. Jain Publishers.

Hering, Constantine. *Guiding Symptoms to Our Materia Medica,* 10 vols. New Delhi: B. Jain Publishers, 1879–91. A ten-volume set. The best for animals. From the provings, you'll often find your specific animal symptoms.

Kent, James. *Repertory of the Homeopathic Materia Medica with Word Index.* New Delhi, India: B. Jain Publishers, 1993. The most popular index of symptoms, affordable and a must for prescribing.

Kunzli, J., M.D. *Kent's Repertorium Generale.* New Delhi, India: B. Jain Publishers, 1987. An expanded Kent, with many new additions. If you can, get this one instead of Kent.

Macleod, G., M.R.C.M.V.S. *A Veterinary Materia Medica and Clinical Repertory with a Materia Medica of the Nosodes.* Saffron Walden, England: C. W. Daniel Co., 1983.

Mac Repertory. Kent Homeopathic Associates, P.O. Box 39, Fairfax, CA, 1986. A repertory for Macintosh computer that helps homeopaths repertorize their cases. Free info packet available: (415) 457-0678. Morrisson, Roger. *Desktop Guide to Keynotes and Confirmatory Symptoms.* Albany, Calif.: Hahnemann Clinic, 1993. Modern, concise.

Murphy, Robin. *Homeopathic Medical Repertory: A Modern Alphabetic Repertory.* Pagosa Springs, Colo.: Hahnemann Academy of North America, 1993. An even more modern repertory, with many new additions. Some people like it much more, some much less. Slightly cumbersome for animal work, but sometimes gives critical, additional remedies.

Phatak, S. R. *Concise Repertory of Homeopathic Medicines.* New Delhi, India: B. Jain Publishers.

Schuessler, W. H., M.D. *Materia Medica.* An abridged therapy manual on the biochemic treatment of diseases.

Wolff, H. G., D.V.M. *Veterinary Materia Medica and Clinical Repertory.* Saffron Walden, England: C. W. Daniel Co., Ltd., 1983.

On Vaccinations and Nosodes

Bastide, M. et al. "Immunoinodulator Activity of Very Low Doses of Thymulin in Mice." *International Journal of Immunotherapy* 3 (1987).

Boiron, J., J. Abecassis, and P. Belon. *Aspects of Research in Homeopathy,* vol. 1. Paris: Editions Boiron, 1983.

Burnett, J. Compton, M.D. *Vaccinosis and Its Cure by Thuja with Remarks on Homeoprophlaxis,* London, 1884.

Day, C. E. I, "Isopathic Prevention of Kennel Cough—Is Vaccination Justified?" *Journal of the International Association for Veterinary Homeopathy* 2, no. 1, 45.

———. "Isopathic Prevention of Kennel Cough—Is Vaccination Justified?" Clarification of kennel cough article in vol. 2, no. 1, *Journal of the International Association for Veterinary Homeopathy* 2, no. 2.

———. "Clinical Trials in Bovine Mastitis Using Nosodes for Prevention." *Journal of the International Association for Veterinary Homeopathy* 1 (1986); *British Homeopathic Journal* (1986).

———. *The Homeopathic Treatment of Small Animals: Principles and Practice.* London: Wigmere Publishing, 1984.

Dodds, Jean W. "Vaccine Safety and Efficacy." *Kennel Healthline* 3, no. 2 (February 1991).

———. "Vaccine Safety and Efficacy Revisited. Autoimmune and Allergic Disease on the Rise." *Veterinary Forum,* May 1993.

———. "More on Vaccines." *AKC Gazette,* March 1994.

———. "Killed Versus Modified Live Virus Vaccines." *AKC Gazette,* August 1991.

Frick, O. L. and D. L. Brooks. "Immunoglobulin E Antibodies to Pollen Augmented in Dogs by Virus Vaccines." *American Journal of Veterinary Research* 44, no. 3 (March 1983).

Julian, A. O., *Materia Medica of New Homeopathic Remedies.* Beaconsfield, England: Beaconsfield Publications, Ltd., 1979.

Karougby, Y. et al. "Immunostimulating and Antitumoral Properties of Thuyone." *Immunology* 173 (1986).

McDonald, I. J. "Factors That Can Undermine the Success of Routine Vaccination Protocols." *Veterinary Medicine,* March 1992.

Oehen, S., H. Hengartner, and R. Ziukernagel. "Vaccination for Disease." *Science* 251, (January 1991).

Phillips, T. R., and R. D. Schultz. "Canine and Feline Vaccinations." In *Current Veterinary Therapy* Vol. 11 Robert W. Kirk, ed. Philadelphia: W. B. Saunders, 1986.

Phillips, T. R., et al. "Effects of Vaccines on the Canine Immune System." *Canine Journal of Veterinary Research* 53 (1989).

Pitcairn, R. H. "Homeopathic Alternatives to Vaccines." *Proceedings of the American Holistic Veterinary Medicine Association,* 1993.

Ray, W. J. "Vaccine Safety and Efficacy Revisited." *Veterinary Forum,* August 1993.

Rude, T., et al. "Safety, Efficacy Heart of Vaccine Use; Experts Discuss Pros and Cons." *DVM Magazine,* December 1988.

Singh, Gupta Girish. "Antiviral Efficacy of Homeopathic Drugs Against Animal Viruses." *British Homeopathic Journal* 74, no. 3 (July 1985).

Tizard, I. "Risks Associated with Use of Live Vaccines." *JAVMA* 196, no. 11, (June 1990).

Wilford, Christine. "Vaccines Revisited." *AKC Gazette* 3, no. 1 (January 1994).

Index

Index

Index

Index

Index